Shifting the Therapeutic Paradigm for Children with Neuromotor Disabilities to Maximizing Development

Shifting the Therapeutic Paradigm for Children with Neuromotor Disabilities to Maximizing Development

Editors

Stephanie C. DeLuca
Jill C. Heathcock

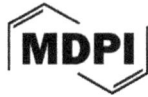

Basel • Beijing • Wuhan • Barcelona • Belgrade • Novi Sad • Cluj • Manchester

Editors
Stephanie C. DeLuca
Fralin Biomedical Research
Institute, Virginia Tech
Blacksburg, VA
USA

Jill C. Heathcock
The Ohio State University
Columbus, OH
USA

Editorial Office
MDPI
St. Alban-Anlage 66
4052 Basel, Switzerland

This is a reprint of articles from the Special Issue published online in the open access journal *Behavioral Sciences* (ISSN 2076-328X) (available at: https://www.mdpi.com/journal/behavsci/special_issues/N7KMODX1J4).

For citation purposes, cite each article independently as indicated on the article page online and as indicated below:

Lastname, A.A.; Lastname, B.B. Article Title. *Journal Name* **Year**, *Volume Number*, Page Range.

ISBN 978-3-7258-0455-9 (Hbk)
ISBN 978-3-7258-0456-6 (PDF)
doi.org/10.3390/books978-3-7258-0456-6

Cover image courtesy of Penna Thomason

© 2024 by the authors. Articles in this book are Open Access and distributed under the Creative Commons Attribution (CC BY) license. The book as a whole is distributed by MDPI under the terms and conditions of the Creative Commons Attribution-NonCommercial-NoDerivs (CC BY-NC-ND) license.

Contents

About the Editors vii

Preface ix

Alyssa LaForme Fiss, Ragnhild Barclay Håkstad, Julia Looper, Silvana Alves Pereira, Barbara Sargent, Jessica Silveira, et al.
Embedding Play to Enrich Physical Therapy
Reprinted from: *Behav. Sci.* **2023**, *13*, 440, doi:10.3390/bs13060440 1

Noelle G. Moreau, Kathleen M. Friel, Robyn K. Fuchs, Sudarshan Dayanidhi, Theresa Sukal-Moulton, Marybeth Grant-Beuttler, et al.
Lifelong Fitness in Ambulatory Children and Adolescents with Cerebral Palsy I: Key Ingredients for Bone and Muscle Health
Reprinted from: *Behav. Sci.* **2023**, *13*, 539, doi:10.3390/bs13070539 13

Susan V. Duff, Justine D. Kimbel, Marybeth Grant-Beuttler, Theresa Sukal-Moulton, Noelle G. Moreau and Kathleen M. Friel
Lifelong Fitness in Ambulatory Children and Adolescents with Cerebral Palsy II: Influencing the Trajectory
Reprinted from: *Behav. Sci.* **2023**, *13*, 504, doi:10.3390/bs13060504 29

Stephanie C. DeLuca, Mary Rebekah Trucks, Dorian Wallace and Sharon Landesman Ramey
Evidence for Using ACQUIRE Therapy in the Clinical Application of Intensive Therapy: A Framework to Guide Therapeutic Interactions
Reprinted from: *Behav. Sci.* **2023**, *13*, 484, doi:10.3390/bs13060484 47

Samuel W. Logan, Bethany M. Sloane, Lisa K. Kenyon and Heather A. Feldner
Powered Mobility Device Use and Developmental Change of Young Children with Cerebral Palsy
Reprinted from: *Behav. Sci.* **2023**, *13*, 399, doi:10.3390/bs13050399 59

Julia Mazzarella, Daniel Richie, Ajit M. W. Chaudhari, Eloisa Tudella, Colleen K. Spees and Jill C. Heathcock
Task-Related Differences in End-Point Kinematics in School-Age Children with Typical Development
Reprinted from: *Behav. Sci.* **2023**, *13*, 528, doi:10.3390/bs13070528 77

Kimberly Kascak, Everette Keller and Cindy Dodds
Use of Goal Attainment Scaling to Measure Educational and Rehabilitation Improvements in Children with Multiple Disabilities
Reprinted from: *Behav. Sci.* **2023**, *13*, 625, doi:10.3390/bs13080625 88

Sudha Srinivasan, Nidhi Amonkar, Patrick Kumavor, Kristin Morgan and Deborah Bubela
Outcomes Associated with a Single Joystick-Operated Ride-on-Toy Navigation Training Incorporated into a Constraint-Induced Movement Therapy Program: A Pilot Feasibility Study
Reprinted from: *Behav. Sci.* **2023**, *13*, 413, doi:10.3390/bs13050413 113

Ka Lai K. Au, Julie L. Knitter, Susan Morrow-McGinty, Talita C. Campos, Jason B. Carmel and Kathleen M. Friel
Combining Unimanual and Bimanual Therapies for Children with Hemiparesis: Is There an Optimal Delivery Schedule?
Reprinted from: *Behav. Sci.* **2023**, *13*, 490, doi:10.3390/bs13060490 132

Shailesh S. Gardas, Christine Lysaght, Amy Gross McMillan, Shailesh Kantak, John D. Willson, Charity G. Patterson and Swati M. Surkar
Bimanual Movement Characteristics and Real-World Performance Following Hand–Arm Bimanual Intensive Therapy in Children with Unilateral Cerebral Palsy
Reprinted from: *Behav. Sci.* **2023**, *13*, 681, doi:10.3390/bs13080681 143

Nancy Lennon, Carrie Sewell-Roberts, Tolulope Banjo, Denver B. Kraft, Jose J. Salazar-Torres, Chris Church and M. Wade Shrader
Preoperative Biopsychosocial Assessment and Length of Stay in Orthopaedic Surgery Admissions of Youth with Cerebral Palsy
Reprinted from: *Behav. Sci.* **2023**, *13*, 383, doi:10.3390/bs13050383 159

Thais Invencao Cabral, Xueliang Pan, Tanya Tripathi, Jianing Ma and Jill C. Heathcock
Manual Abilities and Cognition in Children with Cerebral Palsy: Do Fine Motor Skills Impact Cognition as Measured by the Bayley Scales of Infant Development?
Reprinted from: *Behav. Sci.* **2023**, *13*, 542, doi:10.3390/bs13070542 169

Christiana D. Butera, Shaaron E. Brown, Jennifer Burnsed, Jodi Darring, Amy D. Harper, Karen D. Hendricks-Muñoz, et al.
Factors Influencing Receipt and Type of Therapy Services in the NICU
Reprinted from: *Behav. Sci.* **2023**, *13*, 481, doi:10.3390/bs13060481 181

Julie M. Orlando, Andrea B. Cunha, Zainab Alghamdi and Michele A. Lobo
Information Available to Parents Seeking Education about Infant Play, Milestones, and Development from Popular Sources
Reprinted from: *Behav. Sci.* **2023**, *13*, 429, doi:10.3390/bs13050429 192

About the Editors

Stephanie C. DeLuca

Stephanie C. DeLuca, PhD, has a passion for serving children with disabilities. She has served as PI on numerous randomized controlled trials (RCTs), all of which have had a goal of using science to investigated complex bio-behavioral interventions aimed at helping children maximize their development. Currently, she serves as a lead investigator on a 13-site Phase III clinical trial, serves as a Site-PI for Virginia Tech, and directs the Treatment Implementation Core for this trial. She leads the Neuromotor Research Clinic at the Fralin Biomedical Research Institute where she works to develop novel therapeutics for children with a wide array of diagnoses, including many with rare diseases. In addition, she heads the Didactic Interactions Core for the National Pediatric Rehabilitation Resource Center (C-PROGRESS). This center is part of the Medical Rehabilitation Resource Research (MR 3) Network, and is designed to improve and increase funded pediatric rehabilitation trials that can have immediate and lasting impact in the field of pediatric rehabilitation. Dr DeLuca continues to work towards the development of the field of pediatric rehabilitation across multiple efforts because she has personally witnessed the transformative power of evidence-based rehabilitation practices.

Jill C. Heathcock

Jill C. Heathcock leads the Techniques Development Core and is an Associate Professor at The Ohio State University, School of Health and Rehabilitation Sciences, and Director of the Pediatric and Rehabilitation Laboratory (PEARL Lab). She studies (1) typical and atypical features of upper and lower extremity movements in children; (2) neurodevelopmental impairments in infant populations at high-risk for motor delay; and (3) neurorehabilitation for pediatric populations with an emphasis on dosing. Her research focuses on the development of targeted assessment and interventions for pediatric populations with cognitive and motor disability. Dr Heathcock is also part of the Center for Perinatal Research at Nationwide Children's Hospital. Dr Heathcock has several currently funded projects including one with The National Institutes of Health to determine the optimal doses of physical therapy for infants with severe motor delay and cerebral palsy; and one with the Patient-Centered Outcomes Research Institute (PCORI) to understand the effectiveness of usual weekly and high-intensity periodic therapy regimens for children with cerebral palsy. She is a member of the American Physical Therapy Association (APTA), the American Academy of Developmental Medicine and Child Neurology (AACPDM), and the International Congress for Infant Studies (ICIS).

Preface

We started this special issue with the overarching premise from the United Nations Rights to Children that "Every child with a disability should enjoy the best possible life in society. Governments should remove all obstacles for children with disabilities to become independent and to participate actively in the community." The specific focus was on neuromotor disabilities and to seek a better understanding of what it means for a child with a neuromotor disability to enjoy the best life possible by maximizing independence and societal participation in order to maximize development.

Globally, the likelihood of a child having a disability before their fifth birthday is ten times higher than dying. In the United States, alone there are more than 300,000 children with disabilities which points to the need for effective evidence-based rehabilitation. While these numbers represent all types of disabilities, this edition focused its efforts on children with neuromotor impairments. Many different neurological etiologies can lead to motor impairments, Cerebral Palsy (CP) is by far the leading cause with recent prevalence rates ranging between 1.5-3.4 per 1,000 live births, when considering both high- and low-income countries. What constitutes the most effective type and levels of rehabilitation services for children with neuromotor impairments is highly eclectic across the world. In the United States (U.S.), on average children receive 2–4 Occupational and Physical Therapy sessions per week that last between 30–60 min; still, 1 in 5 children have unmet therapy needs. Many families report mixed experiences with rehabilitation processes, reporting that treatments and therapies need to have more targeted and coordinated practical or real-world outcomes. This request is magnified when you consider that clinical therapy services often fail to correlate with greater such outcomes. The majority of traditional care-delivery rehabilitation systems across the globe provide services for children with neuromotor impairments provide services based on models of care that often lack scientific evidence. All that said, there are many clinicians, scientists, educators, parents, and advocates seeking to change this dynamic. This edition was written in honor of those individual and was designed to provide a platform for challenging existing narratives.

Increasingly, there is widespread recognition that maximizing function, abilities, and community participation minimizes disabilities for children with neuromotor impairments inherently elevating individual, family, and societal outcomes. The edition assembled more than 75 authors who represent a multitude of perspectives including; rehabilitation scientists, clinicians, clinicians-scientists, medical professionals, and people with lived experience. In total, we included 14 manuscripts. Three are classified as perspectives; the first focuses on the concept of play and its importance to development and therapy, and two additional perspectives manuscripts focused on the need to better define, understand and propose how we might increase lifelong fitness in children with CP. The 11 remaining manuscripts were considered original research, although the content and design types varied greatly with one paper offering a therapeutic framework. Topics covered informational sources about developmental milestones, upper extremity kinematics in typically developing children and how they might inform rehabilitation, characteristics of bimanual activities, time of intensive therapy approaches, ride-on toys as a therapeutic adjunct, measuring and obtaining educational goals in children with multiple disabilities, measurement of cognitive abilities and its relationship to fine-motor skills, the use of biopsychosocial assessments to improve operative care, how early mobility improves multiple developmental domains, the limited understanding of NICU therapy services, and a therapeutic framework to improve rehabilitation services. Specifically we found 3 topics of advancement toward functional independence to the best extent possible for children with disabilities.

1. Advancements in technology, assessments, and therapeutic approaches.

Innovation is an important component of research programs and is often a required section of grant applications because it can lead to improved healthcare for children with neuromotor disabilities. Articles in this special edition use innovative outcome measures, novel therapeutic approaches, and evaluations of intervention efficacy.

2. Interconnectedness: Embodied Cognition is still relevant and poorly understood in children with neuromotor disabilities

The link between cognition and motor skill development and how these domains change with intervention has been reported in the literature for more than a century. We are still gaining new knowledge about how to test cognition in a child who has poor motor skills and how motor-based interventions change other developmental domains. Articles in this special issue suggest that there is an interconnectedness of gross motor, fine motor, and cognition. Interventions and measurements of these construct together are necessary because of this interconnectedness. The work in this area suggests that it might be especially important in infancy to understand and promote maximized development.

3. Specialized healthcare settings are just that: *Specialized*.

As the editors, we wish to thank our many colleagues who chose to answer our call for this edition. The breadth and depth of information included is powerful. We believe it is representative of a field that is truly dedicated to the children and families we serve; as well as, an excellent body of work that represents the unique rewards and challenges associated with pediatric rehabilitation. As editors we are partially funded by the National Pediatric Rehabilitation Resource Center, also known as C-PROGRESS. The resource center is dedicated to helping scientists study pediatric rehabilitation. C-PROGRESS stands for the Center for Pediatric Rehabilitation: Growing Research, Education, and Sharing Science, the center's primary objective is to "see progress" in the emerging field of pediatric rehabilitation science. The Center is funded by the Eunice Kennedy Shriver National Institute of Child Health and Human Development, the National Institute of Neurological Disorders and Stroke, and the National Institute of Biomedical Imaging and Bioengineering. Like the mission of C-PROGRESS we believe this edition will serve as a resource for pediatric rehabilitation scientists.

Finally, we would like to thank the children and families that all rehabilitationists serve. Maximizing development for children concerns everyone, and provides an elevation for all lives. The picture on the cover was the winner of the 2023 Life Shots award from the American Academy of Cerebral Palsy and Developmental Medicine. The photo was titled "I win" and shows an exuberant child with CP racing in a wheeled walker ahead of a roller-skater. As the picture suggests and as this edition suggests "We all win" by maximizing the life course of children with neuromotor impairments.

Stephanie C. DeLuca and Jill C. Heathcock
Editors

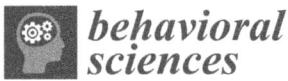

Perspective

Embedding Play to Enrich Physical Therapy

Alyssa LaForme Fiss [1], Ragnhild Barclay Håkstad [2,*], Julia Looper [3], Silvana Alves Pereira [4], Barbara Sargent [5], Jessica Silveira [6], Sandra Willett [7] and Stacey C. Dusing [5]

1. School of Physical Therapy, Texas Woman's University, Dallas, TX 75235, USA; afiss@twu.edu
2. Department of Health and Care Sciences, Faculty of Health Sciences, UiT The Arctic University of Norway, 9037 Tromsoe, Norway
3. School of Physical Therapy, University of Puget Sound, Tacoma, WA 98416, USA; jlooper@pugetsound.edu
4. Department of Physiotherapy, Universidade Federal do Rio Grande do Norte, Natal 59078970, Brazil; silvana.alves@ufrn.br
5. Division of Biokinesiology and Physical Therapy, Herman Ostrow School of Dentistry, University of Southern California, Los Angeles, CA 90033, USA; bsargent@pt.usc.edu (B.S.); stacey.dusing@pt.usc.edu (S.C.D.)
6. Department of Physical Therapy, Texas State University, Round Rock, TX 78665, USA; jm2049@txstate.edu
7. Munroe-Meyer Institute, University of Nebraska Medical Center, Omaha, NE 68198, USA; swillett@unmc.edu
* Correspondence: ragnhild.hakstad@uit.no; Tel.: +47-77660711

Abstract: Play is an active process by which an individual is intrinsically motivated to explore the self, the environment, and/or interactions with another person. For infants and toddlers, engaging in play is essential to support development across multiple domains. Infants and toddlers with or at risk of motor delays may demonstrate differences in play or challenges with engaging in play activities compared to typically developing peers. Pediatric physical therapists often use play as a modality to engage children in therapeutic assessment and interventions. Careful consideration of the design and use of physical therapy that embeds play is needed. Following a 3-day consensus conference and review of the literature, we propose physical therapy that embeds play should consider three components; the child, the environment, and the family. First, engage the child by respecting the child's behavioral state and following the child's lead during play, respect the child's autonomous play initiatives and engagements, use activities across developmental domains, and adapt to the individual child's needs. Second, structure the environment including the toy selection to support using independent movements as a means to engage in play. Allow the child to initiate and sustain play activities. Third, engage families in play by respecting individual family cultures related to play, while also providing information on the value of play as a tool for learning. Partner with families to design an individualized physical therapy routine that scaffolds or advances play using newly emerging motor skills.

Keywords: play; physical therapy; infants; toddlers

1. Introduction

Children, defined here as those under the age of 3, rely on parents or caregivers to provide a safe, dependable, and calm environment in which to live, grow, and learn. This environment is impacted by the child's ability to self-direct their movements, engage with objects, and lead interaction with their caregivers. This often takes on the shape of play. In this paper, we define play as an active process by which an individual is intrinsically motivated to explore the self, the environment, and/or interactions with another person. It is enjoyable with a natural flow individually or between participants. Play is valued for its own sake; the means are more valuable than the ends. This definition was developed during a 3-day consensus conference, organized and hosted by the Motor Development Lab at the University of Southern California.

Multiple organizations have highlighted the importance of play in the developmental continuum. The United Nations Convention on the Rights of the Child recognizes the right "to engage in play and recreational activities appropriate to the age of the child" as a fundamental right for every child [1] (Article 31). Likewise UNICEF highlights the importance of "playing to learn" as an important piece of early childhood education and childcare [2]. The American Academy of Pediatrics (AAP) suggests pediatricians concerned about a child's development write the family a prescription to play with their child, as play may be as powerful as any medication [3].

2. Importance of Play in Early Childhood

Play is essential to support the development of multiple developmental domains: motor, language, cognition, social-emotional, and adaptive behavior [3–5]. Play allows children to learn about themselves and their environment [3,5,6]. Early reciprocal caregiver interactions such as eye contact, smiling, and mimicking sounds are some of the earliest forms of play, laying a foundation for future socialization and language development [7]. As the child ages, exploring the environment during play provides opportunities for children to learn what their body can do and to practice skills that support the development of new abilities [8,9]. For example, an infant may see an interesting toy out of reach, and through repeated attempts to obtain the toy, develop new motor skills such as rolling or crawling. As motor skills advance, new opportunities for exploration further facilitate cognitive growth.

2.1. Play in Pediatric Physical Therapy

Pediatric physical therapists, who traditionally serve children and youth from birth to 21 years of age, and early childhood service providers use play as a modality to assess development and to engage children in intervention [5,10]. Physical therapists design play involving activities representative of the child's developmental stage and gradually adapt the environment to introduce novelty and challenge [11]. Active play during therapeutic intervention in the first 3 years of life is crucial to maximize participation and function, affect positive neuroplasticity, and promote the development of a sense of self. The intentional use of play increases motivation, a critical modulator of neuroplasticity and engagement in physical therapy [12,13]. Recent research on interventions to support early development, including Supporting Play Exploration and Early Developmental Intervention (SPEEDI) [13] and Goal Activity Motor Enrichment (GAME) [14] studies, incorporate principles of play as important components of the intervention, yet define play differently, highlighting the importance and need for additional consideration of play. Additionally, when Håkstad and colleagues [11] observed pediatric physical therapy (PT) sessions with a focus on play, they noted that the therapists occasionally interrupted or prematurely redirected infant play focusing instead on specific therapeutic goals or therapeutic handling. Similarly, in a study comparing two PT intervention approaches, variations on the amount of "help" provided to the child and how the toys were used clearly distinguished the approaches [15]. Because of the importance of play, we encourage thoughtful reflection on the use of play in pediatric PT to ensure the therapist is aware of and sensitive to the child's cues and responses to facilitate ongoing, interactive play.

2.2. Play of Infants and Toddlers with or at Risk of Motor Delays

There is a relative paucity of research on the play of children with or at risk of motor delays to inform PT strategies and family coaching. This lack of research is concerning since young children with motor delays require a supportive environment to fully engage in play. This environment may include adaptive toys, adaptive equipment, and high levels of parent and caregiver responsiveness and support [16,17]. Family coaching on ways to support play is critical since parent and caregiver involvement in a child's play can enhance the complexity, duration, and frequency of more advanced play behaviors [18].

Due to their underlying medical or developmental condition, children with motor delays may demonstrate differences in play relative to their peers with typical development. For example, infants with autism spectrum disorder demonstrate differences in exploratory play, including atypical use of objects for sensory stimulation, more repetitive interactions with objects, and prolonged visual inspection of objects from odd angles [19–21]. Toddlers with autism spectrum disorder are also less likely to engage in symbolic play [22]. As infants, children with Down syndrome demonstrate differences in exploratory play that are associated with a lack of object mastery and decreased attention to objects [18], and as toddlers they tend to repeat the same play schemes more often than their peers with typical development [23]. For young children with cerebral palsy, higher playfulness has been associated with higher gross motor function, more effective adaptive behavior, and less impact of their health conditions on daily life [24]. An understanding of the impact of a child's condition on their play is an important consideration when designing intervention programs and family coaching to meet therapeutic goals.

3. Embedding Play to Enrich and Individualize Physical Therapy
3.1. Engaging the Child
3.1.1. Respecting the Child's Behavioral State and Cues

Engaging the child in PT that embeds play entails respecting the child's behavioral state and following the child's lead by attending to the child's vocalizations, prompts, and other behavior cues. Infants engage in coordinated adult–child interactions from birth, and by 3 months of age they already have expectations of mutuality with reciprocal receptions of and reactions to cues during turn taking [25,26]. Adults can facilitate and increase a child's participation in interactions by creating structured, rhythmic turn taking sequences that are well synchronized with the child's responses [27,28]. Within this synchronization, it is important that the adult provides pauses to allow the child to process information, respond or make choices, or even take a break, if needed [28,29]. Salient, unambiguous prompts, and allowing the child ample response time expands the child's opportunities for exploration and mutuality during interaction [25,30]. This is especially important when working with children with motor delays or multiple disabilities since high frequencies of prompts can be overwhelming [29,30]. These children may need increased time for information processing due to deficits across steps of attention, recognition, recall, encoding, integration, and/or motor planning [30–33].

Children with motor delays may also present with expressive impairments that limit their ability to communicate during play and make it more challenging for the adult to pick up on the child's intentional acts and signs of engagement or distress [34]. Synchrony in interaction requires the adult to learn about and understand the child's less obvious communicative signals (i.e., eye movements, breathing patterns, gestures, vocalizations, and protesting behaviors), then support the child's relaying of these messages and appropriately interpret whether these signals indicate child engagement, dis-engagement, or distress during play [35].

Tactile stimulation and touch are integral within adult–child play interactions. For children with motor delays, tactile stimuli both increase and disturb a child's attention during social play [36]. Given the individual variations in sensory processing among children with motor delays, it is important to determine the appropriate amount and type of tactile stimulation beneficial to the individual child, and to elucidate when such stimuli become overwhelming, leading to dis-engagement or distress [36]. Provenzi et al. [36] classified maternal touch into categories including: affective, playful, facilitating, and holding. Among these, playful touch such as tickling, squeezing, moving, or flexing the child's body was associated with increased attentiveness during social play [36]. Such touch might also increase a child's attention during PT that embeds play. A study of therapeutic touch in pediatric PT shows that flexible, subtle handling during play can awaken the child's curiosity and facilitate new motor explorations [37].

3.1.2. Respecting the Child's Autonomous Play Initiatives and Engagements

Children develop autonomous exploratory behavior as part of their ongoing spontaneous play which is guided by perceptual input, motor output, and the consequences of actions that the child attends to [38]. Infants as young as 2 months of age demonstrate exploratory play engagement by gazing at activities only when they result in interesting consequences [38]. By 7 to 9 months of age, infants engage with more solitary object exploration [8,25], and by 10 months, infants tend to be more responsive and engaged in joint attention during free play compared to semi-structured play [39]. When adults provide directions during play, simple and structured directions best maintain the children's exploratory behavior, as opposed to unstructured or more complex directions [40]. In a study of 3- to 14-month-old infants born preterm, Håkstad et al. [11] noted that to uphold the child's play engagement during therapy sessions, physical therapists need to engage in mutual play and coordinate their actions with the child's play intentions and goals. These findings underscore the importance of allowing children to discover and direct play and to decide the extent of time spent with a play activity, without intrusiveness from the adult play partner.

3.1.3. Including Activities across Developmental Domains

PT that embeds play should include activities that facilitate development across domains. Facilitation of perceptual-motor exploratory behavior, or motor-based problem-solving, along with socioemotional support to help children self-regulate and manage frustrations, is a priority [29]. Play interactions can provide a substrate for rich language and social environments. As adults narrate play activities (e.g., naming objects, describing actions, or counting objects), children learn about shared attention and turn taking, begin to understand that objects have names and actions, and that their body's actions interact with the world to make things happen [29,41]. The use of motor skills such as sitting and reaching, or self-initiated mobility during play, create developmental cascades in language, social, visual-perceptual, and/or cognitive skills as the child engages with the environment or others.

3.1.4. Supporting a Child's Engagement in Play

Mirroring and supporting a child's use of toys assists in engaging the child in play. Mimicry, vocal cues, and pointing support attention maintenance, joint attention, and joint interaction [29,42,43]. Mimicry allows the formation of a social connection and facilitates future interactions. Eighteen-month-old children are more likely to invite an adult when the adult has previously mimicked the child's use of a toy [42]. Mimicry activates the mirror neuron system as the child observes the adult play partner imitate the child's actions. This supports language, social, and emotional development, and observational learning [44]. Vocal cues also support sustained infant attention during play with objects [43] and joint attention in toddlers [45]. Deak and colleagues [45] found that 15- and 21-month-olds responded more to parental gaze-shifting with pointing or with directed language than gaze-shifting alone, highlighting the importance of vocal cues and gesturing during play. In early infancy prior to gaining locomotion, infants are reliant on adults to present toys and objects for exploration; adults organize the infant's interaction. These interactions are often rhythmic, providing structure and facilitating the infant's play with both the object and the adult play partner [28].

Creating the "just right challenge" during play is essential for child engagement during PT that embeds play. If an activity is too challenging, either from a motor or cognitive perspective, the therapist risks losing the child's interest. Conversely, an activity that is too easy may not provide the therapeutic effects intended by the therapist [46]. The activity should engage and motivate the child, and the child should be able to master the skill with their "focused effort" [47]. Physical therapists can scaffold the "just right challenge" by grading motor or cognitive aspects of the task to meet the child's abilities and adapting the activity to the appropriate level for the child [48,49]. The START-Play intervention incorporated the "just right challenge" to scaffold blended motor/cognitive skills, and to engage families in brainstorming about how to increase the difficulty of activities through small, achievable increments. These small increments support advances in motor and cognitive skills. The position of the child during play is an important consideration when creating a "just right challenge". Increased motor demand may reduce opportunity for social interaction and reduce the child's cognitive capacity for motor-based problem solving [50].

Attraction to novel stimuli is an adaptive behavior that intrinsically motivates a child to explore their environment [51,52]. Infants demonstrate a desire to explore in the first weeks of life [53] and a preference for novel stimuli, habituating to what is regular or expected and paying particular attention to what is unusual [51,54,55]. Using novel stimuli to elicit exploration requires ensuring an appropriate familiarization time with the previous stimulus [56]. Rose and colleagues [56] found that infants demonstrate a preference for familiar stimuli when a shortened familiarization period is given. Increased familiarization time is required for younger infants due to slower processing speeds and when introducing complex stimuli [51]. This concept is pertinent for therapists practicing PT that embeds play. Inadvertently switching from one novel activity to another without appropriate familiarization time for the child may lead to a child's preference to return to a previous task and disengage from the new task. This is especially key when working with children who have known cognitive impairments, as they may require more time to explore and process a new object or task due to decreased processing speed [51,54].

3.1.5. Adapting Play to Individual Child Differences

PT that embeds play requires clinicians to consider individual differences in play based on the child's cognitive and sensory-motor abilities. Physical therapists may need to identify alternative stimuli to initiate play, incorporate adaptive toys, use external supportive equipment, and systematically alter activities to find the "just right challenge" for each child. Alternative stimuli may be necessary for children who have sensory deficits such as visual impairments. For example, Hughes [57] encouraged clinicians to create a "sensory-rich play environment" for children with visual impairments. This includes incorporating sensory cues to guide exploration such as changes in the texture of flooring to provide tactile input to a mobile infant with visual impairments. Clinicians also are encouraged to consider the tactile and/or auditory properties of a toy rather than the appearance alone when choosing toys. Allowing a child with sensory impairment to safely explore their environment rather than deterring them is important to ensure continual development of intrinsically motivated locomotion. Finally, beginning with one play partner, perhaps a familiar adult, prior to increasing the number of play participants is important to not overwhelm a child with sensory impairments [57]. A PT who embeds play can support and facilitate play while allowing the parent or caregiver to be the play partner for the child to avoid overwhelming the child and risking subsequent child disengagement from the activity.

Using a strength-based approach is important to motivate the child and family to participate in play. A clinician who engages in a strength-based approach focuses on the child's strengths and assets, rather than their deficits, and incorporates play activities accordingly [58]. Not only does the strength-based focus allow clinicians to identify areas to facilitate development, it also can increase parental well-being and positive interactions between the parent and child. Steiner and colleagues [59] found that using a strength-based approach with families of children with autism spectrum disorder improved parent affect and parent–child interactions, with significant findings for increased physical affection and positive affect as compared to those who received a deficit-based approach.

3.2. Focus, Environment, and Toy Use

3.2.1. The Focus of Play

In PT that embeds play, the child's movement is a means to engage in play, not the primary focus of the child's attention. When focusing primarily on movement patterns or repetitions, physical therapists may inadvertently interrupt or limit a child's play. This inclination away from play and exploration towards movement repetitions becomes frustrating for children who are able to recognize that an adult is intentionally withholding a toy [60]. In contrast, children learn better when adults recognize and respond to the child's communicative gestures and allow the child to be actively engaged in acquiring information that is salient to them [61]. Allowing the child to select how to play within a PT session may remove control from the physical therapist but provides autonomy to the child, leading to decreased frustration and improved learning.

3.2.2. The Environmental Set-Up

A key role of the physical therapist is to set up the environment and materials in a way that allows the child to initiate play and then to explain to parents and caregivers about why and how we do this. Similarly to setting up the "just right challenge" for any task, physical therapists must consider the "just right environment" [62]. It is important to consider the physical and psychosocial environment to ensure the child has the opportunity to explore and engage in complex interactions [53]. Additionally, the therapist or caregiver can guide and enable the child's play behavior within this environment [62]. One factor that affects a child's ability to interact with the environment is body position. A child in prone plays differently than a child in sitting or in supine due to the constraints of the position [53]. A child who has balance difficulties in standing may support themselves with two hands and not engage with toys or may discover the possibility of leaning on the support surface to free their arms to engage [63]. A physical therapist can assess how the child's position impacts their ability to play and interact with the environment to determine if increased support is needed or if a different position is warranted.

The position of the therapist or caregiver and how much support they provide a child also has an impact on the child's ability to explore [63].. For example, children in supported sitting, particularly those who are not well supported, do not touch or reach for objects in their environment as much as independent sitters [64]. Modulating support to match the child's motor and cognitive needs is an important aspect of play within a PT context. Additionally, face-to-face interactions are important so that the caregiver can read the child's behavioral and visual cues and vice versa [65]. In many supported play positions, the caregiver is behind the child, leading to decreased joint attention to an object and to each other's cues, and to a decreased ability for the caregiver to facilitate and scaffold the child's play behavior [66]. The use of an external support may allow a caregiver to move to a position that allows for eye contact and increased quality and scaffolding of play.

3.2.3. The Use of Toys

Play can occur with or without toys. Social games such as Peak-a-boo are play opportunities that have a clear recurring structure that young infants recognize [67] and enjoy as long as the established routine is followed [68]. Physical therapists can use social games to establish a playful atmosphere even with very young infants. Play can also occur as a child actively explores and interacts with toys and objects, discovering and exploring movement possibilities, environmental opportunities, and their own autonomy [69–71]. Physical therapists can interrupt or limit a child's play by using toys as bait to encourage movement repetitions without allowing the child to fully explore the toy before it is moved again. This not only removes autonomy from the child, but also leads to frustration and missed opportunities to learn through exploration. Therapists may help extend the play with the toy that the child is interested in and support movement when the child is ready to transition to a new activity. As few as four to five toys [72] may be appropriate to support movement as larger numbers of toys may create less focus and less creative play [72,73].

3.3. Engaging Families in Play

3.3.1. Understanding a Family's Play Culture

Play is deeply enculturated. Who plays, how they play, why they play and what they play with is influenced by societal, geographical, sociodemographic, familial, and individual belief systems and values [74]. Adult eye contact, expression of emotion, use of narratives, and physical proximity or touch during play differs across cultures and across families, parents, and children based on child temperament, gender, and/or birth order [75–77]. Play in Western cultures largely is defined as a child-initiated, child-led learning activity focusing on self-discovery, object exploration, and/or social interaction [70,75,78]. Families of higher socioeconomic status link play to resources: safe, physical indoor and outdoor play spaces, a wide variety of play materials, and caregivers who have the time for and understanding of developmental play [79]. Families in low-income settings are less likely to have access to these resources. Perceived gender or social roles, of both the parent and the child, interact with the players' individual temperaments and beliefs, shaping overt play behaviors [80]. The reasons, or why of play, and the materials used, or what is played with, are similarly related to cultural factors [74,79]. Some families do not value play and view it as frivolous; while others value it as an opportunity to scaffold learning and development [78,81,82]. Some prioritize physical activity; others prioritize cognitive, social-emotional or fine motor skills as predictors of success at school age [75,76]. What is played with can vary widely based on custom, resources, or preference. Sicart [83] argues that anything (a toy, a household item, another person) may become a 'plaything' or object of relational interaction. From such perspective, it is not what is played with but how the child interacts with the 'plaything' that matters.

Finally, parents' perceptions of child well-being or capabilities influence all the above aspects of play. Children with multiple medical conditions or diagnosed with motor delays are more likely to be perceived by their families as vulnerable [80]. Parents with this perception are less likely to introduce play behaviors that involve risk and are less likely to choose play items or motor activities that appropriately challenge their children [84,85]. They are also more likely to underestimate their child's physical, developmental or play abilities and to interrupt or control play activities [84,85]. If physical therapists fail to probe for, acknowledge, or attend family play culture, they risk designing intervention or play programs of little practical value.

3.3.2. Partnering with Families

Partnering is a multi-faceted, family-centered process that promotes family engagement in intervention programs [86,87]. It implies 'co-construction' of the therapeutic relationship: shared observation of child and family strengths/needs, shared development of therapy goals and outcomes, and shared conceptualization of the role of intervention in the child's development [88,89]. It acknowledges that the primary agent for a child's developmental change is the parent–child relationship [86,90,91]. A parent's contingent responsiveness, or ability to read and respond to their child's cues, is related to both secure relationships and the degree to which very young children explore their environments [91–93]. Responsive parents extend play and promote early learning through attentive but non-directive interactions [93]. These carefully nuanced interactions enhance the child's mastery motivation, tolerance to frustration, and focused attention: all skills associated with stronger cognitive, communication, and self-regulatory/adaptive developmental outcomes [92,93]. Partnering between professionals and parents implies transparency, equality in decision making, and absolute 'presence' [87].

Presence may be considered physical proximity. Anecdotally, therapists and parents often comment that parental presence in the PT session is distracting to the young child. However, motor learning suggests that behaviors observed during therapist–child interactions are capacity-related and not true performance [94]. There is no guarantee of carry-over into daily routines if parents are not actively involved. Additionally, children rely on familiar caregivers to understand the context of any social interaction. When separated from their parents, they are not as likely to read the subtle shifts in gaze or to respond to the tactile cues that familiar caregivers use to direct, attenuate, and shift attention [92,93,95] needed for both social-emotional regulation and learning [93,96].

Presence may be considered attentional. In the therapeutic relationship, attentional demands are complex, dynamic and triadic (parent-child-therapist) [88,91]. Parents' and therapists' attention at any given moment is potentially fragmented by many things: other responsibilities, worries about the immediate and distant future, and constant technoference, defined as cell or smart-phone disruptions during social interactions [97]. In the parent–child relationship, these interruptions can lead to increased child distress, disrupted infant social-emotional regulation, lowered child inhibitory responses, and impaired contingency-related learning of both language and social cues [97–99]. Simply put, attentional disruptions interfere with the ability to recognize and respond to a child's cues during play or any therapeutic interaction.

Engaged parents extend the reach and dose of any intervention, including play by embedding therapeutic activities into daily routines [89,90]. Parents who participate in play-based intervention programs report gaining an understanding of quality play time, spending more time with their child during play activities, and having a greater understanding of the developmental impact of play [100]. Multiple frameworks for engaging families exist. King et al. [87,88] propose four key principles for family engagement: (1) the personalizing principle, or 'knowing the client'; (2) the individual variation principle, or knowing that clients differ in how they demonstrate engagement and what engages them; (3) the relationship principle, or that engagement is cultivated through interpersonal relationships; and (4) the monitoring principle, or staying attuned to the child's and the parent's level of engagement from moment-to-moment and from session-to-session. Practical strategies for family engagement as described by Marvin et al. include open communication, encouraging parent–child interaction during sessions, overtly linking play behaviors to developmental or motor outcomes and modeling, suggesting and practicing play behaviors in action and together. Therapists can invite parents to play, describe the purpose and learning opportunities embedded in play, and affirm parents in their parent–child play interactions. For children with motor impairments, this may include teaching parents to 'wait', to allow their child opportunities for trial and error and to support their child's focused attention during play.

4. Conclusions

PT that embeds play has the potential to support acquisition of skills across the developmental continuum. In this framework, therapists work to engage the child in play, to facilitate optimal environmental set-up and toy selection, and to engage the family in play interactions with their child. Consideration of these components ensures the therapist is supporting play and development and is not disrupting or interfering with the play of children.

Currently, a gap exists in our understanding of PT that embeds play. Research suggests there may be differences in how physical therapists interpret and implement play in the design of PT sessions with children [11,15]. Additional information on if and how physical therapists intentionally incorporate play within their assessment and intervention sessions should be examined in greater depth. Educational guidelines for how physical therapists should be prepared to incorporate and support the play of children with or at high risk of motor delays are lacking, which may contribute to variation and a disconnect between effective strategies and clinical practice trends.

Future research should explore perceptions of both clinicians and of parents related to PT that embeds play. Greater understanding of therapist beliefs related to the importance of play in facilitating developmental skills, their own playfulness during therapy, and their comfort and skill in supporting the parent's ability to play with their child is needed. Additionally, the perceptions of parents related to play and how best to facilitate their interactions with their children should be explored. Together, this information may inform additional guidelines or research to inform how best to support optimal play and overall development of infants and toddlers with or at risk of motor delays.

Author Contributions: Conceptualization, A.L.F., R.B.H., J.L., S.A.P., B.S., J.S., S.W. and S.C.D.; writing—original draft preparation, A.L.F., R.B.H., J.L., S.A.P., B.S., J.S., S.W. and S.C.D.; writing—review and editing, A.L.F.; project administration, S.C.D.; funding acquisition, S.C.D. and R.B.H. All authors have read and agreed to the published version of the manuscript.

Funding: The consensus conference that led to this paper was funded by the Sykes Chair of Pediatric Physical Therapy, Health and Development Endowment at the University of Southern California. Researchers time was supported by 2 awards from the Eunice Kennedy Shriver National Institute of Child Health and Human Development; R01HD093624 (S.C.D.), and R01HD101900 (S.C.D., S.W., B.S).

Institutional Review Board Statement: Not applicable.

Informed Consent Statement: Not applicable.

Data Availability Statement: Not applicable.

Conflicts of Interest: The authors declare no conflict of interest.

References

1. UNICEF. Convention on the Rights of the Child. *Treaty Ser.* **1989**, *1577*, 3.
2. UNICEF. Learning through Play: Strengthening Learning through Play in Early Childhood Education Programs. 2018. Available online: https://www.unicef.org/sites/default/files/2018-12/UNICEF-Lego-Foundation-Learning-through-Play.pdf (accessed on 9 April 2023).
3. Ginsburg, K.R.; American Academy of Pediatrics Committee on Communications; American Academy of Pediatrics Committee on Psychosocial Aspects of Child and Family Health. The Importance of Play in Promoting Healthy Child Development and Maintaining Strong Parent-Child Bonds. *Pediatrics* **2007**, *119*, 182–191. [CrossRef] [PubMed]
4. Herzberg, O.; Fletcher, K.K.; Schatz, J.L.; Adolph, K.E.; Tamis-LeMonda, C.S. Infant exuberant object play at home: Immense amounts of time-distributed, variable practice. *Child Dev.* **2022**, *93*, 150–164. [CrossRef] [PubMed]
5. Lifter, K.; Mason, E.J.; Barton, E.E. Children's Play: Where We Have Been and Where We Could Go. *J. Early Interv.* **2011**, *33*, 281–297. [CrossRef]
6. Rossmanith, N.; Costall, A.; Reichelt, A.F.; LÃ3pez, B.; Reddy, V. Jointly structuring triadic spaces of meaning and action: Book sharing from 3 months on. *Front. Psychol.* **2014**, *5*, 1390. [CrossRef]
7. Yogman, M.; Garner, A.; Hutchinson, J.; Hirsh-Pasek, K.; Golinkoff, R.M.; Committee on Psychosocial Aspects of Child and Family Health; Council on Communications and Media; Baum, R.; Gambon, T.; Lavin, A.; et al. The Power of Play: A Pediatric Role in Enhancing Development in Young Children. *Pediatrics* **2018**, *142*, e20182058. [CrossRef]
8. Henricks, T. The nature of play: An overview. *Am. J. Play.* **2008**, *1*, 157–180.
9. Muentener, P.; Herrig, E.; Schulz, L. The Efficiency of Infants' Exploratory Play Is Related to Longer-Term Cognitive Development. *Front. Psychol.* **2018**, *9*, 635. [CrossRef]
10. Chiarello, L.A.; Palisano, R.J.; Bartlett, D.J.; McCoy, S.W. A Multivariate Model of Determinants of Change in Gross-Motor Abilities and Engagement in Self-Care and Play of Young Children With Cerebral Palsy. *Phys. Occup. Ther. Pediatr.* **2011**, *31*, 150–168. [CrossRef]
11. Håkstad, R.B.; Obstfelder, A.; Øberg, G.K. Let's play! An observational study of primary care physical therapy with preterm infants aged 3–14 months. *Infant Behav. Dev.* **2017**, *46*, 115–123. [CrossRef]
12. Majnemer, A. Importance of Motivation to Children's Participation: A Motivation to Change. *Phys. Occup. Ther. Pediatr.* **2011**, *31*, 1–3. [CrossRef] [PubMed]
13. Dusing, S.C.; Tripathi, T.; Marcinowski, E.C.; Thacker, L.R.; Brown, L.F.; Hendricks-Muñoz, K.D. Supporting play exploration and early developmental intervention versus usual care to enhance development outcomes during the transition from the neonatal intensive care unit to home: A pilot randomized controlled trial. *BMC Pediatr.* **2018**, *18*, 46. [CrossRef] [PubMed]
14. Morgan, C.; Novak, I.; Dale, R.C.; Guzzetta, A.; Badawi, N. GAME (Goals—Activity—Motor Enrichment): Protocol of a single blind randomised controlled trial of motor training, parent education and environmental enrichment for infants at high risk of cerebral palsy. *BMC Neurol.* **2014**, *14*, 203. [CrossRef]
15. An, M.; Nord, J.; Koziol, N.A.; Dusing, S.C.; Kane, A.E.; Lobo, M.A.; Mccoy, S.W.; Harbourne, R.T. Developing a fidelity measure of early intervention programs for children with neuromotor disorders. *Dev. Med. Child Neurol.* **2021**, *63*, 97–103. [CrossRef]
16. Lynch, H.; Moore, A. Play as an occupation in occupational therapy. *Br. J. Occup. Ther.* **2016**, *79*, 519–520. [CrossRef]
17. Hamm, E.M. Playfulness and the Environmental Support of Play in Children with and without Developmental Disabilities. *OTJR Occup. Particip. Health* **2006**, *26*, 88–96. [CrossRef]
18. Venuti, P.; de Falco, S.; Giusti, Z.; Bornstein, M.H. Play and emotional availability in young children with Down syndrome. *Infant Ment. Health J.* **2008**, *29*, 133–152. [CrossRef]

19. Miller, M.; Sun, S.; Iosif, A.-M.; Young, G.S.; Belding, A.; Tubbs, A.; Ozonoff, S. Repetitive behavior with objects in infants developing autism predicts diagnosis and later social behavior as early as 9 months. *J. Abnorm. Psychol.* **2021**, *130*, 665–675. [CrossRef]
20. Westby, C. Playing to Pretend or "Pretending" to Play: Play in Children with Autism Spectrum Disorder. *Semin. Speech Lang.* **2022**, *43*, 331–346. [CrossRef]
21. Williams, E. A Comparative Review of Early Forms of Object-Directed Play and Parent-Infant Play in Typical Infants and Young Children with Autism. *Autism* **2003**, *7*, 361–374. [CrossRef]
22. Perzolli, S.; Bentenuto, A.; Bertamini, G.; Venuti, P. Play with Me: How Fathers and Mothers Play with Their Preschoolers with Autism. *Brain Sci.* **2023**, *13*, 120. [CrossRef] [PubMed]
23. Venuti, P.; de Falco, S.; Esposito, G.; Bornstein, M.H. Mother–Child Play: Children with Down Syndrome and Typical Development. *Am. J. Intellect. Dev. Disabil.* **2009**, *114*, 274–288. [CrossRef] [PubMed]
24. Chiarello, L.A.; Bartlett, D.J.; Palisano, R.J.; McCoy, S.W.; Jeffries, L.; Fiss, A.L.; Wilk, P. Determinants of playfulness of young children with cerebral palsy. *Dev. Neurorehabilit.* **2019**, *22*, 240–249. [CrossRef]
25. Brigham, N.B.; Yoder, P.J.; Jarzynka, M.A.; Tapp, J. The Sequential Relationship Between Parent Attentional Cues and Sustained Attention to Objects in Young Children with Autism. *J. Autism Dev. Disord.* **2010**, *40*, 200–208. [CrossRef]
26. Sugden, D. Handbook of Developmental Disabilities—Edited by Samual Odom, Robert Horner, Martha Snell and Jan Blacher. *Br. J. Spec. Educ.* **2008**, *35*, 188–189. [CrossRef]
27. Fantasia, V.; Galbusera, L.; Reck, C.; Fasulo, A. Rethinking Intrusiveness: Exploring the Sequential Organization in Interactions Between Infants and Mothers. *Front. Psychol.* **2019**, *10*, 1543. [CrossRef]
28. Moreno-Núñez, A.; Rodríguez, C.; Del Olmo, M.J. Rhythmic ostensive gestures: How adults facilitate infants' entrance into early triadic interactions. *Infant Behav. Dev.* **2017**, *49*, 168–181. [CrossRef] [PubMed]
29. Committee on the Science of Children Birth to Age 8: Deepening and Broadening the Foundation for Success; Board on Children, Youth, and Families; Institute of Medicine; National Research Council; Allen, L.R.; Kelly, B.B. (Eds.) Child Development and Early Learning. In *Transforming the Workforce for Children Birth through Age 8*; National Academies Press (US): Washington, DC, USA, 2015.
30. Rose, S.A.; Feldman, J.F.; Jankowski, J.J. Information processing in toddlers: Continuity from infancy and persistence of preterm deficits. *Intelligence* **2009**, *37*, 311–320. [CrossRef]
31. Smith, K.E.; Swank, P.R.; Denson, S.E.; Landry, S.H.; Baldwin, C.D.; Wildin, S. The Relation of Medical Risk and Maternal Stimulation with Preterm Infants' Development of Cognitive, Language and Daily Living Skills. *J. Child Psychol. Psychiatry* **1996**, *37*, 855–864. [CrossRef]
32. Johnson, N.; Parker, A.T. Effects of Wait Time when Communicating with Children who have Sensory and Additional Disabilities. *J. Vis. Impair. Blind.* **2013**, *107*, 363–374. [CrossRef]
33. Niutanen, U.; Harra, T.; Lano, A.; Metsäranta, M. Systematic review of sensory processing in preterm children reveals abnormal sensory modulation, somatosensory processing and sensory-based motor processing. *Acta Paediatr.* **2020**, *109*, 45–55. [CrossRef] [PubMed]
34. Cress, C.J.; Grabast, J.; Jerke, K.B. Contingent Interactions Between Parents and Young Children With Severe Expressive Communication Impairments. *Commun. Disord. Q.* **2013**, *34*, 81–96. [CrossRef]
35. Sigafoos, J.; Woodyatt, G.; Keen, D.; Tait, K.; Tucker, M.; Roberts-Pennell, D.; Pittendreigh, N. Identifying Potential Communicative Acts in Children with Developmental and Physical Disabilities. *Commun. Disord. Q.* **2000**, *21*, 77–86. [CrossRef]
36. Provenzi, L.; Rosa, E.; Visintin, E.; Mascheroni, E.; Guida, E.; Cavallini, A.; Montirosso, R. Understanding the role and function of maternal touch in children with neurodevelopmental disabilities. *Infant Behav. Dev.* **2020**, *58*, 101420. [CrossRef]
37. Håkstad, R.B.; Øberg, G.K.; Girolami, G.L.; Dusing, S.C. Enactive explorations of children's sensory-motor play and therapeutic handling in physical therapy. *Front. Rehabilit. Sci.* **2022**, *3*, 994804. [CrossRef]
38. Gibson, E.J. Exploratory Behavior in the Development of Perceiving, Acting, and the Acquiring of Knowledge. *Annu. Rev. Psychol.* **1988**, *39*, 1–42. [CrossRef]
39. Mateus, V.; Martins, C.; Osório, A.; Martins, E.C.; Soares, I. Joint attention at 10 months of age in infant–mother dyads: Contrasting free toy-play with semi-structured toy-play. *Infant Behav. Dev.* **2013**, *36*, 176–179. [CrossRef]
40. Clearfield, M.W. Play for Success: An intervention to boost object exploration in infants from low-income households. *Infant Behav. Dev.* **2019**, *55*, 112–122. [CrossRef]
41. Lobo, M.A.; Harbourne, R.T.; Dusing, S.C.; McCoy, S.W. Grounding Early Intervention: Physical Therapy Cannot Just Be About Motor Skills Anymore. *Phys. Ther.* **2013**, *93*, 94–103. [CrossRef]
42. Fawcett, C.; Liszkowski, U. Mimicry and play initiation in 18-month-old infants. *Infant Behav. Dev.* **2012**, *35*, 689–696. [CrossRef]
43. Parise, E.; Cleveland, A.; Costabile, A.; Striano, T. Influence of vocal cues on learning about objects in joint attention contexts. *Infant Behav. Dev.* **2007**, *30*, 380–384. [CrossRef] [PubMed]
44. Cattaneo, L.; Rizzolatti, G. The Mirror Neuron System. *Arch. Neurol.* **2009**, *66*, 557–560. [CrossRef] [PubMed]
45. Deák, G.O.; Walden, T.A.; Kaiser, M.Y.; Lewis, A. Driven from distraction: How infants respond to parents' attempts to elicit and re-direct their attention. *Infant Behav. Dev.* **2008**, *31*, 34–50. [CrossRef]
46. Ayres, A.J.; Robbins, J. *Sensory Integration and the Child: Understanding Hidden Sensory Challenges*, 25th anniversary ed.; WPS: Los Angeles, CA, USA, 2005; ISBN 978-0-87424-437-3.

47. Santha, J.C. *Occupational Therapy for Children and Adolescents*, 7th ed.; Case-Smith, J., O'Brien, J.C., Eds.; Elsevier: St. Louis, MI, USA, 2015; ISBN 978-0-323-16925-7.
48. Fiss, A.L.; Chiarello, L.A.; Hsu, L.-Y.; McCoy, S.W. Adaptive behavior and mastery motivation in children with physical disabilities. *Physiother. Theory Pract.* 2023, 39, 1–12. [CrossRef]
49. American Occupational Therapy Association. Occupational Therapy Practice Framework: Domain and Process—Fourth Edition. *Am. J. Occup. Ther.* 2020, 74, 7412410010p1–7412410010p87. [CrossRef] [PubMed]
50. O'Grady, M.G.; Dusing, S.C. Assessment Position Affects Problem-Solving Behaviors in a Child with Motor Impairments. *Pediatr. Phys. Ther.* 2016, 28, 253–258. [CrossRef]
51. Mather, E. Novelty, attention, and challenges for developmental psychology. *Front. Psychol.* 2013, 4, 491. [CrossRef]
52. Shinskey, J.L.; Munakata, Y. Something old, something new: A developmental transition from familiarity to novelty preferences with hidden objects. *Dev. Sci.* 2010, 13, 378–384. [CrossRef]
53. Lobo, M.A.; Kokkoni, E.; de Campos, A.C.; Galloway, J.C. Not just playing around: Infants' behaviors with objects reflect ability, constraints, and object properties. *Infant Behav. Dev.* 2014, 37, 334–351. [CrossRef]
54. Roder, B.J.; Bushneil, E.W.; Sasseville, A.M. Infants' Preferences for Familiarity and Novelty During the Course of Visual Processing. *Infancy* 2000, 1, 491–507. [CrossRef]
55. Sheets-Johnstone, M. *The Primacy of Movement*, Expanded 2nd ed.; John Benjamins Pub. Co: Amsterdam, The Netherlands, 2011; ISBN 978-90-272-5218-0.
56. Rose, S.A.; Gottfried, A.W.; Melloy-Carminar, P.; Bridger, W.H. Familiarity and novelty preferences in infant recognition memory: Implications for information processing. *Dev. Psychol.* 1982, 18, 704–713. [CrossRef]
57. Hughes, F.P. *Children, Play, and Development*, 4th ed.; Sage: Los Angeles, CA, USA, 2010; ISBN 978-1-4129-6769-3.
58. Wehmeyer, M.L.; Singh, N.N.; Shogren, K.A. (Eds.) *Handbook of Positive Psychology in Intellectual and Developmental Disabilities: Translating Research into Practice*; Springer: Cham, Switzerland, 2017; ISBN 978-3-319-86540-9.
59. Steiner, A.M. A Strength-Based Approach to Parent Education for Children With Autism. *J. Posit. Behav. Interv.* 2011, 13, 178–190. [CrossRef]
60. Behne, T.; Carpenter, M.; Call, J.; Tomasello, M. Unwilling Versus Unable: Infants' Understanding of Intentional Action. *Dev. Psychol.* 2005, 41, 328–337. [CrossRef] [PubMed]
61. Begus, K.; Gliga, T.; Southgate, V. Infants Learn What They Want to Learn: Responding to Infant Pointing Leads to Superior Learning. *PLoS ONE* 2014, 9, e108817. [CrossRef] [PubMed]
62. Lynch, H. Infant Places, Spaces and Objects: Exploring the Physical in Learning Environments for Infants Under Two. Ph.D. Thesis, Technological University Dublin, Dublin, Ireland, 2011. [CrossRef]
63. Looper, J.; Ulrich, D. Does Orthotic Use Affect Upper Extremity Support During Upright Play in Infants With Down Syndrome? *Pediatr. Phys. Ther.* 2011, 23, 70–77. [CrossRef]
64. Rachwani, J.; Santamaria, V.; Saavedra, S.L.; Wood, S.; Porter, F.; Woollacott, M.H. Segmental trunk control acquisition and reaching in typically developing infants. *Exp. Brain Res.* 2013, 228, 131–139. [CrossRef]
65. Kretch, K.S.; Marcinowski, E.C.; Hsu, L.; Koziol, N.A.; Harbourne, R.T.; Lobo, M.A.; Dusing, S.C. Opportunities for learning and social interaction in infant sitting: Effects of sitting support, sitting skill, and gross motor delay. *Dev. Sci.* 2022, 26, e13318. [CrossRef]
66. Bigelow, A.E.; MacLean, K.; Proctor, J. The role of joint attention in the development of infants' play with objects. *Dev. Sci.* 2004, 7, 518–526. [CrossRef]
67. Stern, D.N. *The First Relationship: Infant and Mother*; Harvard University Press: Cambridge, MA, USA, 2002; ISBN 978-0-674-00783-3.
68. Fantasia, V.; Fasulo, A.; Costall, A.; LÃ³pez, B. Changing the game: Exploring infants' participation in early play routines. *Front. Psychol.* 2014, 5, 522. [CrossRef]
69. Lewthwaite, R.; Chiviacowsky, S.; Drews, R.; Wulf, G. Choose to move: The motivational impact of autonomy support on motor learning. *Psychon. Bull. Rev.* 2015, 22, 1383–1388. [CrossRef]
70. Swirbul, M.S.; Herzberg, O.; Tamis-LeMonda, C.S. Object play in the everyday home environment generates rich opportunities for infant learning. *Infant Behav. Dev.* 2022, 67, 101712. [CrossRef] [PubMed]
71. Smith, L.B. Cognition as a dynamic system: Principles from embodiment. *Dev. Rev.* 2005, 25, 278–298. [CrossRef]
72. Dauch, C.; Imwalle, M.; Ocasio, B.; Metz, A.E. The influence of the number of toys in the environment on toddlers' play. *Infant Behav. Dev.* 2018, 50, 78–87. [CrossRef] [PubMed]
73. Koşkulu, S.; Küntay, A.C.; Liszkowski, U.; Uzundag, B.A. Number and type of toys affect joint attention of mothers and infants. *Infant Behav. Dev.* 2021, 64, 101589. [CrossRef]
74. Gosso, Y.; Carvalho, A. Play and cultural context. *Encycl. Early Child. Dev.* 2013, 1, 1–7.
75. Holden, E.; Buryn-Weitzel, J.C.; Atim, S.; Biroch, H.; Donnellan, E.; Graham, K.E.; Hoffman, M.; Jurua, M.; Knapper, C.V.; Lahiff, N.J.; et al. Maternal attitudes and behaviours differentially shape infant early life experience: A cross cultural study. *PLoS ONE* 2022, 17, e0278378. [CrossRef]
76. Rochanavibhata, S.; Marian, V. Culture at Play: A Cross-Cultural Comparison of Mother-Child Communication during Toy Play. *Lang. Learn. Dev.* 2022, 18, 294–309. [CrossRef]
77. Moon-Seo, S.K.; Munsell, S.E.; Kim, N. Mothers' and Fathers' Perceptions of Children's Play. *Early Child. Educ. J.* 2023, 51, 1–13. [CrossRef]

78. Schmidt, W.J.; Keller, H.; Coto, M.R. The cultural specificity of parent-infant interaction: Perspectives of urban middle-class and rural indigenous families in Costa Rica. *Infant Behav. Dev.* **2023**, *70*, 101796. [CrossRef] [PubMed]
79. Prioreschi, A.; Wrottesley, S.V.; Slemming, W.; Cohen, E.; Norris, S.A. A qualitative study reporting maternal perceptions of the importance of play for healthy growth and development in the first two years of life. *BMC Pediatr.* **2020**, *20*, 428. [CrossRef]
80. Stillianesis, S.; Spencer, G.; Villeneuve, M.; Sterman, J.; Bundy, A.; Wyver, S.; Tranter, P.; Naughton, G.; Ragen, J.; Beetham, K.S. Parents' perspectives on managing risk in play for children with developmental disabilities. *Disabil. Soc.* **2022**, *37*, 1272–1292. [CrossRef]
81. Keller, H.; Lohaus, A.; Kuensemueller, P.; Abels, M.; Yovsi, R.; Voelker, S.; Jensen, H.; Papaligoura, Z.; Rosabal-Coto, M.; Kulks, D.; et al. The Bio-Culture of Parenting: Evidence From Five Cultural Communities. *Parenting* **2004**, *4*, 25–50. [CrossRef]
82. Metaferia, B.K.; Futo, J.; Takacs, Z.K. Parents' Views on Play and the Goal of Early Childhood Education in Relation to Children's Home Activity and Executive Functions: A Cross-Cultural Investigation. *Front. Psychol.* **2021**, *12*, 646074. [CrossRef] [PubMed]
83. Sicart, M. Playthings. *Games Cult.* **2022**, *17*, 140–155. [CrossRef]
84. Stern, M.; Karraker, K.H.; Sopko, A.M.; Norman, S. The prematurity stereotype revisited: Impact on mothers' interactions with premature and full-term infants. *Infant Ment. Health J.* **2000**, *21*, 495–509. [CrossRef]
85. Tallandini, M.A.; Morsan, V.; Gronchi, G.; Macagno, F. Systematic and Meta-Analytic Review: Triggering Agents of Parental Perception of Child's Vulnerability in Instances of Preterm Birth. *J. Pediatr. Psychol.* **2015**, *40*, 545–553. [CrossRef]
86. Pellecchia, M.; Beidas, R.S.; Mandell, D.S.; Cannuscio, C.C.; Dunst, C.J.; Stahmer, A.C. Parent empowerment and coaching in early intervention: Study protocol for a feasibility study. *Pilot Feasibility Stud.* **2020**, *6*, 22. [CrossRef]
87. King, G.; Chiarello, L.A.; Ideishi, R.; D'Arrigo, R.; Smart, E.; Ziviani, J.; Pinto, M. The Nature, Value, and Experience of Engagement in Pediatric Rehabilitation: Perspectives of Youth, Caregivers, and Service Providers. *Dev. Neurorehabil.* **2020**, *23*, 18–30. [CrossRef]
88. King, G.; Chiarello, L.A.; McLarnon, M.J.W.; Ziviani, J.; Pinto, M.; Wright, F.V.; Phoenix, M. A measure of parent engagement: Plan appropriateness, partnering, and positive outcome expectancy in pediatric rehabilitation sessions. *Disabil. Rehabil.* **2022**, *44*, 3459–3468. [CrossRef]
89. Sheridan, S.; Marvin, C.; Knoche, L.; Edwards, C. Getting ready: Promoting school readiness through a relationship-based partnership model. *Early Child. Serv. Interdiscip. J. Eff.* **2008**, *2*, 149–172.
90. Nix, R.L.; Bierman, K.L.; Motamedi, M.; Heinrichs, B.S.; Gill, S. Parent engagement in a Head Start home visiting program predicts sustained growth in children's school readiness. *Early Child. Res. Q.* **2018**, *45*, 106–114. [CrossRef]
91. Knoche, L.L.; Edwards, C.P.; Sheridan, S.M.; Kupzyk, K.A.; Marvin, C.A.; Cline, K.D.; Clarke, B.L. Getting Ready: Results of a Randomized Trial of a Relationship-Focused Intervention on the Parent-Infant Relationship in Rural Early Head Start. *Infant Ment. Health J.* **2012**, *33*, 669. [CrossRef] [PubMed]
92. Tomalski, P.; Pérez, D.L.; Radkowska, A.; Malinowska-Korczak, A. Dyadic interactions during infant learning: Exploring infant-parent exchanges in experimental eye-tracking studies. *Infant Behav. Dev.* **2022**, *69*, 101780. [CrossRef] [PubMed]
93. Schroer, S.E.; Yu, C. The real-time effects of parent speech on infants' multimodal attention and dyadic coordination. *Infancy* **2022**, *27*, 1154–1178. [CrossRef] [PubMed]
94. Holsbeeke, L.; Ketelaar, M.; Schoemaker, M.M.; Gorter, J.W. Capacity, Capability, and Performance: Different Constructs or Three of a Kind? *Arch. Phys. Med. Rehabil.* **2009**, *90*, 849–855. [CrossRef] [PubMed]
95. Suarez-Rivera, C.; Schatz, J.L.; Herzberg, O.; Tamis-LeMonda, C.S. Joint engagement in the home environment is frequent, multimodal, timely, and structured. *Infancy* **2022**, *27*, 232–254. [CrossRef] [PubMed]
96. Custode, S.A.; Tamis-LeMonda, C. Cracking the code: Social and contextual cues to language input in the home environment. *Infancy* **2020**, *25*, 809–826. [CrossRef]
97. Carson, V.; Kuzik, N. The association between parent–child technology interference and cognitive and social–emotional development in preschool-aged children. *Child. Care Health Dev.* **2021**, *47*, 477–483. [CrossRef]
98. Morris, A.J.; Filippetti, M.L.; Rigato, S. The impact of parents' smartphone use on language development in young children. *Child Dev. Perspect.* **2022**, *16*, 103–109. [CrossRef]
99. Myruski, S.; Gulyayeva, O.; Birk, S.; Pérez-Edgar, K.; Buss, K.A.; Dennis-Tiwary, T.A. Digital disruption? Maternal mobile device use is related to infant social-emotional functioning. *Dev. Sci.* **2018**, *21*, e12610. [CrossRef]
100. Duch, H.; Marti, M.; Wu, W.; Snow, R.; Garcia, V. CARING: The Impact of a Parent–Child, Play-Based Intervention to Promote Latino Head Start Children's Social–Emotional Development. *J. Prim. Prev.* **2019**, *40*, 171–188. [CrossRef] [PubMed]

Disclaimer/Publisher's Note: The statements, opinions and data contained in all publications are solely those of the individual author(s) and contributor(s) and not of MDPI and/or the editor(s). MDPI and/or the editor(s) disclaim responsibility for any injury to people or property resulting from any ideas, methods, instructions or products referred to in the content.

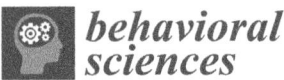

Perspective

Lifelong Fitness in Ambulatory Children and Adolescents with Cerebral Palsy I: Key Ingredients for Bone and Muscle Health

Noelle G. Moreau [1,*], Kathleen M. Friel [2], Robyn K. Fuchs [3], Sudarshan Dayanidhi [4], Theresa Sukal-Moulton [5], Marybeth Grant-Beuttler [6], Mark D. Peterson [7], Richard D. Stevenson [8] and Susan V. Duff [9]

1. Department of Physical Therapy, School of Allied Health Professions, Louisiana State University Health Sciences Center, New Orleans, LA 70112, USA
2. Burke Neurological Institute, Weill Cornell Medicine, White Plains, NY 10605, USA; kaf3001@med.cornell.edu
3. Division of Biomedical Science, College of Osteopathic Medicine, Marian University, Indianapolis, IN 46222, USA; rfuchs@marian.edu
4. Shirley Ryan Ability Lab, Chicago, IL 60611, USA; sdayanidhi@sralab.org
5. Department of Physical Therapy & Human Movement Sciences, Northwestern University, Chicago, IL 60611, USA; theresa-moulton@northwestern.edu
6. Department of Physical Therapy, Oregon Institute of Technology, Klamath Falls, OR 97601, USA; marybeth.grantbeuttler@oit.edu
7. Department of Physical Medicine and Rehabilitation, Michigan Medicine, University of Michigan, Ann Arbor, MI 48109, USA; mdpeterz@med.umich.edu
8. Division of Neurodevelopmental and Behavioral Pediatrics, Department of Pediatrics, School of Medicine, University of Virginia, Charlottesville, VA 22903, USA; rds8z@uvahealth.org
9. Department of Physical Therapy, Crean College of Health and Behavioral Sciences, Chapman University, Irvine, CA 92618, USA; duff@chapman.edu
* Correspondence: nmorea@lsuhsc.edu

Abstract: Physical activity of a sufficient amount and intensity is essential to health and the prevention of a sedentary lifestyle in all children as they transition into adolescence and adulthood. While fostering a fit lifestyle in all children can be challenging, it may be even more so for those with cerebral palsy (CP). Evidence suggests that bone and muscle health can improve with targeted exercise programs for children with CP. Yet, it is not clear how musculoskeletal improvements are sustained into adulthood. In this perspective, we introduce key ingredients and guidelines to promote bone and muscle health in ambulatory children with CP (GMFCS I–III), which could lay the foundation for sustained fitness and musculoskeletal health as they transition from childhood to adolescence and adulthood. First, one must consider crucial characteristics of the skeletal and muscular systems as well as key factors to augment bone and muscle integrity. Second, to build a better foundation, we must consider critical time periods and essential ingredients for programming. Finally, to foster the sustainability of a fit lifestyle, we must encourage commitment and self-initiated action while ensuring the attainment of skill acquisition and function. Thus, the overall objective of this perspective paper is to guide exercise programming and community implementation to truly alter lifelong fitness in persons with CP.

Keywords: muscle strength; muscle power; resistance training; bone health; lifelong fitness

1. Current Physical Activity Guidelines for Children and Adolescents

The World Health Organization (WHO) [1] and the American College of Sports Medicine (ACSM) [2] recommend that children and adolescents achieve a minimum of 60 min of physical activity per day at a moderate to vigorous intensity to maintain health. Both groups recommend involvement in vigorous-intense aerobic activities three times per week to support the integrity of the developing musculoskeletal and cardiopulmonary systems. Despite these published guidelines and benefits, many children and adolescents who are typically developing (TD) fall below recommended levels [3], and those with

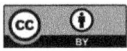

neurodevelopmental conditions such as cerebral palsy (CP) are at even greater risk for achieving insufficient physical activity [4,5]. We believe that these data, demonstrating deficient physical activity, should serve as a call to action for fostering lifelong fitness in all children, particularly adolescents at risk for the secondary effects of a sedentary lifestyle, such as those with CP.

Physical activity is linked to quality of life and happiness [6,7]; thus, strategies to enhance adherence to programming should be holistic in nature and salient to the individual performer [8]. Empowering children and adolescents to be self-directed in their choice of activities is a powerful link to sustaining change and preventing a sedentary lifestyle. Long-term adherence to physical activity can also strengthen the musculoskeletal (MSK) system and sustain the shorter-term gains in MSK health seen during focused fitness programs. The positive impact of interventions targeting bone and muscle health demonstrated in children with CP further amplifies the need for opportunities to participate in activities that benefit these body systems. The purpose of this perspective paper is to identify key ingredients for interventions targeting the MSK system and provide guidelines for promoting bone and muscle health that are essential to programming for achieving the goal of lifelong fitness for persons with CP across the Gross Motor Function Classification Scale (GMFCS), particularly those who are ambulatory (GMFCS levels I–III). Further, embedding a framework of lifestyle intervention into programming could help empower children to be self-directed, fostering motivation and habit formation essential to sustaining change in the MSK system and preventing a sedentary lifestyle as they move into adolescence and adulthood [9].

2. Musculoskeletal (MSK) System

Adults living with CP and other pediatric-onset disabilities that target the MSK system have a significantly higher prevalence of common psychological, cardiometabolic, and musculoskeletal morbidity and multimorbidity as compared to adults without CP [10–12]. Changes in the muscular system contribute to the onset of sedentary behavior, which is pervasive in children and adolescents with CP—even those at higher levels on the GMFCS [4,13,14]. Therefore, it is important to consider the characteristics of the MSK system and related functions in persons with CP during the design of programs to augment the integrity of this system and improve function in this group at risk.

The health of the MSK system is influenced by insufficient physical activity, especially during the transition from adolescence to adulthood. The risk of progressive, age-and activity-related declines in MSK health is even greater for persons with CP [15–17]. Changes in bone and muscle integrity and associated function are well documented in those with CP, particularly during development and into adulthood [18–24]. A reduction in muscle growth has been found as early as 15 months of age [25]. As children move into adolescence and adulthood, suboptimal nutritional and mechanical factors can negatively influence the integrity of the MSK system, thereby reducing tolerance to physical activity [24,26].

2.1. Skeletal System

Bone mass, cross-sectional bone size, and bone strength increase rapidly in childhood and peak in adolescence for TD persons, as shown in Figure 1. Individuals that attain optimal peak bone mass have a reduced risk of developing osteoporosis and sustaining a low-trauma fracture [27]. The development and maintenance of bone mass require adequate mechanical loading to stimulate structural and mineral adaptations. Engaging in moderate- to high-level physical activity during childhood and adolescence contributes to optimizing peak bone mass and the ability to sustain it into adulthood [28,29].

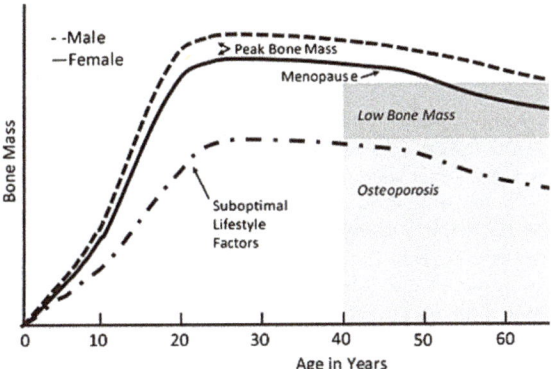

Figure 1. Bone mass across the lifespan with optimal and suboptimal lifestyle choices. Reproduced with permission from Weaver et al. [30].

Gunter and colleagues [31] stress that activities that have the greatest effect on developing bone mass are those with a high magnitude of force applied at a rapid rate. Figure 2 depicts the ground reaction force (GRF) in units of bodyweight and the time to peak force for low- and high-impact activities performed by a representative 10-year-old girl. The authors report that activities with the most osteogenic potential have GRFs greater than 3.5 times body weight (per leg), with peak force occurring in less than 0.1 s. Jumping activities from a 100 cm box had GRFs of 8.5 times body weight and were found to improve hip bone mass in children [32,33].

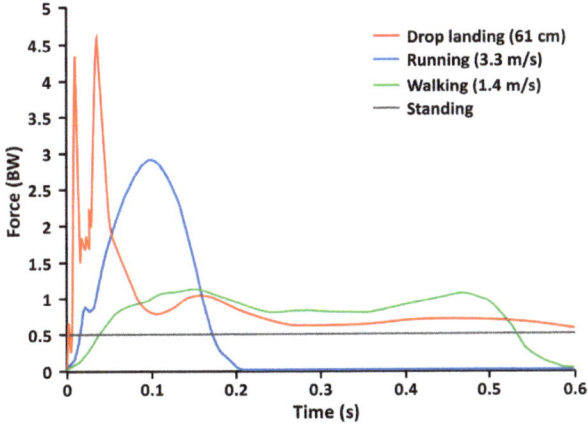

Figure 2. Ground reaction forces and rates of loading for **(1)** drop landings from a 61-cm box with a peak force of 4.5 BW/leg (red); **(2)** running at a speed of 3.3 m/s resulting in a peak force of 3 BW/leg (blue); **(3)** w at a speed of 1.4 m/s resulting in a peak force of 1 BW/leg (green); and **(4)** quiet standing resulting in a static load of 0.5 BW/leg (gray). This illustration of unpublished data by Jeremy J. Bauer was adapted and used with his permission [34].

Inactivity in childhood has been linked to an increased incidence of osteoporosis and osteoarthritis later in life [31,35,36]. The National Osteoporosis Foundation advocates for high physical activity and the intake of calcium (~1000–1300 mg/d) and vitamin D (600 IU/d) in childhood and adolescence to enhance bone health [30,37]. A decrease in activity and mobility in persons with CP reduces mechanical loading vital for bone integrity [24,38]. Yet, it is important to consider whether children and adolescents with

CP who have alterations in skeletal alignment and strength can tolerate sufficient impact loading on an ongoing basis to improve and sustain bone health. It is also unknown whether a lower-impact activity could provide adequate osteogenic potential to augment bone integrity in persons with CP. Therefore, it is important to consider individualized exercise prescriptions that safely expand impact loading through physical activity in persons with CP across the GMFCS levels I–III. Further, prescriptions that safely target all GMFCS levels to increase bone mass and sustain bone health into adulthood must be investigated.

Adolescents who are TD accumulate 25% of their adult bone mass during the two years after peak height velocity, occurring from about 11.8 to 13.4 years of age [36]. Bone minerals accrue in those with CP during adolescence and young adulthood but remain significantly below those of the general population [39]. Deficiencies in bone mineral accrual are multifactorial and include inadequate nutrition and suboptimal physical activity [40]. By the time those with CP enter adulthood, their mean bone density may be greater than 2 standard deviations below the mean for age and sex, depending on GMFCS levels [41]. The impact on bone mass is also dependent on the severity of CP, with children that have limited mechanical loading having lower bone health compared to TD children and those with a lower GMFCS level [39,42,43]. Moderate to severe impairment in persons with CP, along with inactivity [5], contribute to the higher prevalence of fractures [36,44,45]. To have a positive influence on long-term bone health requires the targeted intervention at critical time points during development, with optimal gains in bone mass and size prior to late childhood and early adolescence to take advantage of the accrual associated with pubertal growth [46].

Skeletal maturation and integrity vary within and across GMFCS levels. Henderson et al. [47] found that in children and adolescents 2.6 to 21 years of age with moderate to severe CP, skeletal age closely approximated chronological age. However, deficiencies in skeletal maturation were found to be associated with delays in height, low lumbar bone density, and poor nutrition status. Clinically, these could be used as markers to evaluate the risk of low bone mass in children with CP across all GMFCS levels. Chen et al. [48] examined skeletal integrity in children with CP with a range in severity and found lower limb bone density to be correlated with increasing GMFCS level. Vertebral fracture risk is increased in children with GMFCS levels IV/V, with those children at GMFCS levels I–III having a similar incidence of fracture as TD children [49,50]. Paying close attention to the integrity of the skeletal system before and during intense physical activity and impact loading is vital to preventing injury during any training program, regardless of GMFCS level.

2.2. Muscular System

The properties of healthy muscle, including architecture, elasticity, connective tissue, and sarcomeres, typically adapt to functional demands and use [51]. As children grow, muscle strength and motor skills progressively increase [52]. Sufficient muscle development, strength, power, and adaptability are essential before engaging in demanding physical activities and specific motor skills (e.g., sports). Thus, those who lack sufficient strength and skill may be less competent and confident in their performance abilities, leading to less frequent engagement in physical activity. To ensure safety, muscle integrity must be considered before attempting to augment muscle function with demanding physical activity.

Atypical muscle growth contributes to altered physiology and MSK integrity [18,25,53–55]. Muscle volume and passive mechanical properties of those with CP have been reported to differ from those who are TD as early as 1–3 years of age [25,54]. Multiple factors contribute to variable growth, passive stiffness, and the onset of muscle contracture. At a cellular level, muscle myofiber areas in persons with CP do not appear to develop at the same rate as in those who are TD (Figure 3) [53]. Muscle sarcomeres typically increase in series in response to chronic stretching, including during postnatal development [56–58]. Yet, muscle contractures in persons with CP demonstrate overstretched muscles and fewer serial sarcomeres [59,60], suggesting an inability to add sarcomeres during growth. In CP, muscle contractures and a reduction in muscle stem cells (satellite cells) with abnormalities in their function are reported, along with an increase in the extracellular matrix [53,61–64]. Importantly, this might not be true for all muscles or at younger ages [65]. The muscle substrate of those with CP has also been found to have a reduction in mitochondrial function and content, which is important for energy production [66,67]. Interestingly, the onset of fat infiltration can alter the ability of affected muscles to generate adequate force [68–70]. These multiple alterations in muscle for those with CP are important to consider during training since sufficient loading is essential for muscle plasticity and muscle performance.

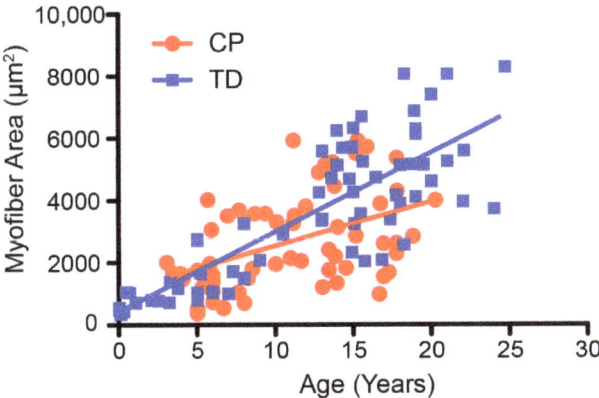

Figure 3. Change in mean myofiber area for age in TD children (squares, $n = 67$) and those with CP (circles, $n = 58$). Data were extracted based on published cross-sectional studies.

At the macroscopic level, measures of muscle size, such as muscle volume, cross-sectional area, and muscle thickness, are significantly decreased in children and adolescents with CP as compared to TD peers [18,19,23,71,72]. Muscle size is a strong predictor of force output, but force-generating capacity is also negatively impacted by changes in both passive and active mechanical properties that were discussed previously. Moreover, diminished muscle size is a significant contributor to decreased muscular strength and is strongly influenced by mobility levels as measured by the GMFCS [73]. While deficits in voluntary activation are present in CP and do play a role, these deficits appear to be more pronounced in the plantarflexors as compared to the quadriceps [74].

During typical development, muscle strength increases until it peaks between 20 and 30 years of age, then slowly declines. In persons with CP, muscle strength and power increase at a lower rate, peak at an earlier age, and are hypothesized to contribute to a faster decline with age than those without CP [75] (Figure 4). This loss of strength and muscular reserve is believed to result in early and rapid age-related decreases in function. This time period also corresponds to a period of ambulatory decline as individuals with CP transition into adolescence and adulthood [76–79].

In addition to muscular strength, Moreau [80] stresses the importance of muscle power for the performance of functional activities. Muscle power and a sufficient rate of force development (RFD) are essential for motor transitions during gait, stairclimbing, and other functional tasks such as transfers and are also important for reducing fall risk. Moreau reported that muscle power is more significantly impaired than strength in persons with CP compared to those who are TD [81,82]. In addition, while knee extensor muscle power increases linearly with age in persons who are TD, the rate of increase is lower for those with CP as they move from childhood to young adulthood [83] (Figure 5). Investigations into the neuromuscular adaptations that occur in response to specific activity and exercise have been examined in CP [81,83,84], yet further work is needed across the GMFCS spectrum.

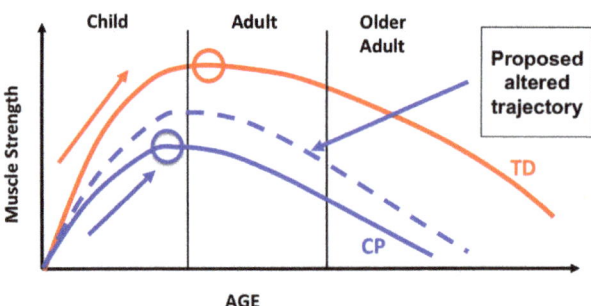

Figure 4. Age-related changes in muscle strength for TD individuals (red line) and those with CP (blue line). Circles signify peak muscle strength for TD (red) and CP (blue). The dashed blue line denotes a proposed altered trajectory of age-related decline with targeted intervention during the pre-adolescent critical period, including lifelong changes in fitness, health, and function.

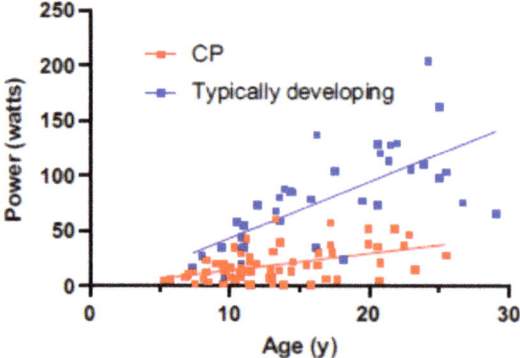

Figure 5. Relationship between knee extensor power and age in a TD (blue circles) cohort (*n* = 42; ages 7–29 y) and in a cohort with CP (red circles) (*n* = 66; ages 5–25 y). Data compiled from unpublished and published cross-sectional data. Reproduced with permission from Moreau and Lieber, 2022.

In a recent review article, Faigenbaum et al. [85] remarks on the decline in muscular fitness in 7-year-old TD children and adolescents. This decline and the incidence of suboptimal physical activity levels place children and adolescents at risk for injury and adverse health conditions. Faigenbaum et al. [85] advocate for early resistance training and postulate that strength gains after training are often related to neural and muscular adaptations. Given the high degree of neuroplasticity in pre-adolescence, the development of muscular strength, power, and motor skill performance should be emphasized in childhood in preparation for projected gains in adolescence [86,87]. In addition to the neuromuscular and musculoskeletal benefits of resistance training, there is longstanding literature documenting the robust association between strength and cardiometabolic health among children and adolescents [88,89].

3. Building a Better Foundation for MSK Health in Children with CP

Despite the risk of progressive declines in fitness, health, and function in persons with CP, the optimal age and key program ingredients essential to ensuring a long-lasting level of fitness, health, and function are largely unknown. However, current and related data can be leveraged to begin program design and monitoring. Creating a strong physical health foundation that supports optimal MSK development should include critical considerations, as reviewed below.

3.1. Critical Time Periods

Given the number of factors contributing to atypical MSK growth and development in persons with CP [47], it is vital to intervene early enough and at an adequate intensity and dose to have a long-lasting effect on muscle and bone integrity. Targeted intervention at critical time points during development is needed, particularly in childhood and early adolescence, to optimize peak bone mineral accrual associated with pubertal growth. Ideally, this would occur prior to peak height velocity in order to significantly influence muscle and bone health [36,39], allowing for successful participation in fitness and leisure activities of interest. This is also the optimal period for building a strong muscular reserve, as muscular strength peaks in early adulthood before slowly declining. In children with CP, the rate of increase in muscular strength during growth is less than TD, thus reaching peak strength earlier and potentially contributing to an earlier decline in muscular strength and function over the lifespan (Figure 4). Therefore, intervening during childhood and pre-adolescence is necessary to potentially restore the natural history of strength optimization early in life and attenuate the decline that occurs in adulthood. In Figure 4, we propose an altered trajectory of age-related decline secondary to targeted interventions delivered during the pre-adolescent critical period.

3.2. Key Ingredients

Programs that aim to improve and sustain MSK integrity require specific physical activities to target key components of morphology and functional capacity. Recommended guidelines for exercise and physical activity in persons with CP have been proposed [45,80]. In addition, we suggest that programs include activities aimed at improving bone and muscle integrity as well as cardiorespiratory reserve tailored to GMFCS level with consideration of tolerance as well as level of interest.

3.2.1. Targeted Musculoskeletal Intervention

- Augmenting Bone Health. Sufficient physical activity that provides muscular stimulus and impact forces that target osteogenesis could prevent osteoporosis and reduce the risk of fracture. Yet, to ensure that the skeletal system of a person with CP can tolerate force-related and impact loading activities, pre-testing of bone density is required. Bone mineral content (BMC; g) and areal bone mineral density (BMD); g/cm^2) are two clinical measures of bone health that can be assessed with dual X-ray absorptiometry (DXA). Knowing the patient's bone health will ensure that precautions are taken to ensure a child at risk can begin to safely engage in physical activity. For children with low bone mass based on calculated Z-scores, it is still safe to exercise. For example, a child with a higher GMFCS level may have low bone mass, but if placed in a harness or assisted with the exercises, the individual can still benefit from the exercise while minimizing fall risk. Ultimately, fractures are primarily caused by an impact force from a fall or landing that exceeds the failure properties of the bone tissue [90]. Given the limited data in children on the risk of fracture during exercise and what the skeleton can tolerate, we can glean some insight from exercise interventions in osteoporotic women who are performing high-intensity exercise. In these studies, women with osteoporosis were able to handle high impact loads and did not fracture [91].

    Based on published and unpublished data [32,34] by Bauer et al. and Gunter et al. [31], GRFs per body weight (BW) for activities performed by a TD child are about 1.0 times BW for walking, 2.9 times BW for running, and 4.6 times BW for drop landing (see Figure 2). The GRFs per BW for activities performed by a child with CP are less widely known and may be strongly influenced by select impairments such as ligamentous laxity, joint deformity, body malalignment, inadequate passive and active range-of-motion, and insufficient eccentric muscular control. Quick, high-load tasks that a child with CP at GMFCS levels I–III may tolerate could include jumping rope, hopscotch, or jump downs off a bench. Individuals with mobility at GMFCS level III may require the use of a harness or walker for support and balance during loading tasks. Tasks with a low impact load, such as jumps on a mini-trampoline, may be safer, but they may not provide sufficient GRFs per BW to influence changes in bone mass and structure. It may be best to have a child participate in circuit training, which may include intermittent impact loading, allowing for periodic monitoring of safety and tolerance. For example, the sequence of a course could be: (1) hopscotch; (2) jump rope; (3) crawling through tubes; and (4) jump downs. Further study is needed to ascertain the types of loads safely tolerated by persons with CP at all levels of the GMFCS.

- Enhancing Muscle Performance. As reviewed, there are important age-related changes in the muscles of persons with CP that differ from those who are TD. Despite these differences, muscle hypertrophy, force production, and power can increase in children and adolescents with CP who undergo targeted training at a sufficient dosage [81,92]. Because muscle architecture can differentially adapt in response to different types of resistance training [81], the type of training and dosing essential to altering muscle function must be incorporated into programming (Section 3.2.2. Dosing Parameters).

Strength training is recommended to build a strong muscular foundation, promote muscle hypertrophy, and provide a synergistic stimulus for bone health. Yet, the effects of traditional strength training have not been shown to carry over to activities such as gait and functional mobility in those with CP [93,94]. Power training, which involves training at moderate to high loads at a higher concentric velocity of movement, is recommended for better carryover to gait and functional activities. Targeted high-velocity training may not only increase muscle power but also induce muscle architectural adaptations, such as an increase in fascicle length and cross-sectional area, and promote a right-ward shift of the torque-angle curve, increasing torque production at higher velocity [81,83].

Traditional resistive training equipment (i.e., free weights and isotonic machines) is readily available in most gyms and clinics and can easily be used for strength and power training. Basic bodyweight exercises can also be used, especially in very young children, and can be progressed to free weights, machines, or other loaded exercises. Other modifications for children at GMFCS level III may include the use of support walkers for balance and to encourage hands-free positioning in standing while promoting weightbearing through the lower limbs. Regardless of GMFCS level, the advantages of using weight machines are that the child can be supported and single or multiple joints can be isolated while preventing or discouraging compensatory patterns and unwanted movements. For example, an inclined leg press can be used to train and target multiple lower extremity muscle groups while safely supporting the trunk and body [95,96]. In this supported position, the muscles can be loaded in a safe manner to a greater extent than if the same movement was attempted as an upright standing squat.

While there are selected types of equipment that provide precise measures of velocity and force, such as isokinetic equipment, these are not necessary for resistance training purposes. Power training can be feasibly conducted on most equipment by moving a constant load while decreasing the amount of time allowed to produce the concentric contraction (i.e., increasing the velocity). For example, a power leg press can be performed on an inclined leg press machine and would train and target the hip and knee extensors and ankle plantarflexors with a single exercise [95]. Typical verbal instructions include "Push, pull, or press as fast as possible" and "lower slow and controlled", referring to the concentric and eccentric portions of the motion, respectively. Once a sufficient velocity is reached, the load should be increased. Instrumented versions can also be used to reliably measure power output while performing a power leg press [95]. Another example of equipment that can be used for power training is flywheel ergometers. The equipment can be in the mode of a bike, rower, or ski machine that couples resistance from the device with the speed of active motion while providing digital power output. In a randomized crossover study by Moreau and colleagues [97] in persons with CP, 7 to 24 years of age, power output in the upper extremities significantly increased after 15 training sessions using an upper extremity flywheel ergometer (Concept2 SkiErg™, Morrisville, VT, USA). Use of the device at home or in school strengthened adherence.

Community-based training alternatives are also important for promoting mobility-based participation. RaceRunning (or Frame Running), which uses a three-wheeled running frame, is an example of how children within GMFCS levels I–IV can successfully engage in community-based sports programming if provided with adaptation [98]. Further, muscle hypertrophy and an increase in cardiorespiratory endurance were observed after a 12-week program across a wide age range (9 to 29 years) and mobility levels (GMFCS I–IV) [99]. Training alternatives to improve muscle and bone health while fostering engagement should continue to expand, allowing greater access to this type of programming in various settings.

Despite the success of resistance training programs for persons with CP, there are some risks of pain and injury. However, no serious adverse events have been reported for resistance training interventions in children and adolescents with CP. A few studies have reported mild adverse events, such as joint or muscle soreness [100,101]. It is highly recommended that those participating in any resistive or power training program be supervised and monitored closely by a trained professional [80]. Safety and tolerance are key factors for all programs to augment muscle integrity and function.

3.2.2. Dosing Parameters

Exercise prescription includes the parameters of frequency, intensity, volume, duration, and velocity. Frequency considers the number of training sessions per week. Volume refers to the number of sets and repetitions within one session. Intensity indicates the relative load used and is often defined as a percentage of the one-repetition maximum (1RM) or percentage of body weight [80,96]. The duration is the full length of the training program. Velocity refers to the rate and direction in which an exercise is performed. Exercise guidelines differ for bone and muscle, yet both should be strongly considered when designing programs.

- Dosing for Bone. Dosing parameters used to guide interventions to improve bone health are often based on guidelines to increase peak bone mass and prevent osteoporosis [27,102], which may be an important consideration for those with CP given the risk factors. General guidelines for TD children have been advocated by Gunter et al. [31]. These guidelines have been framed within the dosing parameters of frequency and volume (Table 1). The authors propose that children engage in 40–60 min of daily weight-bearing activity to target hip structure and strength [103]. Based on their own findings, they recommend 10–15 min of jumping 3 times per week to augment bone mass and structure [33,104]. This frequency and volume equate to 100 jumps from a two-foot height with GRFs at least 3.5 BW and higher). Table 1 includes examples of bone-building exercises that could be performed in children across all GMFCS levels, with associated ideas for how to modify activities. Since tolerance to skeletal loading varies across the GMFCS spectrum, methods to augment bone health in persons with CP must consider the individual integrity of the skeletal system and monitor safety and tolerance throughout the training program.
- Dosing for Muscle. Recommended optimal dosing guidelines for progressive resistance training have been assembled as shown in Table 2, specific to muscle strengthening vs. power training [80]. Novice lifters should begin training at a lower intensity (percentage of 1RM) as described in Moreau [80] in more detail and then progress up to the optimal dosage provided in Table 2 in order to maximize muscle plasticity. For example, a novice may begin power training at 40% of 1RM and focus on form and speed, then progress to a higher percentage of 1RM after successful completion of the target reps at the higher concentric velocity. Of note is that intensity, volume,

and speed differ between the two training paradigms. It is important that a 1RM test be performed to adequately dose the intensity of the intervention and the progression of the intensity throughout the intervention period. The safety, feasibility, and protocol for performing a 1RM in youth with CP have recently been published by Pontiff and Moreau [96]. Although a multiple repetition maximum test may be used to predict 1RM values, the prediction is less accurate for repetition ranges greater than 10 [105]. Regardless of what muscle performance parameter is being targeted, the recommended frequency for resistance training is 2 to 3 times per week on nonconsecutive days for a duration of 8 to 20 weeks (refer to Moreau, 2020 for more details) [80]. A recent review article by Moreau and Lieber [83] on resistance training interventions for youth with CP showed that if the optimal dosing guidelines were adhered to, then muscle plasticity was observed at the macroscopic structural level (i.e., increases in cross-sectional area, muscle thickness, volume, or fascicle lengths).

Table 1. Recommended optimal dosing guidelines for bone health. Examples of different types of exercises that dynamically load the skeleton to stimulate osteogenesis. The duration required to stimulate a bone response is longer.

Intensity *	Volume	Skeletal Site †	Speed	Duration #	Rest
Body weight	100 jumps of boxes of varying heights up to 24 inches.	Hip, spine	Controlled, landing with both feet	3–6 m	15–30 s between jumps
Body weight	100 jump circuit (hopscotch, jump ups, skips, side jumps) from floor height.	Hip, spine	Controlled landing with both feet	3–6 m	15–30 s between jumps
Body weight	Jump roping, 5–10 min (~50 jumps/min)	Hip, spine	Controlled, landing with both feet	3–6 m	

* These could be performed using a harness system for children with higher GMFCS levels to provide added support. Some studies have had participants add a weighted vest for added loading, with weights between 1 and 3 kg. † Only the bones that are mechanically loaded will respond. # Evaluate changes in bone by DXA after 6–12 months.

Table 2. Optimal dosing parameters for strength vs. power training.

Parameter	Intensity	Volume	Speed	Frequency	Duration	Rest
Muscle strength	70% to 85% of 1RM	3 sets of 6 to 10 repetitions	Slow and controlled to moderate (concentric and eccentric)	2–3 × per week (nonconsecutive days)	8–20 weeks	1–2 min. between sets; 48 h between sessions
Muscle power	60% to 80% of 1RM	3–6 sets of 1 to 6 repetitions	Concentric: As fast as possible Eccentric: Slow and controlled over 2–3 s	2–3 × per week (nonconsecutive days)	8–20 weeks	1–2 min. between sets; 48 h between sessions

From Moreau (2020); 1RM: one repetition maximum.

3.3. Maximizing Engagement and Addressing Barriers

Youth are significantly influenced by environmental factors, including relationships with peers and mentors. Sport-based youth development is a strategy that aims to promote healthy behaviors in conjunction with social confidence [106] through athletic games, team building, and emotional learning opportunities. These principles can be adjusted to sports or activities of interest to children of different ability levels. It is important to offer various types of activities that may be of interest to lay a strong foundation of MSK health that could be maintained over a lifetime.

Fortunately, the variety of physical activities available to children with CP is expanding. Grant–Beuttler and colleagues [107] delivered a Balanced Families Dance Program for children with CP and other disabling conditions. They have shown that a child with diplegic CP at GMFCS Level II was able to improve his scores on the GMFM through ongoing engagement in the Dance Program. Sukal–Moulton and colleagues [98] similarly showed an improvement in self-efficacy and self-perception in an adolescent with diplegia following participation in a running program using a running frame for aerobic training, including engagement in a community race. At the conclusion of training, the participant stated, "we are a family of runners now" in reference to joining her parents and younger brother in running for fitness; this was followed by a study where group level differences were found [98]. The inclusion of psychosocial features into any program designed to increase physical activity while augmenting bone and muscle health may significantly contribute to immediate and long-term sustainability and enrich quality of life [108].

Despite the fact that physical activity and exercise are essential to enhance and maintain bone and muscle health, barriers to engagement in fitness activities for children include disinterest, transportation, cost, and time [109]. There are additional barriers to these that significantly impact participation in fitness centers and sports for persons with CP and other disabling conditions. In a study by Wright et al. [110], the key barriers identified by youth with disabilities were the lack of accessible and inclusive opportunities. Even if fitness centers are considered inclusive, Nikolajsen et al. [111] reported that patrons still encounter issues of ableism and disablism from staff and members. *Albeism* places value on self-sufficiency, autonomy, and independence, which can lead to the exclusion of people with disabilities where the diversity of physical form is not represented. *Disablism* refers to the psychosocial oppression that persons with disabilities may experience directly due to negative interactions from staff or club members and indirectly due to structural barriers. Nikolajsen et al. [112] found that while able-bodied members at inclusive fitness centers held the desire for persons with disabilities to feel welcome, the notions of direct and indirect psychosocial disablism did have an influence. These societal constructs and barriers are also seen in youth sports programs, where participation is too often limited to those with a specific set of physical skills and the ability to navigate a variety of environments. Specific barriers for people with disabilities include not being physically capable but also societal attitudes, frustration, and loss of confidence. Bringing fitness and social opportunities to the home setting via tele-rehabilitation may address transportation needs and inclusion but may not offer the maximal engagement and positive encouragement that have been shown to be vital to increasing the confidence and skills of participants [109]. These offerings, as well as other options for virtual exercise, may reduce the burden by eliminating the need for travel. Virtual exercise can be effective and engaging, though it is important to determine which specific types and doses of exercises are best suited to a particular individual at their current level of abilities. Programs focused on inclusion must consider many elements of access, including activities, physical spaces, understanding participant needs, and intentional actions to shift attitudes and expectations of anyone interacting with the program.

4. Sustaining Gains

Introducing sustainable physical activity options at an early age that could augment MSK health is essential for persons with CP. To ensure that fitness is maintained into adolescence and adulthood, programs must be engaging and fit into one's interests and lifestyle [9]. We propose that a comprehensive, individualized multi-modal exercise program introduced in pre-adolescence may provide the optimal stimulus to enhance the integrity of multiple systems, prevent the acquisition of a sedentary lifestyle, and contribute to positive gains in self-efficacy.

5. Conclusions

The recent initiative to improve physical activity in children and adolescents with CP requires attention to key ingredients and dosing parameters to augment muscle and bone health. The dosing guidelines and recommendations put forth here can guide designers in planning multi-modal exercise programs that include impact loading and resistance training for individuals with CP at a sufficient but safe level. Based on research evidence, we recommend building a strong foundation of MSK health in pre-adolescence through participation in individualized exercise activities that are engaging, enjoyable, and promote skill acquisition. Sustaining fitness requires the integration of healthy habits into one's lifestyle. With a strong MSK foundation merged into a healthy lifestyle, lifelong fitness can be achievable for persons with CP.

Author Contributions: N.G.M., R.D.S., S.V.D. and K.M.F.: Conceptualization; N.G.M., K.M.F., R.K.F., S.D. and S.V.D.: writing—original draft preparation; N.G.M., K.M.F., R.K.F., S.D., T.S.-M., M.G.-B., M.D.P., R.D.S. and S.V.D.: writing—review and editing; S.V.D., N.G.M. and K.M.F.: funding acquisition. All authors have read and agreed to the published version of the manuscript.

Funding: This research within this paper was funded by the Academy of Pediatric Physical Therapy—Planning Grant.

Institutional Review Board Statement: Not applicable.

Informed Consent Statement: Not applicable.

Data Availability Statement: Not applicable.

Acknowledgments: Conceptualization of the ideas presented in this paper was initiated at Research Summit V sponsored by the Academy of Pediatric Physical Therapy.

Conflicts of Interest: The authors declare no conflict of interest.

References

1. Word Health Organization. Physical Activity. Available online: https://www.who.int/news-room/fact-sheets/detail/physical-activity (accessed on 13 April 2021).
2. American College of Sports Medicine. Physical Activity Guidelines. Available online: https://www.acsm.org/read-research/trending-topics-resource-pages/physical-activity-guidelines (accessed on 13 April 2021).
3. Gunter, K.B.; Nader, P.A.; John, D.H. Physical activity levels and obesity status of Oregon Rural Elementary School children. *Prev. Med. Rep.* **2015**, *2*, 478–482. [CrossRef] [PubMed]
4. Bjornson, K.F.; Belza, B.; Kartin, D.; Logsdon, R.; McLaughlin, J.F. Ambulatory physical activity performance in youth with cerebral palsy and youth who are developing typically. *Phys. Ther.* **2007**, *87*, 248–257. [CrossRef]
5. Bratteby Tollerz, L.U.; Forslund, A.H.; Olsson, R.M.; Lidstrom, H.; Holmback, U. Children with cerebral palsy do not achieve healthy physical activity levels. *Acta Paediatr.* **2015**, *104*, 1125–1129. [CrossRef]
6. Maher, C.A.; Toohey, M.; Ferguson, M. Physical activity predicts quality of life and happiness in children and adolescents with cerebral palsy. *Disabil. Rehabil.* **2016**, *38*, 865–869. [CrossRef]
7. Marker, A.M.; Steele, R.G.; Noser, A.E. Physical activity and health-related quality of life in children and adolescents: A systematic review and meta-analysis. *Health Psychol.* **2018**, *37*, 893–903. [CrossRef] [PubMed]
8. Van Wely, L.; Balemans, A.C.; Becher, J.G.; Dallmeijer, A.J. Physical activity stimulation program for children with cerebral palsy did not improve physical activity: A randomised trial. *J. Physiother.* **2014**, *60*, 40–49. [CrossRef] [PubMed]
9. Duff, S.V.; Kimbel, J.D.; Grant-Beuttler, M.; Sukal-Moulton, T.; Moreau, N.G.; Friel, K.M. Lifelong Fitness for Ambulatory Children and Adolescents with Cerebral Palsy II: Influencing the Trajectory. *Behav. Sci.* **2023**; *accepted*.
10. Peterson, M.D.; Ryan, J.M.; Hurvitz, E.A.; Mahmoudi, E. Chronic Conditions in Adults with Cerebral Palsy. *JAMA* **2015**, *314*, 2303–2305. [CrossRef]
11. Ryan, J.M.; Peterson, M.D.; Ryan, N.; Smith, K.J.; O'Connell, N.E.; Liverani, S.; Anokye, N.; Victor, C.; Allen, E. Mortality due to cardiovascular disease, respiratory disease, and cancer in adults with cerebral palsy. *Dev. Med. Child Neurol.* **2019**, *61*, 924–928. [CrossRef] [PubMed]
12. Smith, K.J.; Peterson, M.D.; O'Connell, N.E.; Victor, C.; Liverani, S.; Anokye, N.; Ryan, J.M. Risk of Depression and Anxiety in Adults with Cerebral Palsy. *JAMA Neurol.* **2019**, *76*, 294–300. [CrossRef]
13. Carlon, S.L.; Taylor, N.F.; Dodd, K.J.; Shields, N. Differences in habitual physical activity levels of young people with cerebral palsy and their typically developing peers: A systematic review. *Disabil. Rehabil.* **2013**, *35*, 647–655. [CrossRef]

14. Maher, C.A.; Williams, M.T.; Olds, T.; Lane, A.E. Physical and sedentary activity in adolescents with cerebral palsy. *Dev. Med. Child Neurol.* **2007**, *49*, 450–457. [CrossRef] [PubMed]
15. Keawutan, P.; Bell, K.L.; Oftedal, S.; Davies, P.S.; Ware, R.S.; Boyd, R.N. Habitual Physical Activity in Children with Cerebral Palsy Aged 4 to 5 Years Across All Functional Abilities. *Pediatr. Phys. Ther.* **2017**, *29*, 8–14. [CrossRef] [PubMed]
16. Krakovsky, G.; Huth, M.M.; Lin, L.; Levin, R.S. Functional changes in children, adolescents, and young adults with cerebral palsy. *Res. Dev. Disabil.* **2007**, *28*, 331–340. [CrossRef] [PubMed]
17. Lauruschkus, K.; Westbom, L.; Hallstrom, I.; Wagner, P.; Nordmark, E. Physical activity in a total population of children and adolescents with cerebral palsy. *Res. Dev. Disabil.* **2013**, *34*, 157–167. [CrossRef]
18. Barber, L.; Hastings-Ison, T.; Baker, R.; Barrett, R.; Lichtwark, G. Medial gastrocnemius muscle volume and fascicle length in children aged 2 to 5 years with cerebral palsy. *Dev. Med. Child Neurol.* **2011**, *53*, 543–548. [CrossRef] [PubMed]
19. Barber, L.A.; Read, F.; Lovatt Stern, J.; Lichtwark, G.; Boyd, R.N. Medial gastrocnemius muscle volume in ambulant children with unilateral and bilateral cerebral palsy aged 2 to 9 years. *Dev. Med. Child Neurol.* **2016**, *58*, 1146–1152. [CrossRef]
20. Hanna, S.E.; Rosenbaum, P.L.; Bartlett, D.J.; Palisano, R.J.; Walter, S.D.; Avery, L.; Russell, D.J. Stability and decline in gross motor function among children and youth with cerebral palsy aged 2 to 21 years. *Dev. Med. Child Neurol.* **2009**, *51*, 295–302. [CrossRef]
21. Johnson, D.C.; Damiano, D.L.; Abel, M.F. The evolution of gait in childhood and adolescent cerebral palsy. *J. Pediatr. Orthop.* **1997**, *17*, 392–396. [CrossRef]
22. Noble, J.J.; Fry, N.; Lewis, A.P.; Charles-Edwards, G.D.; Keevil, S.F.; Gough, M.; Shortland, A.P. Bone strength is related to muscle volume in ambulant individuals with bilateral spastic cerebral palsy. *Bone* **2014**, *66*, 251–255. [CrossRef]
23. Noble, J.J.; Fry, N.R.; Lewis, A.P.; Keevil, S.F.; Gough, M.; Shortland, A.P. Lower limb muscle volumes in bilateral spastic cerebral palsy. *Brain Dev.* **2014**, *36*, 294–300. [CrossRef]
24. Whitney, D.G.; Hurvitz, E.A.; Devlin, M.J.; Caird, M.S.; French, Z.P.; Ellenberg, E.C.; Peterson, M.D. Age trajectories of musculoskeletal morbidities in adults with cerebral palsy. *Bone* **2018**, *114*, 285–291. [CrossRef] [PubMed]
25. Herskind, A.; Ritterband-Rosenbaum, A.; Willerslev-Olsen, M.; Lorentzen, J.; Hanson, L.; Lichtwark, G.; Nielsen, J.B. Muscle growth is reduced in 15-month-old children with cerebral palsy. *Dev. Med. Child Neurol.* **2016**, *58*, 485–491. [CrossRef]
26. Warden, S.; Fuchs, R. Physical Activity to Promote Bone Health in Adolescents. In *A Practical Approach to Adolescent Bone Health*; Pitts, S., Gordon, C., Eds.; Springer: Cham, Switzerland, 2018; pp. 53–76. [CrossRef]
27. Warden, S.J.; Fuchs, R.K. Exercise and bone health: Optimising bone structure during growth is key, but all is not in vain during ageing. *Br. J. Sports Med.* **2009**, *43*, 885–887. [CrossRef] [PubMed]
28. Linden, C.; Alwis, G.; Ahlborg, H.; Gardsell, P.; Valdimarsson, O.; Stenevi-Lundgren, S.; Besjakov, J.; Karlsson, M.K. Exercise, bone mass and bone size in prepubertal boys: One-year data from the pediatric osteoporosis prevention study. *Scand. J. Med. Sci. Sports* **2007**, *17*, 340–347. [CrossRef] [PubMed]
29. Valdimarsson, O.; Sigurdsson, G.; Steingrímsdóttir, L.; Karlsson, M.K. Physical activity in the post-pubertal period is associated with maintenance of pre-pubertal high bone density—A 5-year follow-up. *Scand. J. Med. Sci. Sports* **2005**, *15*, 280–286. [CrossRef] [PubMed]
30. Weaver, C.M.; Gordon, C.M.; Janz, K.F.; Kalkwarf, H.J.; Lappe, J.M.; Lewis, R.; O'Karma, M.; Wallace, T.C.; Zemel, B.S. The National Osteoporosis Foundation's position statement on peak bone mass development and lifestyle factors: A systematic review and implementation recommendations. *Osteoporos. Int.* **2016**, *27*, 1281–1386. [CrossRef] [PubMed]
31. Gunter, K.B.; Almstedt, H.C.; Janz, K.F. Physical activity in childhood may be the key to optimizing lifespan skeletal health. *Exerc. Sport Sci. Rev.* **2012**, *40*, 13–21. [CrossRef]
32. Bauer, J.; Fuchs, R.; Smith, G.; Snow, C. Quantifying Force Magnitude and Loading Rate from Drop Landings That Induce Osteogenesis. *J. Appl. Biomech.* **2001**, *17*, 142–152. [CrossRef]
33. Fuchs, R.K.; Bauer, J.J.; Snow, C.M. Jumping improves hip and lumbar spine bone mass in prepubescent children: A randomized controlled trial. *J. Bone Miner. Res.* **2001**, *16*, 148–156. [CrossRef]
34. Bauer, J. Ground reaction forces and rates of loading. **2001**, *unplublished work*.
35. O'Connell, N.E.; Smith, K.J.; Peterson, M.D.; Ryan, N.; Liverani, S.; Anokye, N.; Victor, C.; Ryan, J.M. Incidence of osteoarthritis, osteoporosis and inflammatory musculoskeletal diseases in adults with cerebral palsy: A population-based cohort study. *Bone* **2019**, *125*, 30–35. [CrossRef]
36. Whitney, D.G.; Alford, A.I.; Devlin, M.J.; Caird, M.S.; Hurvitz, E.A.; Peterson, M.D. Adults with Cerebral Palsy have Higher Prevalence of Fracture Compared with Adults without Cerebral Palsy Independent of Osteoporosis and Cardiometabolic Diseases. *J. Bone Miner. Res.* **2019**, *34*, 1240–1247. [CrossRef]
37. Golden, N.H.; Abrams, S.A.; Committee on Nutrition; Daniels, S.R.; Abrams, S.A.; Corkins, M.R.; Schwarzenberg, S.J. Optimizing bone health in children and adolescents. *Pediatrics* **2014**, *134*, e1229–e1243. [CrossRef] [PubMed]
38. Gannotti, M.E.; Liquori, B.M.; Thorpe, D.E.; Fuchs, R.K. Designing Exercise to Improve Bone Health Among Individuals with Cerebral Palsy. *Pediatr. Phys. Ther.* **2021**, *33*, 50–56. [CrossRef] [PubMed]
39. Trinh, A.; Wong, P.; Fahey, M.C.; Brown, J.; Strauss, B.J.; Ebeling, P.R.; Fuller, P.J.; Milat, F. Longitudinal changes in bone density in adolescents and young adults with cerebral palsy: A case for early intervention. *Clin. Endocrinol.* **2019**, *91*, 517–524. [CrossRef]
40. Jesus, A.O.; Stevenson, R.D. Optimizing Nutrition and Bone Health in Children with Cerebral Palsy. *Phys. Med. Rehabil. Clin.* **2020**, *31*, 25–37. [CrossRef]
41. Won, J.H.; Jung, S.H. Bone Mineral Density in Adults with Cerebral Palsy. *Front. Neurol.* **2021**, *12*, 733322. [CrossRef]

42. Duran, I.; Katzmann, J.; Martakis, K.; Stark, C.; Semler, O.; Schoenau, E. Individualized evaluation of lumbar bone mineral density in children with cerebral palsy. *Arch. Osteoporos.* **2018**, *13*, 120. [CrossRef]
43. Marciniak, C.; Gabet, J.; Lee, J.; Ma, M.; Brander, K.; Wysocki, N. Osteoporosis in adults with cerebral palsy: Feasibility of DXA screening and risk factors for low bone density. *Osteoporos. Int.* **2016**, *27*, 1477–1484. [CrossRef]
44. Stevenson, R.D.; Conaway, M.; Barrington, J.W.; Cuthill, S.L.; Worley, G.; Henderson, R.C. Fracture rate in children with cerebral palsy. *Pediatr. Rehabil.* **2006**, *9*, 396–403. [CrossRef]
45. Verschuren, O.; Smorenburg, A.R.P.; Luiking, Y.; Bell, K.; Barber, L.; Peterson, M.D. Determinants of muscle preservation in individuals with cerebral palsy across the lifespan: A narrative review of the literature. *J. Cachexia Sarcopenia Muscle* **2018**, *9*, 453–464. [CrossRef]
46. Liquori, B.M.; Gannotti, M.E.; Thorpe, D.E.; Fuchs, R.K. Characteristics of Interventions to Improve Bone Health in Children with Cerebral Palsy: A Systematic Review. *Pediatr. Phys. Ther.* **2022**, *34*, 163–170. [CrossRef] [PubMed]
47. Henderson, R.C.; Gilbert, S.R.; Clement, M.E.; Abbas, A.; Worley, G.; Stevenson, R.D. Altered skeletal maturation in moderate to severe cerebral palsy. *Dev. Med. Child. Neurol.* **2005**, *47*, 229–236. [CrossRef] [PubMed]
48. Chen, C.L.; Ke, J.Y.; Wang, C.J.; Wu, K.P.; Wu, C.Y.; Wong, A.M. Factors associated with bone density in different skeletal regions in children with cerebral palsy of various motor severities. *Dev. Med. Child. Neurol.* **2011**, *53*, 131–136. [CrossRef]
49. Uddenfeldt Wort, U.; Nordmark, E.; Wagner, P.; Düppe, H.; Westbom, L. Fractures in children with cerebral palsy: A total population study. *Dev. Med. Child. Neurol.* **2013**, *55*, 821–826. [CrossRef] [PubMed]
50. Martínez de Zabarte Fernández, J.M.; Ros Arnal, I.; Peña Segura, J.L.; García Romero, R.; Rodríguez Martínez, G. Bone health impairment in patients with cerebral palsy. *Arch. Osteoporos.* **2020**, *15*, 91. [CrossRef]
51. Lieber, R.L.; Roberts, T.J.; Blemker, S.S.; Lee, S.S.M.; Herzog, W. Skeletal muscle mechanics, energetics and plasticity. *J. Neuroeng. Rehabil.* **2017**, *14*, 108. [CrossRef]
52. Tveter, A.T.; Holm, I. Influence of thigh muscle strength and balance on hop length in one-legged hopping in children aged 7–12 years. *Gait Posture* **2010**, *32*, 259–262. [CrossRef] [PubMed]
53. Dayanidhi, S.; Dykstra, P.B.; Lyubasyuk, V.; McKay, B.R.; Chambers, H.G.; Lieber, R.L. Reduced satellite cell number in situ in muscular contractures from children with cerebral palsy. *J. Orthop. Res.* **2015**, *33*, 1039–1045. [CrossRef] [PubMed]
54. Willerslev-Olsen, M.; Lorentzen, J.; Sinkjaer, T.; Nielsen, J.B. Passive muscle properties are altered in children with cerebral palsy before the age of 3 years and are difficult to distinguish clinically from spasticity. *Dev. Med. Child Neurol.* **2013**, *55*, 617–623. [CrossRef]
55. Zogby, A.M.; Dayanidhi, S.; Chambers, H.G.; Schenk, S.; Lieber, R.L. Skeletal muscle fiber-type specific succinate dehydrogenase activity in cerebral palsy. *Muscle Nerve* **2017**, *55*, 122–124. [CrossRef]
56. Boakes, J.L.; Foran, J.; Ward, S.R.; Lieber, R.L. Muscle adaptation by serial sarcomere addition 1 year after femoral lengthening. *Clin. Orthop. Relat. Res.* **2007**, *456*, 250–253. [CrossRef] [PubMed]
57. Williams, P.E.; Goldspink, G. Longitudinal growth of striated muscle fibres. *J. Cell. Sci.* **1971**, *9*, 751–767. [CrossRef] [PubMed]
58. Williams, P.E.; Goldspink, G. The effect of immobilization on the longitudinal growth of striated muscle fibres. *J. Anat.* **1973**, *116*, 45–55. [PubMed]
59. Mathewson, M.A.; Ward, S.R.; Chambers, H.G.; Lieber, R.L. High resolution muscle measurements provide insights into equinus contractures in patients with cerebral palsy. *J. Orthop. Res.* **2015**, *33*, 33–39. [CrossRef]
60. Smith, L.R.; Lee, K.S.; Ward, S.R.; Chambers, H.G.; Lieber, R.L. Hamstring contractures in children with spastic cerebral palsy result from a stiffer extracellular matrix and increased in vivo sarcomere length. *J. Physiol.* **2011**, *589*, 2625–2639. [CrossRef] [PubMed]
61. Domenighetti, A.A.; Mathewson, M.A.; Pichika, R.; Sibley, L.A.; Zhao, L.; Chambers, H.G.; Lieber, R.L. Loss of myogenic potential and fusion capacity of muscle stem cells isolated from contractured muscle in children with cerebral palsy. *Am. J. Physiol. Cell. Physiol.* **2018**, *315*, C247–C257. [CrossRef]
62. Sibley, L.A.; Broda, N.; Gross, W.R.; Menezes, A.F.; Embry, R.B.; Swaroop, V.T.; Chambers, H.G.; Schipma, M.J.; Lieber, R.L.; Domenighetti, A.A. Differential DNA methylation and transcriptional signatures characterize impairment of muscle stem cells in pediatric human muscle contractures after brain injury. *FASEB J.* **2021**, *35*, e21928. [CrossRef]
63. Smith, L.R.; Chambers, H.G.; Lieber, R.L. Reduced satellite cell population may lead to contractures in children with cerebral palsy. *Dev. Med. Child Neurol.* **2013**, *55*, 264–270. [CrossRef]
64. Von Walden, F.; Gantelius, S.; Liu, C.; Borgstrom, H.; Bjork, L.; Gremark, O.; Stal, P.; Nader, G.A.; Ponte, N.E. Muscle contractures in patients with cerebral palsy and acquired brain injury are associated with extracellular matrix expansion, pro-inflammatory gene expression, and reduced rRNA synthesis. *Muscle Nerve* **2018**, *58*, 277–285. [CrossRef]
65. Corvelyn, M.; De Beukelaer, N.; Duelen, R.; Deschrevel, J.; Van Campenhout, A.; Prinsen, S.; Gayan-Ramirez, G.; Maes, K.; Weide, G.; Desloovere, K.; et al. Muscle Microbiopsy to Delineate Stem Cell Involvement in Young Patients: A Novel Approach for Children with Cerebral Palsy. *Front. Physiol.* **2020**, *11*, 945. [CrossRef]
66. Dayanidhi, S.; Buckner, E.H.; Redmond, R.S.; Chambers, H.G.; Schenk, S.; Lieber, R.L. Skeletal muscle maximal mitochondrial activity in ambulatory children with cerebral palsy. *Dev. Med. Child Neurol.* **2021**, *63*, 1194–1203. [CrossRef] [PubMed]
67. von Walden, F.; Vechetti, I.J., Jr.; Englund, D.; Figueiredo, V.C.; Fernandez-Gonzalo, R.; Murach, K.; Pingel, J.; McCarthy, J.J.; Stal, P.; Ponten, E. Reduced mitochondrial DNA and OXPHOS protein content in skeletal muscle of children with cerebral palsy. *Dev. Med. Child Neurol.* **2021**, *63*, 1204–1212. [CrossRef]

68. Choi, S.J.; Files, D.C.; Zhang, T.; Wang, Z.M.; Messi, M.L.; Gregory, H.; Stone, J.; Lyles, M.F.; Dhar, S.; Marsh, A.P.; et al. Intramyocellular Lipid and Impaired Myofiber Contraction in Normal Weight and Obese Older Adults. *J. Gerontol. A Biol. Sci. Med. Sci.* **2016**, *71*, 557–564. [CrossRef]
69. Johnson, D.L.; Miller, F.; Subramanian, P.; Modlesky, C.M. Adipose tissue infiltration of skeletal muscle in children with cerebral palsy. *J. Pediatr.* **2009**, *154*, 715–720. [CrossRef] [PubMed]
70. Whitney, D.G.; Singh, H.; Miller, F.; Barbe, M.F.; Slade, J.M.; Pohlig, R.T.; Modlesky, C.M. Cortical bone deficit and fat infiltration of bone marrow and skeletal muscle in ambulatory children with mild spastic cerebral palsy. *Bone* **2017**, *94*, 90–97. [CrossRef]
71. Elder, G.C.; Kirk, J.; Stewart, G.; Cook, K.; Weir, D.; Marshall, A.; Leahey, L. Contributing factors to muscle weakness in children with cerebral palsy. *Dev. Med. Child Neurol.* **2003**, *45*, 542–550. [CrossRef] [PubMed]
72. Lampe, R.; Grassl, S.; Mitternacht, J.; Gerdesmeyer, L.; Gradinger, R. MRT-measurements of muscle volumes of the lower extremities of youths with spastic hemiplegia caused by cerebral palsy. *Brain Dev.* **2006**, *28*, 500–506. [CrossRef]
73. Moreau, N.G.; Simpson, K.N.; Teefey, S.A.; Damiano, D.L. Muscle architecture predicts maximum strength and is related to activity levels in cerebral palsy. *Phys. Ther.* **2010**, *90*, 1619–1630. [CrossRef] [PubMed]
74. Stackhouse, S.K.; Binder-Macleod, S.A.; Lee, S.C. Voluntary muscle activation, contractile properties, and fatigability in children with and without cerebral palsy. *Muscle Nerve* **2005**, *31*, 594–601. [CrossRef] [PubMed]
75. Pontiff, M.R.T.; Connick, B.; Robertson, M.; Moreau, N.G. Age related changes in muscle size and strength across the lifespan in individuals with cerebral palsy. *Dev. Med. Child Neurol.* **2018**, *60*, 34–35.
76. Andersson, C.; Mattsson, E. Adults with cerebral palsy: A survey describing problems, needs, and resources, with special emphasis on locomotion. *Dev. Med. Child Neurol.* **2001**, *43*, 76–82. [CrossRef]
77. Jahnsen, R.; Villien, L.; Egeland, T.; Stanghelle, J.K.; Holm, I. Locomotion skills in adults with cerebral palsy. *Clin. Rehabil.* **2004**, *18*, 309–316. [CrossRef] [PubMed]
78. Murphy, K.P.; Molnar, G.E.; Lankasky, K. Medical and functional status of adults with cerebral palsy. *Dev. Med. Child Neurol.* **1995**, *37*, 1075–1084. [CrossRef] [PubMed]
79. Opheim, A.; Jahnsen, R.; Olsson, E.; Stanghelle, J.K. Walking function, pain, and fatigue in adults with cerebral palsy: A 7-year follow-up study. *Dev. Med. Child Neurol.* **2009**, *51*, 381–388. [CrossRef]
80. Moreau, N.G. Muscle Performance in Children and Youth with Cerebral Palsy: Implications for Resistance Training. In *Cerebral Palsy*; Miller, F., Bachrach, S., Lennon, N., O'Neil, M., Eds.; Springer: Cham, Switzerland, 2020; pp. 2629–2640. [CrossRef]
81. Moreau, N.G.; Holthaus, K.; Marlow, N. Differential adaptations of muscle architecture to high-velocity versus traditional strength training in cerebral palsy. *Neurorehabil. Neural Repair* **2013**, *27*, 325–334. [CrossRef] [PubMed]
82. Moreau, N.G. Muscle structural adaptation in cerebral palsy and its relationship to function. In *A Handbook of Pediatric Constraint-Induced Movement Therapy (P-CIMT): A Guide for Occupational and Physical Therapists, Researchers, and Clinicians*; Ramey, S., Coker-Bolt, P., DeLuca, S., Eds.; American Occupational Therapy Association Press: Bethesda, MD, USA, 2013.
83. Moreau, N.G.; Lieber, R.L. Effects of voluntary exercise on muscle structure and function in cerebral palsy. *Dev. Med. Child Neurol.* **2022**, *64*, 700–708. [CrossRef]
84. Gillett, J.G.; Boyd, R.N.; Carty, C.P.; Barber, L.A. The impact of strength training on skeletal muscle morphology and architecture in children and adolescents with spastic cerebral palsy: A systematic review. *Res. Dev. Disabil.* **2016**, *56*, 183–196. [CrossRef] [PubMed]
85. Faigenbaum, A.D.; Lloyd, R.S.; Myer, G.D. Youth resistance training: Past practices, new perspectives, and future directions. *Pediatr. Exerc. Sci.* **2013**, *25*, 591–604. [CrossRef]
86. Faigenbaum, A.D.; Bush, J.A.; McLoone, R.P.; Kreckel, M.C.; Farrell, A.; Ratamess, N.A.; Kang, J. Benefits of Strength and Skill-based Training During Primary School Physical Education. *J. Strength Cond. Res.* **2015**, *29*, 1255–1262. [CrossRef]
87. Zwolski, C.; Quatman-Yates, C.; Paterno, M.V. Resistance Training in Youth: Laying the Foundation for Injury Prevention and Physical Literacy. *Sports Health* **2017**, *9*, 436–443. [CrossRef]
88. Peterson, M.D.; Saltarelli, W.A.; Visich, P.S.; Gordon, P.M. Strength capacity and cardiometabolic risk clustering in adolescents. *Pediatrics* **2014**, *133*, e896–e903. [CrossRef]
89. Peterson, M.D.; Zhang, P.; Saltarelli, W.A.; Visich, P.S.; Gordon, P.M. Low Muscle Strength Thresholds for the Detection of Cardiometabolic Risk in Adolescents. *Am. J. Prev. Med.* **2016**, *50*, 593–599. [CrossRef]
90. Fuchs, R.K.; Kersh, M.E.; Carballido-Gamio, J.; Thompson, W.R.; Keyak, J.H.; Warden, S.J. Physical Activity for Strengthening Fracture Prone Regions of the Proximal Femur. *Curr. Osteoporos. Rep.* **2017**, *15*, 43–52. [CrossRef] [PubMed]
91. Watson, S.L.; Weeks, B.K.; Weis, L.J.; Harding, A.T.; Horan, S.A.; Beck, B.R. High-Intensity Resistance and Impact Training Improves Bone Mineral Density and Physical Function in Postmenopausal Women with Osteopenia and Osteoporosis: The LIFTMOR Randomized Controlled Trial. *J. Bone Miner. Res.* **2018**, *33*, 211–220. [CrossRef] [PubMed]
92. McNee, A.E.; Gough, M.; Morrissey, M.C.; Shortland, A.P. Increases in muscle volume after plantarflexor strength training in children with spastic cerebral palsy. *Dev. Med. Child Neurol.* **2009**, *51*, 429–435. [CrossRef]
93. Moreau, N.G.; Bodkin, A.W.; Bjornson, K.; Hobbs, A.; Soileau, M.; Lahasky, K. Effectiveness of Rehabilitation Interventions to Improve Gait Speed in Children with Cerebral Palsy: Systematic Review and Meta-analysis. *Phys. Ther.* **2016**, *96*, 1938–1954. [CrossRef]
94. Ryan, J.M.; Cassidy, E.E.; Noorduyn, S.G.; O'Connell, N.E. Exercise interventions for cerebral palsy. *Cochrane Database Syst. Rev.* **2017**, *6*, CD011660. [CrossRef] [PubMed]

95. Pontiff, M.; Li, L.; Moreau, N.G. Reliability, Validity and Minimal Detectable Change of a Power Leg Press Test in Individuals with Cerebral Palsy. *Phys. Occup. Ther. Pediatr.* 2023; in press. [CrossRef]
96. Pontiff, M.; Moreau, N.G. Safety and Feasibility of 1-Repetition Maximum (1-RM) Testing in Children and Adolescents with Bilateral Spastic Cerebral Palsy. *Pediatr. Phys. Ther.* **2022**, *34*, 472–478. [CrossRef]
97. Colquitt, G.; Kiely, K.; Caciula, M.; Li, L.; Vogel, R.L.; Moreau, N.G. Community-Based Upper Extremity Power Training for Youth with Cerebral Palsy: A Pilot Study. *Phys. Occup. Ther. Pediatr.* **2020**, *40*, 31–46. [CrossRef]
98. Sukal-Moulton, T.; Egan, T.; Johnson, L.; Lein, C.; Gaebler-Spira, D. Use of Frame Running for Adolescent Athletes with Movement Challenges: Study of Feasibility to Support Health and Participation. *Front. Sports Act. Living* **2022**, *4*, 830492. [CrossRef]
99. Hjalmarsson, E.; Fernandez-Gonzalo, R.; Lidbeck, C.; Palmcrantz, A.; Jia, A.; Kvist, O.; Pontén, E.; von Walden, F. RaceRunning training improves stamina and promotes skeletal muscle hypertrophy in young individuals with cerebral palsy. *BMC Musculoskelet. Disord.* **2020**, *21*, 193. [CrossRef] [PubMed]
100. Mockford, M.; Caulton, J.M. Systematic review of progressive strength training in children and adolescents with cerebral palsy who are ambulatory. *Pediatr. Phys. Ther.* **2008**, *20*, 318–333. [CrossRef] [PubMed]
101. Park, E.Y.; Kim, W.H. Meta-analysis of the effect of strengthening interventions in individuals with cerebral palsy. *Res. Dev. Disabil.* **2014**, *35*, 239–249. [CrossRef]
102. Koshy, F.S.; George, K.; Poudel, P.; Chalasani, R.; Goonathilake, M.R.; Waqar, S.; George, S.; Jean-Baptiste, W.; Yusuf Ali, A.; Inyang, B.; et al. Exercise Prescription and the Minimum Dose for Bone Remodeling Needed to Prevent Osteoporosis in Postmenopausal Women: A Systematic Review. *Cureus* **2022**, *14*, e25993. [CrossRef]
103. Janz, K.F.; Burns, T.L.; Levy, S.M.; Torner, J.C.; Willing, M.C.; Beck, T.J.; Gilmore, J.M.; Marshall, T.A. Everyday activity predicts bone geometry in children: The Iowa bone development study. *Med. Sci. Sports Exerc.* **2004**, *36*, 1124–1131. [CrossRef] [PubMed]
104. Gunter, K.; Baxter-Jones, A.D.; Mirwald, R.L.; Almstedt, H.; Fuchs, R.K.; Durski, S.; Snow, C. Impact exercise increases BMC during growth: An 8-year longitudinal study. *J. Bone Miner. Res.* **2008**, *23*, 986–993. [CrossRef]
105. Faigenbaum, A.D.; Milliken, L.A.; Westcott, W.L. Maximal strength testing in healthy children. *J. Strength Cond. Res.* **2003**, *17*, 162–166. [CrossRef] [PubMed]
106. Curran, T.; Wexler, L. School-Based Positive Youth Development: A Systematic Review of the Literature. *J. Sch. Health* **2017**, *87*, 71–80. [CrossRef] [PubMed]
107. Santos, J.W.D.; McCauley, C.; Grant-Beuttler, M. Assessing Functional Outcomes in Children with Disabilities through a Community Dance Program. *Pediatr. Phys. Ther.* **2021**, *34*, 97–140. [CrossRef]
108. Wiart, L. How do we ensure sustainable physical activity options for people with disabilities? *Dev. Med. Child Neurol.* **2016**, *58*, 788. [CrossRef]
109. Shields, N.; Synnot, A. Perceived barriers and facilitators to participation in physical activity for children with disability: A qualitative study. *BMC Pediatr.* **2016**, *16*, 9. [CrossRef] [PubMed]
110. Wright, A.; Roberts, R.; Bowman, G.; Crettenden, A. Barriers and facilitators to physical activity participation for children with physical disability: Comparing and contrasting the views of children, young people, and their clinicians. *Disabil. Rehabil.* **2019**, *41*, 1499–1507. [CrossRef] [PubMed]
111. Nikolajsen, H.; Richardson, E.V.; Sandal, L.F.; Juul-Kristensen, B.; Troelsen, J. Fitness for all: How do non-disabled people respond to inclusive fitness centres? *BMC Sports Sci. Med. Rehabil.* **2021**, *13*, 81. [CrossRef] [PubMed]
112. Nikolajsen, H.; Sandal, L.F.; Juhl, C.B.; Troelsen, J.; Juul-Kristensen, B. Barriers to, and Facilitators of, Exercising in Fitness Centres among Adults with and without Physical Disabilities: A Scoping Review. *Int. J. Environ. Res. Public Health* **2021**, *18*, 7341. [CrossRef]

Disclaimer/Publisher's Note: The statements, opinions and data contained in all publications are solely those of the individual author(s) and contributor(s) and not of MDPI and/or the editor(s). MDPI and/or the editor(s) disclaim responsibility for any injury to people or property resulting from any ideas, methods, instructions or products referred to in the content.

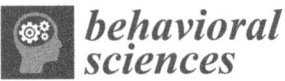

Perspective

Lifelong Fitness in Ambulatory Children and Adolescents with Cerebral Palsy II: Influencing the Trajectory

Susan V. Duff [1,*], Justine D. Kimbel [1], Marybeth Grant-Beuttler [2], Theresa Sukal-Moulton [3], Noelle G. Moreau [4] and Kathleen M. Friel [5]

1. Department of Physical Therapy, Crean College of Health and Behavioral Sciences, Chapman University, Irvine, CA 92618, USA; jkimbel@chapman.edu
2. Department of Physical Therapy, Oregon Institute of Technology, Klamath Falls, OR 97601, USA; marybeth.grantbeuttler@oit.edu
3. Department of Physical Therapy & Human Movement Sciences, Northwestern University, Chicago, IL 60611, USA; theresa-moulton@northwestern.edu
4. Department of Physical Therapy, Louisiana State University Health Sciences Center, New Orleans, LA 70112, USA; nmorea@lsuhsc.edu
5. Burke Neurological Institute, Weill Cornell Medicine, White Plains, NY 10605, USA; kaf3001@med.cornell.edu
* Correspondence: duff@chapman.edu

Abstract: Physical activity of at least moderate intensity in all children contributes to higher levels of physical and psychological health. While essential, children with cerebral palsy (CP) often lack the physical capacity, resources, and knowledge to engage in physical activity at a sufficient intensity to optimize health and well-being. Low levels of physical activity place them at risk for declining fitness and health, contributing to a sedentary lifestyle. From this perspective, we describe a framework to foster a lifelong trajectory of fitness in ambulatory children with CP (GMFCS I–III) as they progress into adolescence and adulthood, implemented in conjunction with a training program to augment bone and muscle health. First, we recommend that altering the fitness trajectory of children with CP will require the use of methods to drive behavioral change prior to adolescence. Second, to promote behavior change, we suggest embedding lifestyle intervention into fitness programming while including meaningful activities and peer socialization to foster self-directed habit formation. If the inclusion of lifestyle intervention to drive behavior change is embedded into fitness programs and found to be effective, it may guide the delivery of targeted programming and community implementation. Participation in comprehensive programming could alter the long-term trajectory of musculoskeletal health while fostering strong self-efficacy in persons with CP.

Keywords: cerebral palsy; motor learning; lifestyle intervention; lifelong fitness

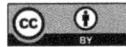

1. Introduction

Exercise and fitness are key elements of lifelong physical and psychological well-being and have been referred to as "the fountain of youth" [1]. Multiple public health and professional organizations recommend that children and adolescents from 6 to 17 years of age engage in moderate to vigorous exercise for 60 min per day at least 3 times per week, including activities for bone and muscle strengthening and aerobic conditioning [2–4]. Physical activity in this context refers to the bodily movements performed by skeletal muscles that result in energy expenditure [5]. Exercise can be considered a subset of physical activity, particularly when the aim is physical fitness and the activity is structured, planned, repetitive, and goal-directed.

The amount and intensity of physical activity strongly influence physical and psychosocial health in typical and atypically developing children. Daily physical activity has been found to improve a child's self-esteem, social interactions, and stress management [6]. In a study of over 4000 typically developing (TD) children 8–10 years of age, Vella and colleagues [7,8] found that ongoing participation in organized extracurricular sports was associated with higher levels of social and emotional health by age 10. Conversely, children who are inactive may be at higher risk for chronic health conditions such as cardiovascular disease and diabetes, which negatively influence physical and psychological well-being as they age [9]. These risks are even higher for those with physical disabilities such as cerebral palsy (CP), with the effects of inactivity compounding as they progress through adolescence into adulthood [10–12].

The purpose of this perspective paper is to describe a framework of lifestyle intervention designed to foster autonomy, motivation, social engagement, and personal habits to run in conjunction with a program aimed at promoting bone and muscle health in children with CP at GMFCS levels I–III [13]. To aid the identification of key ingredients essential to successful fitness programming for children, we surveyed youth with and without CP who participate in physical activity regularly and one parent each to gain their perspectives. The themes generated from the surveys are reviewed below. With sufficient evidence regarding methods to safely augment bone and muscle health among children at GMFCS levels IV–V and how to best engage children of varying intellectual capacities, we hope to expand our program to include a wider range of children with CP. It is our view that if children with CP at any level can feasibly establish an active, self-directed, fit lifestyle by adolescence, it could foster the development of healthy personal habits that may extend to adulthood.

2. Physical Activity and Fitness

In general, children with CP have lower levels of physical activity than TD children [6,14]. Individuals at levels IV–V, based on the Gross Motor Function Classification System (GMFCS), have much lower levels of physical activity than those at GMFCS levels I–III who can ambulate with or without an assistive device [15]. Based on data gathered from 3 days of wearing wrist and ankle accelerometers and self-reported daily logs, children with CP at GMFCS levels II–III were found to have lower levels of daily active energy expenditure in comparison to children who were TD [6]. In another study [14], walking activity was tracked in persons 10–13 years of age with CP at levels GMFCS levels I–II and youth who were developing typically. Data were gathered from all participants for 7 days while they wore a StepWatch monitor (Mountlake Terrace, WA, USA) unilaterally on one ankle. The authors found that the youth with CP were significantly less active than their TD peers [14]. Yoon and colleagues [15] assessed physical activity in children with CP, aged 4–18 years of age, across GMFCS levels I–V with varying comorbidities. The participants wore a GT3X+ (ActiGraph, Pensacola, FL, USA) accelerometer on the waist for 7 days. The findings revealed that non-ambulatory children at GMFCS levels IV–V spent significantly less time in moderate to vigorous activity than ambulatory children at GMFCS levels I–III. Decreased physical activity was also associated with lower physical quality of life (QOL). These data represent an overall trend of decreased activity that contributes to secondary health conditions [16,17], even as the lifespan of persons with CP continues to expand [18]. Therefore, to best promote a healthy lifestyle that could minimize the development of chronic conditions we need to better understand the pace at which motor function decreases [17] and how to successfully engage children in fitness at a young age, to promote long-term adherence to physical activity.

There are many challenges that children with CP may face when striving to reach sufficient physical activity and fitness. These concerns must be addressed in programming to ensure adherence and engagement. First, given their physical disability, they are often less active and more reliant on external resources to facilitate participation in sports and other activities, making self-advocacy more onerous while placing an additional burden on parents. Second, bias from others and a lack of program accommodations can limit their inclusion in extracurricular sports programs, even for those at higher functioning GMFCS levels compared to age-matched peers without physical disabilities. Finally, without clear personal choice and access, children with CP may feel disconnected and isolated from their community [19], leading to underdeveloped social skills and insufficient resilience to stress. As these children move into adolescence, these effects may contribute to lower levels of self-efficacy [6,20], defined as an individual's confidence that they will be able to perform actions that bring about desired task outcomes [21]. These and other barriers often limit the establishment of healthy habits essential to the development of an active, fit lifestyle [8,19]. However, if these barriers were minimized and meaningful skills were developed, self-efficacy may improve. While overcoming challenges and promoting fitness habits to minimize the adoption of a sedentary lifestyle are key, it is important to consider how programs that aim to augment bone and muscle health with lifestyle intervention embedded in them can be successfully implemented.

3. Altering the Fitness Trajectory of Children with CP

Investigating the factors that affect an individual's willingness to participate and adopt positive fitness habits is vital to long-term adherence. González-Hernández and colleagues [22] showed that vigorous consistent exercise and the pursuit of perfectionism in teenagers who engaged in sport-centered or recreational exercise resulted in increased self-efficacy and psychological well-being. This so-called adaptive perfectionism may encourage adherence to regular fitness activity due at least in part to the positive outcomes that result. In a longitudinal study of 8–10-year-old TD children, Vella et al. [7,8] found that organized, consistent, and developmentally appropriate sports and physical activity were linked with higher levels of health-related QOL. Positive outcomes that result from successful participation often encourage frequent engagement in regular fitness activity and higher overall levels of well-being.

There is no physiological reason to anticipate that these same results would not be possible in children with CP who are able to increase their level of physical activity. Fortunately, the availability of participation-based community exercise programs for persons with CP is increasing, particularly for those at GMFCS levels I–III, and positive outcomes are being reported [20,23–26]. Cleary and colleagues [23] conducted an aerobic training study for youth with CP in a school setting, showing evidence of high adherence and significant gains in cardiovascular markers with no adverse events for the exercise group. Thorpe et al. [25], evaluated the outcomes of a treadmill training or aquatic exercise program held at a community center for adolescents with CP at GMFCS levels I–III. The authors found increases in walking distance, leg muscle mass, and self-perception of function among all participants. A 6-week ballet program was run for youth with CP, aged 9–14 years, at GMFCS levels I–III [26]. The results revealed improvements in select gait parameters including decreased time of ambulation and increases in step and stride length [26]. The evidence for successful outcomes from community programs for children with CP continues to expand but adherence and the prevention of a sedentary lifestyle remain challenges that must be addressed.

The development of the key ingredients for successful long-term participation in fitness activities should begin in childhood. In addition to the inclusion of methods to enhance bone and muscle health, programs could incorporate components to drive behavioral change, fostered through lifestyle intervention (see Figure 1). With strong evidence and clinical expertise, practical program guidelines can be designed to improve specific outcomes while assessing for effectiveness and adherence in children with CP across all GMFCS levels of classification [27,28].

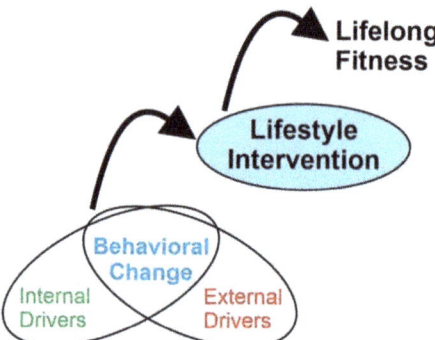

Figure 1. Framework for changing behavior via lifestyle intervention to achieve lifelong fitness. Internal drivers—system integrity, self-determination, and skill acquisition. External drivers—opportunity and relationships. With lifestyle interventions embedded into meaningful program activity and socialization, self-initiated habits could contribute to lifelong fitness.

3.1. Internal Drivers of Behavioral Change

Despite the challenges, most persons with CP do wish to be active, fit, and socially connected [29]. Altering the fitness trajectory of children with CP may require attention to the internal or individual drivers of behavioral change. Studies stemming from select psychological theories and motor learning principles can serve to guide this aspect of program design to bolster long-term adherence to physical activity and fitness.

Self-determination theory: This theory proposes that intrinsic motivation is fostered when three basic psychological needs are met: autonomy, competence, and relatedness [30,31]. According to self-determination theory (SDT), *autonomy* refers to a sense of initiative and choice; *competence* signifies a feeling of mastery or success; *relatedness* denotes a sense of belonging or connection [31]. Autonomous forms of motivation can positively predict the likelihood and duration of exercise participation [32]. Feelings of competence stemming from experiences of mastery clearly influence overall well-being and the ability to sustain behavior change. Relatedness acquired through accepting environments and meaningful personal relationships can strongly motivate participation. Conversely, external control, harsh internal or external critiques of performance, and an inability to relate to other participants or coaches can limit behavior change and negatively influence participation. Therefore, to foster motivation using SDT, participants should make activity choices and task demands that are achievable with minimal negative feedback within programs that are positive and accepting. Fostering a child's social connections while promoting skill development and active learning can strengthen engagement in fitness programs, which promote behavior change [19]. Since motivation is an important aspect of behavioral change, incorporating aspects of self-determination theory within programming may be essential [33].

Skill acquisition: Skills are actions that demonstrate consistency, efficiency, and flexibility [34]. *Consistency* refers to the repeatability of a task or skill over time. *Efficiency* refers to the optimization of energy resources from the musculoskeletal and cardiovascular systems. *Flexibility* or transferability refers to the adaptability of task or skill performance to changing environments or conditions. Specific aspects of skill acquisition could be incorporated into training programs to foster motor learning. Considerations include understanding the stage of the learner, structuring the task practice, and the strength of intrinsic and extrinsic feedback, among others.

When designing programs to enhance skill acquisition, one should first consider whether the individual is in the early or later stage of learning a particular sport or activity [35,36]. In the early stage of learning, a child would be developing an understanding of the task goal and the dynamics (i.e., the power required to throw a ball to a target). They would be developing movement strategies and learning to distinguish between the regulatory and non-regulatory features of the environment. Regulatory features are conditions to which the movement must conform, such as the size and speed of a moving baseball when catching. The non-regulatory features are those that can influence skill performance but the body does not have to conform to them, such as the color of the baseball. In the later stage of learning, a child would be refining movements, adapting to changing tasks and environmental demands. They would be learning to perform tasks consistently and efficiently. Improving a physical skill in a context that allows an individual to modify the force used or spatial–temporal requirements to perform the task or skill enhances flexibility or transferability.

Setting up the practice conditions and ensuring that the feedback is sufficient during task performance are elements that can be tailored to any stage of learning [37,38]. The practice conditions for a particular skill or task can differ in their amount, the order of specific components, or whether part or whole practice will be used. The practice could be specific to one task and done in ways that vary the amount a child receives. Practice can be done in one intensive (massed) bout, such as a boot camp type experience, or it could be distributed across time, such as soccer practice for one hour per session, two sessions per week, for many weeks. Practice can be scheduled in a random or blocked order within a day or over a set period of time. Children could practice a full activity, such as playing games of baseball, or could repetitively practice one aspect of the activity, such as throwing a baseball repeatedly. Part-practice should ideally be followed by practice of the whole activity. Preferably, the practice conditions should be individualized.

Feedback can be intrinsic or extrinsic, providing knowledge of performance or knowledge of results. Intrinsic feedback is the sensory experience gained through the movement itself. Extrinsic or augmented feedback can be verbal, visual as with demonstrations, or physical as provided with manual guidance. Biofeedback is an additional form of augmented feedback. Extrinsic feedback can be given concurrently during practice or at the end of performance. It can be provided 100% of the time or less. It may be precise or general. The research suggests that extrinsic feedback should be given intermittently and should lessen over time [39,40]. We propose that to foster physical and behavioral changes that promote long-term adherence to fitness, motor learning principles should be incorporated into programming and measured by retention or transfer tests [34].

The Optimal Theory: This theory introduced by Wulf and Lewthwaite [21] proposes that performance and motor learning can be optimized through intrinsic motivation and attention, linking goals to actions. The three key factors of this theory are *enhancing expectancies* for future performance, *autonomy*, and *an external focus* of attention on motor actions. Theoretically, performance can be enhanced by including statements such as "children who exercise every day often get stronger," encouraging the adoption of consistent physical activity. Autonomy refers to the choices one has, such as allowing the child to choose the sequence of program activities. An external focus of attention refers to attention on a target versus a focus on bodily actions. The authors [21] propose that dopamine responses increase due to the anticipation of positive experiences, which could contribute to motor learning [41,42]. Integrating this theory into programming can help foster motivation, autonomy, and attention.

Instilling self-determination and autonomy is vital to developing and maintaining fitness habits in children with CP as they move through adolescence into adulthood [32]. Palisano et al. [19] noted that the autonomous control of decisions, flexible and individualized approaches, and opportunities for problem-solving at an incremental level are key factors in a self-determined strengths-based approach to fitness participation. The activities should be intentionally designed to promote autonomy while providing the necessary structure and support for successful task completion. A segment of any program could be individualized and self-directed to raise a child's self-efficacy and satisfaction in their own competence. For example, if a child wishes to play soccer, the part-practice of essential aspects of the game followed by whole practice could be integrated into their training program. According to the optimal theory, providing choices aids motivation. Thus, offering a choice regarding the part-practice order, such as between high-velocity power training of the legs, ball passing strategies, or shooting goals, may provide an incentive. Then, after the part-practice of all 3 aspects of soccer, a one-on-one game could be played with a peer or sibling. This type of sport-specific training within a fitness program could encourage the adoption of essential physical skills and learning in a natural environment. Ensuring self-determination and personal choice could aid investment in future goal setting and contribute to a positive fitness trajectory [31–33].

3.2. External Drivers of Behavioral Change

Factors external to the individual often have a strong influence on behavior change. Initially, there must be the opportunity to engage. Then, altering the fitness trajectory of children with CP would require a focus on external drivers of change, such as the task and environment [38] and relationships with parents, peers, and mentors. These external factors must be considered in combination with internal or individual factors.

3.2.1. Opportunity

Challenges or adversity in tasks and the environment can contribute to the development of psychological resilience. Within the environment, one must consider whether it is open or closed. In a closed environment, the environment is stable, as when walking up a standard set of stairs. An open environment has time constraints and involves prediction, such as for the speed and location of moving objects when trying to step up onto an escalator or catch a moving ball. When planning tasks, providing "just the right challenge" [43] is a common phrase used to foster success in training programs for children. Along with this, it is important to consider affordances, defined by Gibson [44] as the reciprocal fit between the person and the environment needed to perform tasks. For example, when learning to catch balls, trainers may start with large balls or large mitts so that the allowable bandwidth of error is wider. Practicing new skills that incorporate participant strengths may reframe challenging tasks and activities from obstacles to opportunities for growth [19].

3.2.2. Relationships

Parents: Parents are a crucial domain of influence in a child's successful participation in physical activities and fitness programs. In a qualitative study interviewing parents of 8–11-year-old children with CP, Lauruschkus et al. [45] reported that parents desire opportunities for their child to have peers with whom they can be physically active. Additionally, they found that parents tend to seek programs where competent persons can provide support for participation. Family culture and attitudes towards fitness, the level of support in facilitating participation, and the feasibility of the program (location and frequency) are important factors to consider in designing a fitness intervention program.

Peers: Sport-based youth development is a program strategy that aims to promote healthy behaviors concurrently with social confidence [46]. This is often achieved through team building and athletic games while increasing resilience and the ability to handle adversity, which are important components for developing social–emotional well-being in children. Peers provide a motivating avenue to participation, adding *"fun"* to activities given the natural flow between children, perhaps because they identify with each other due to having similar interests and communication styles. Encouraging participation in fitness programs in pairs, whether with siblings or age-matched peers, could enhance engagement and foster a sense of belonging, promoting social confidence.

Mentors: The acknowledgement of progress checkpoints toward a larger goal may increase self-driven participation and encourage adherence to that goal, especially in the context of skill-learning and physical ability. Mentors and coaches can also be models for certain tasks, demonstrating feasibility while providing encouragement. Effective interventions involve collaborative goal-setting among the child, family, and coach. Helping children distinguish between where they are now and where they want to be could enhance their motivation to achieve short-term goals as precursors to larger goals [47].

4. Engaged Consumers

While the literature provides a theoretical underpinning of how to promote a positive trajectory, there are practical implications where additional feedback is needed. To better inform the direction of a new program, we surveyed 11 youth, 8 to 18 years of age with and without CP, along with one parent or guardian each to determine their perspectives regarding the most desirable rewards and the feasibility of conducting a fitness program at a sufficient frequency to improve bone and muscle health. We hypothesized that the reward preferences and feasibility would differ between children of different ages, whether the person is TD or has CP, and where they reside. All youth participants were recruited because of their successful participation in physical activities. The children with CP were within GMFCS levels I–II. The youths and parents both completed an online questionnaire (Appendix A) pertaining to internal and external factors of influence to better understand features of motivation and reward as well as obstacles to participation [48].

Participant (youth) results: The survey indicated that 75% of youth participants reported a preference for activities that were not physically active, including computer games or hanging out with friends. However, 62.5% ranked physical activity as "essential" or "very important" for their health. All participants (100%) believed that time spent exercising would result in positive physical changes. Over 62% reported that activity with a goal to improve strength would motivate them to participate in a fitness program, whereas 50% were motivated to participate in programs that improved endurance or coordination. The survey indicated that most children (75%) felt that healthy bones and muscles required activity on a "frequent" basis and every participant indicated they would complete activities that were not fun if it helped them to improve.

Fifty percent of participants reported that physical activities involving friends were a positive motivator to participate. However, twenty-five percent indicated that situations that highlighted their limitations in "keeping up" with others negatively influenced their desire to participate. Additional limiting factors to participating in physical activity included transportation, with most children reporting they would be reliant on a parent to transport them to and from any activity outside of school. Time was also reported as a limiting factor, stating that school and homework were their highest priorities.

Parent results: Nearly 66% of parents were interested in physical activity programs that focused on improving their child's strength, agility, and flexibility. However, this same number of parents reported that they were not aware of the current programming recommendations for bone and muscle health. Fifty percent of parents reported that they had concerns about their child participating in physical activity programs. When asked to elaborate on their concerns, parents reported that they were concerned about the time required to participate in a program, transportation to get their child to the program, and safety for their child's "specific needs". The large majority of parents (87.5%) would be willing to drive their child to a fitness program, with 50% willing to drive to programs run 3 times per week for 3 months or longer.

Our analysis of participant and parent survey responses supported the three main domains of influence regarding the successful participation in physical activity and fitness for these interviewees: the participant, parent, and environment. Based on the literature and our findings from the surveys, we developed a simple yet clear model featuring key domains of influence to participation in children and adolescents with CP (see Figure 2). These domains of influence for participation were given strong consideration in the design of our framework to foster lifelong fitness.

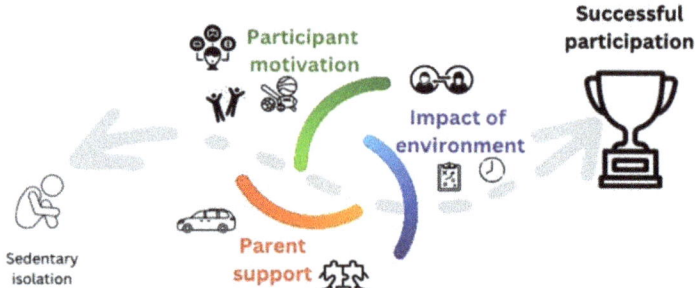

Figure 2. Domains of influence toward successful community participation.

Participant domain: Most of the children who represented successful examples of participation clearly revealed *competence* in their survey responses based on the self-determination theory [31,32]. The responses indicated that they desired to improve their physical skills and that this improvement was important to them, recognizing its positive contribution to long-term performance goals. The participants reported negative feelings of competence when they felt that their physical performance was judged as poorer than their peers. This suggests that self-perception of competence in select activities can be uplifting or manifest as an aversion to failure if a participant believes they will be judged unfairly by others.

Parent domain: Many parents are interested in programs and activities that they perceive as focused on areas of weakness for their children. However, it appears that there is a need to educate parents on current recommendations on bone and muscle health and the need to foster an internal drive in participants. Negative factors for parents include programs that do not "match" their child's physical abilities and require significant time and travel. They often reported feeling hesitant and responsible for providing accessibility for their child. The barrier to a parent's investment in a child's activities [49,50] can be addressed by a supportive community with consideration for the timing of sessions, carpooling options, and convenient facility locations. By supporting the parents and aiding them in overcoming barriers, the child can receive support for their autonomy in participation [49,51].

Environmental domain: The impact of the environment was the third domain of influence brought up by participants. Factors of program frequency and location were the most common influences on activity participation. All youth expressed that they would prefer to participate in outdoor spaces or gyms and would be willing to commit to a program for about three months. The parents expressed that the location of the program matters but most would be willing to support their child's participation even if long commutes are required. The main concerns about participating in a fitness program raised by both youth participants and parents were scheduling conflicts and the level of difficulty. We believe that transitioning the motor skills practiced and learned in a simulated environment to real-world tasks could lead to higher levels of community participation among children with CP.

5. Lifestyle Intervention

Without personal investment in altering one's lifestyle, any changes in activity level and fitness may be short-lived. Lifestyle Redesign® is a therapeutic means of enabling people to actively engage in individualized health-promoting occupations [52–55] while limiting their reliance on external factors. Specifically, the design of an intervention to drive behavior change linked to exercise and physical activity must satisfy the lifestyle needs of the participants and can include education and coaching on themes that are meaningful and important to the participants.

Lifestyle intervention has been successfully used to design programs for improving physical fitness in children with CP [56,57]. In a randomized controlled trial by Slaman et al. [56], adolescents at GMFCS levels I to IV engaged in 3 months of fitness training and 6 months of counseling on daily physical activity and sports participation. The authors found improvements in cardiopulmonary fitness, muscle strength, and body composition after the physical fitness intervention. However, the short-term success in adherence to physical fitness was no longer seen six months after the intervention. Despite the early gains, it is important to consider the missing ingredients in programming. The suggestions for future programming from the authors were to include accelerometry to provide immediate feedback to participants. They also revealed that if parents considered involvement in fitness programming more important than their children did, this led to drop-out. Based on the findings from this study, it seems essential to foster self-determination and personal fitness habits within a lifestyle intervention program to achieve sufficient adherence to training and move toward a positive, long-term fitness trajectory.

Determining which activities are meaningful to children as well as their perceptions of their ability should be assessed from the onset of any fitness training program. Therefore, prior to engaging in any training program, we recommend having children rate their performance and satisfaction on meaningful and desirable skills and fitness using a tool such as the Canadian Occupational Performance Measure (COPM) [58,59]. To measure changes in perceptions of self-competency and self-efficacy among participating individuals, we also recommend the Children's Self-Perceptions of Adequacy in and Predilection for Physical Activity (CSAPPA) [60,61]. A coaching tool such as motivational interviewing (https://motivationalinterviewing.org/) [62,63], which involves active listening, open questions, and affirmations of strengths and past successes, may encourage the child to make decisions based on their own reflections during or after training. Using an approach titled solutions-focused coaching [64–66], Schwellnus et al. [64] found improvements in goal satisfaction, attainment, and performance based on the attainment of participation goals in a group of 12 children with CP at 6–19 years of age. With this relatively small sample size, the authors used quantitative data, the COPM, and the Goal Attainment Scale to evaluate progress on short-term goals. Further research is needed to investigate the effects of the solutions-focused approach on long-term goals, yet the findings suggest that it may be effective in improving participation goals among children with CP [64]. Programs that include personal goals with guidance from program leaders and those that embrace challenges as a link to goal achievement while fostering resilience in facing obstacles should be included to ensure success. Including activities that are meaningful and achievable can aid in the development of key skills inherent in activities or sports of individual interest in any fitness program.

Based on the evidence and results from our survey, we are designing a fitness program that aims to target bone and muscle health through the optimal dosing of training exercises [13,67,68] for children at GMFCS levels I–III, with consideration of internal and external drivers of behavior change fostered through lifestyle intervention. The combination of these important aspects of programming will ideally foster self-directed habit formation with the overarching goal of promoting a positive, lifelong fitness trajectory in these children with CP (see Figure 1). The evidence base is primarily available for the use of these techniques in children who are able to actively participate in higher gross motor skill types of physical activity (GMFCS I–III). However, given the heterogeneity of CP, investigations with a more inclusive range of participants and with respect for their life experience is necessary. With greater evidence and safe guidelines, future research studies and programs such as ours could be more inclusive, with a focus on this underrepresented population.

6. Lifelong Sustainability

Introducing sustainable physical activity options at an early age that could augment musculoskeletal health is essential for persons with CP. To ensure that fitness is maintained into adolescence and adulthood, such programs must also be engaging and fit into one's interests and lifestyle. We propose that a comprehensive, individualized program introduced in pre-adolescence will provide the optimal stimulus to enhance the integrity of multiple systems, prevent the acquisition of a sedentary lifestyle, and contribute to positive self-efficacy. Ideally, programming should be integrated into one's lifestyle and have a positive link to function and skill acquisition. Importantly, building accepting, integrated fitness communities is essential for people with CP and other disabilities. If a person is active in childhood and adolescent fitness programs tailored exclusively to people with disabilities, they may easily become frustrated when they age out of adaptive programs and lack the confidence and tools to interface with non-adaptive programs. As acceptance by the non-disabled community and physical access continue to be quite variable, it is important to teach self-advocacy to young people with disabilities.

Despite the risks of developing a sedentary lifestyle, if the physical activity required to significantly enhance and maintain musculoskeletal health could be incorporated at an earlier age, this trend may be altered. This could begin by having a child or adolescent make the choice regarding which physical activity or sport they wish to be involved in and committing to opportunities to engage in that activity. Choice alone may help to increase the level of engagement and degree of skill acquisition [69]. Since most individuals thrive on socialization and companionship, programs that include these aspects are likely to be more readily accepted. If a personal goal to engage in community programs is known, the ingredients of an exercise program can include the essential motor skills needed to achieve the goal.

While exercise programs can improve motor function, they can also increase the readiness for participation in community-based activities if methods to foster internal motivation are embedded into programming. As cited earlier, Thorpe et al. [25] conducted a treadmill training and aquatic exercise program at a community center for adolescents with CP. The authors found that along with improvements in outcomes, having the program at a community center was beneficial for both the adolescents and the staff/members of the center. The authors believe more research is needed on the role motivation plays in lifelong physical activity for individuals with CP [25]. Another study by Darrah et al. [70] found that a fitness program held at a community center increased muscle strength and perceived confidence in adolescents with CP. By organizing a fitness program into pairs or peer groups, socialization and teamwork become essential and can lift engagement and the readiness to participate in other community activities.

Case Example

A co-author of this manuscript is an adult with CP (K.F.). In her mid-30s, she noticed that her balance, strength, and endurance were decreasing compared to when she was younger. She realized that she needed to increase her activity level to maintain her health. K.F. decided to begin martial arts training and joined the Harlem Tae Kwon Do (TKD) family as its first student with CP. Each class began with stretching and strength-building exercises that are similar to activities she did, unexcitedly, for years as a child and adolescent in physical therapy. By engaging in the same principles of building flexibility, strength, coordination, and balance at a TKD program, she greatly improved her fitness level beyond what she felt as a young adult. In addition, TKD classes are fun, challenging, and build community, and K.F. quickly made friends in the program who offer an added layer of engagement and accountability—if she misses too many classes, she is contacted and encouraged to return! These key ingredients of fun, accountability, community, and a variety of engaging exercises have given K.F. greater flexibility, balance, strength, and confidence in her body. This case shows how it is possible for people with disabilities to harness the ingredients for life-long fitness. By identifying and incorporating these ingredients into programming, K.F.'s successful participation could be replicated by others. As shown, exercise that is valuable and enjoyable could be the 'bridge' to sustained fitness for its physical and psychological benefits.

7. Conclusions

Our framework shown in Figure 1 aims to incorporate the ingredients for lifelong fitness and directly fulfill the psychological needs for autonomy, relatedness, and competence in order to increase self-efficacy and internal motivation. Framing a fitness program as a gateway to a fit and active lifestyle rather than a means to an end, such as receiving a tangible reward, could enhance adherence to fitness. Thus, recognizing opportunities for both physical and psychological growth and improvement are fundamental to fostering a lifestyle of fitness and healthy habits, which could be achieved using a framework of lifestyle intervention.

Improvements in bone and muscle health, motor skills, exercise habits, and the development of internally driven motivation may strongly influence the long-term adherence to fitness in children with CP. Including aspects of our suggested domains of influence toward motivation and participation could increase the adoption of positive fitness habits among children with CP. If children have not been fully engaged in physical activity, they need to find a sport or activity that is desired or gives them the most satisfaction on a social and physical level. While this would ideally be attained in pre-adolescence, it is not always done. An improvement in self-efficacy can provide reference and structure for an active lifestyle that may not have been recognized prior to participation in a targeted fitness program. If found to be feasible and effective, our framework for lifestyle intervention embedded within programs designed to augment bone and muscle health could be implemented into the community before adolescence so that we could truly alter the fitness trajectory of children with CP.

Author Contributions: S.V.D., J.D.K., conceptualization; J.D.K., S.V.D., data collection; M.G.-B., online survey format; J.D.K., M.G.-B., T.S.-M., formal analysis; S.V.D., J.D.K., N.G.M., K.M.F., writing—original draft preparation; S.V.D., J.D.K., M.G.-B., T.S.-M., N.G.M., K.M.F., writing—review and editing; S.V.D., N.G.M., K.M.F., funding acquisition. All authors have read and agreed to the published version of the manuscript.

Funding: This research within this paper was funded by the Academy of Pediatric Physical Therapy–Planning Grant.

Institutional Review Board Statement: The study was conducted in accordance with the Declaration of Helsinki and approved by the Institutional Review Board of Chapman University (IRB-20-187, 4-13-20).

Informed Consent Statement: Informed consent was obtained from all subjects involved in the study.

Data Availability Statement: Requests for survey data can be made to duff@chapman.edu.

Acknowledgments: We thank the youths and parents and caregivers for their contributions to our survey. We also thank Valerie Ann Hill, PhD, MS, OTR/L, for her thoughtful insight on lifestyle intervention.

Conflicts of Interest: The authors declare no conflict of interest.

Appendix A Fitness Program Incentive Questions—Program Ideas

Start of Block: Part 1: Child

Child name (first):_____ Age: _____

1. What is your favorite thing to do outside of school?

    _____
    _____

2. Do you to do things that make you move around and/or breath hard? (Select One)

    _____ Yes (1)
    _____ No (2)

3. What physical activity (sport, dance, martial art, playing outside) do you participate in most outside of school? Why do you like it?

   _____
   _____
   _____

4. Where do you participate in this activity or exercise? At home, school, or somewhere else?

   _____
   _____
   _____

5. If you participate outside your home or school, how do you get there?

   _____
   _____
   _____

6. Was it your idea to start doing this activity or exercise? (Select one)

   _____ Yes (1)
   _____ No (2)

Display: Was it your idea to start doing this activity or exercise? (Select one) = Yes or No

7. If not, who suggested it?

   _____

8. What do you need to get better at this activity or exercise? Select all that apply.

   _____ Move faster
   _____ Be stronger
   _____ Keep moving for longer
   _____ Be more flexible
   _____ Be more coordinated
   _____ Other: _____

9. Do you believe working out will help you get better now or in the future? (Select one)

   _____ Yes (1)
   _____ No (2)

10. Rank the following physical activities in terms of your interests. Drag to rank each item in order 1 (best)–5 (worst):

    _____ Playing outside
    _____ Playing sports
    _____ Strength exercises (push-ups, sit-ups, etc.)
    _____ Dancing
    _____ Martial Arts

11. How important is it to you to be fit or have an active lifestyle (pick one)?

    _____ Essential
    _____ Very important
    _____ Important
    _____ Slightly important
    _____ Not at all important

12. What would you be most excited about if you were able to do a fitness program?

    _____
    _____
    _____

13. Does anything about a fitness program worry you?
    _____
    _____
    _____

14. Do you think having the right type of gear (clothes, water bottles, sneakers, etc.) is important to participate in a fitness program?
    _____

15. Are you willing to do activities that are less fun if they help you get better at sports or activities you like to participate in? (Select one)
    ____ Yes (1)
    ____ No (2)

16. Rank order the list of rewards below by what you would prefer, Rank in order of 1 (best)–7 (worst):
    ____ Free game apps for my phone or computer
    ____ Favorite food treats like
    ____ Free tickets to a movie, play, or concert
    ____ Free entry into an amusement park
    ____ Free months at the gym, dance program, martial arts program or other site
    ____ Free gear for participating in activity of choice
    ____ Other rewards: _____

17. What would motivate you to get more fit? Rank in order of 1 (best motivator)–6 (worst):
    ____ Having a friend or brother/sister do it with me
    ____ Go to a fitness center or site that other kids go to
    ____ Get better at my sport, dance, martial art, or other activity
    ____ Trying new activities
    ____ Receive rewards
    ____ Other

18. How often do you think children should exercise to improve their bone and muscle health?

(Select one)
    ____ Frequently
    ____ Sometimes
    ____ Not frequently

19. How many times per week would you be willing or able to go somewhere outside your home to improve your fitness? Consider other things you do, such as homework or music lessons.
    ____ 1/week
    ____ 2/week
    ____ 3/week
    ____ More

20. Would you be willing to participate in a fitness program for 3 months or more? (Select one)
    ____ Yes (1)
    ____ No (2)

21. What would be the biggest challenge for you to participate for 3 months or more?

    _____
    _____
    _____

22. Other comments:

    _____
    _____

End of Block: Part 1: Child

Start of Block: Part 2: Caretaker

Caretaker Name (first): _____

23. What physical activities or fitness programs would you like your child to be involved in?

    _____
    _____
    _____

24. What is your view of your child's current physical activity or exercise program? How do you support your child's participation in physical activities?

    _____
    _____
    _____

25. Does anything about a fitness program that involves or would involve your child concern you? (Select one)

    ____ Yes (1)
    ____ No (2)

Display: *Does anything about a fitness program that involves or would involve your child concern, you? = Yes or No*

26. If you answered yes to the question above, what would the concern(s) be?

    _____
    _____

27. What would motivate your child to get more fit (rank these)? 1 (best)–6 (worst)

    ____ Having a friend or brother/sister do it with them
    ____ Go to a fitness center or site that other kids go to
    ____ Get better at their sport, dance, martial art, or other activity
    ____ Trying new activities
    ____ Receive rewards
    ____ Other:

28. Rank order the list of rewards your child may prefer: 1 (best)–7 (worst)

    ____ Free game apps for their phone or computer
    ____ Favorite food treats like
    ____ Free tickets to a movie, play, or concert
    ____ Free entry into an amusement park
    ____ Free months at the gym, dance program, martial arts program or other
    ____ Free gear for participating in activity of choice
    ____ Other rewards: _____

29. Would you or a caretaker be willing and able to drive your child to a community-based program?

    (Select one)

    ____ Yes (1)
    ____ No (2)

30. Would it be more feasible for your child to participate in a community-based program if we provided transportation?

    (Select one)

    ____ Yes (1)
    ____ No (2)

31. Do you know what the current recommendation is for your child to exercise to maximize their bone and muscle health?

    ____ Yes (1)
    ____ No (2)

Display: *Do you know what the current recommendation is for your child to exercise to maximize their bone and muscle health = Yes or No*

32. If you answered yes to the question above, what frequency are you aware of?

    _____
    _____

33. How many days per week could your child attend a fitness program, outside your home, considering your schedule, your child's other activities, rides, etc. Rank 1 (most likely)–4 (least likely)

    _____ 1x/week
    _____ 2x/week
    _____ 3x/week
    _____ More

34. What would be your preferred frequency if there were few obstacles such as transportation or other obligations? Rank 1 (best)–4 (worst)

    _____ 1x/week (1)
    _____ 2x/week (2)
    _____ 3/week (3)
    _____ More (4)

35. How long could your child realistically participate given current constraints (rank order)?

    _____ 1 month
    _____ 2 months
    _____ 3 months
    _____ More

36. What is the biggest challenge for your child to participate in a regular fitness program?

    _____
    _____

37. Other Comments:

    _____
    _____
    _____
    _____

End of Block: Part 2: Caretaker

Kimbel, J. D.; Duff, S. V.; Friel, K. M.; Grant-Beuttler M.; Sukal Moulton, T.; Moreau, N. Incentives to Participate in Fitness Programming: Insights From Youth and Parents. *Qualtrics.* **2020**.

References

1. Joyner, M.J.; Barnes, J.N. I Am 80 Going on 18: Exercise and the Fountain of Youth. *J. Appl. Physiol.* **2013**, *114*, 1–2. [CrossRef] [PubMed]
2. Centers for Disease Control and Prevention (CDC). Aerobic, Muscle- and Bone Strengthening: What Counts for School-Aged Children and Adolescents? Available online: https://www.cdc.gov/physicalactivity/basics/children/what_counts.htm (accessed on 21 March 2023).
3. Piercy, K.L.; Troiano, R.P.; Ballard, R.M.; Carlson, S.A.; Fulton, J.E.; Galuska, D.A.; George, S.M.; Olson, R.D. The Physical Activity Guidelines for Americans. *JAMA* **2018**, *320*, 2020–2028. [CrossRef] [PubMed]
4. US Department of Health and Human Services. *Physical Activity Guidelines for Americans*, 2nd ed.; US Dept of Health and Human Services: Washington, DC, USA, 2018.
5. Caspersen, C.J.; Powell, K.E.; Christenson, G.M. Physical Activity, Exercise, and Physical Fitness: Definitions and Distinctions for Health-Related Research. *Public Health Rep.* **1985**, *100*, 126–131. [PubMed]
6. Bratteby Tollerz, L.U.; Forslund, A.H.; Olssom, R.M.; Lindström, H.; Holmbäck, U. Children with Cerebral Palsy Do Not Achieve Healthy Activity Levels. *Acta Paediatr.* **2015**, *104*, 1125–1129. [CrossRef] [PubMed]
7. Vella, S.A.; Cliff, D.P.; Magee, C.A.; Okely, A.D. Sports Participation and Parent-Reported Health-Related Quality of Life in Children: Longitudinal Associations. *J. Pediatr.* **2014**, *164*, 1469–1474. [CrossRef] [PubMed]
8. Vella, S.A.; Cliff, D.P.; Magee, C.A.; Okely, A.D. Associations between Sports Participation and Psychological Difficulties during Childhood: A Two-Year Follow-Up. *J. Sci. Med. Sport* **2015**, *18*, 304–309. [CrossRef]
9. Sonu, S.; Post, S.; Feinglass, J. Adverse Childhood Experiences and the Onset of Chronic Disease in Young Adulthood. *Prev. Med.* **2019**, *123*, 163–170. [CrossRef]
10. Peterson, M.D.; Ryan, J.M.; Hurvitz, E.A.; Mahmoudi, E. Chronic Conditions in Adults with Cerebral Palsy. *JAMA* **2015**, *314*, 2303–2305. [CrossRef]
11. Ryan, J.M.; Peterson, M.D.; Ryan, N.; Smith, K.J.; O'Connell, N.E.; Liverani, S.; Anokye, N.; Victor, C.; Allen, E. Mortality Due to Cardiovascular Disease, Respiratory Disease, and Cancer in Adults with Cerebral Palsy. *Dev. Med. Child Neurol.* **2019**, *61*, 924–928. [CrossRef]
12. Smith, K.J.; Peterson, M.D.; O'Connell, N.E.; Victor, C.; Liverani, S.; Anokye, N.; Ryan, J.M. Risk of Depression and Anxiety in Adults with Cerebral Palsy. *JAMA Neurol.* **2019**, *76*, 294–300. [CrossRef]
13. Moreau, N.G.; Friel, K.M.; Fuchs, R.K.; Dayanidhi, S.; Sukal Moulton, T.; Grant-Beuttler, M.; Peterson, M.; Stevenson, R.; Duff, S.V. Lifelong Fitness for Ambulatory Children and Adolescents with Cerebral Palsy I: Key Ingredients for Bone and Muscle Health. *Behav. Sci.* **2023**, accepted.
14. Bjornson, K.F.; Belza, B.; Kartin, D.; Logsdon, R.; McLaughlin, J.F. Ambulatory Physical Activity Performance in Youth with Cerebral Palsy and Youth Who Are Developing Typically. *Phys. Ther.* **2007**, *87*, 248–257. [CrossRef]
15. Yoon, M.J.; Choi, H.; Kim, J.S.; Lim, S.H.; Yoo, Y.J.; Hong, B.Y. Physical activity, quality of life and parenting stress in children with cerebral palsy. *Pediatr. Int.* **2022**, *64*, e15295. [CrossRef]
16. Cremer, N.; Hurvitz, E.A.; Peterson, M.D. Multimorbidity in Middle-Aged Adults with Cerebral Palsy. *Am. J. Med.* **2017**, *130*, 744.e9–744.e15. [CrossRef]
17. Thorpe, D. The Role of Fitness in Health and Disease: Status of Adults with Cerebral Palsy. *Dev. Med. Child. Neurol.* **2009**, *51* (Suppl. S4), 52–58. [CrossRef]
18. Strauss, D.; Brooks, J.; Rosenbloom, L.; Shavelle, R. Life Expectancy in Cerebral Palsy: An Update. *Dev. Med. Child. Neurol.* **2008**, *50*, 487–493. [CrossRef]
19. Palisano, R.J.; Chiarello, L.A.; King, G.A.; Novak, I.; Stoner, T.; Fiss, A. Participation-Based Therapy for Children with Physical Disabilities. *Disabil. Rehabil.* **2012**, *34*, 1041–1052. [CrossRef]
20. Reedman, S.; Boyd, R.N.; Sakzewski, L. The Efficacy of Interventions to Increase Physical Activity Participation of Children with Cerebral Palsy: A Systematic Review and Meta-Analysis. *Dev. Med. Child Neurol.* **2017**, *59*, 1011–1018. [CrossRef]
21. Wulf, G.; Lewthwaite, R. Optimizing Performance Through Intrinsic Motivation and Attention for Learning: The OPTIMAL Theory of Motor Learning. *Psychon. Bull. Rev.* **2016**, *23*, 1382–1414. [CrossRef]
22. González-Hernández, J.; Gómez-López, M.; Pérez-Turpin, J.A.; Muñoz-Villena, A.J.; Andreu-Cabrera, E. Perfectly Active Teenagers. When Does Physical Exercise Help Psychological Well-Being in Adolescents? *Int. J. Environ. Res. Public Health* **2019**, *16*, 4525. [CrossRef]
23. Cleary, S.L.; Taylor, N.F.; Dodd, K.J.; Shields, N. An Aerobic Exercise Program for Young People with Cerebral Palsy in Specialist Schools: A Phase I Randomized Controlled Trial. *Dev. Neurorehabil.* **2017**, *20*, 331–338. [CrossRef] [PubMed]

24. Shields, N.; van den Bos, R.; Buhlert-Smith, K.; Prendergast, L.; Taylor, N.A. Community-based exercise program to increase participation in physical activities among youth with disability: A feasibility study. *Disabil. Rehabil.* **2019**, *41*, 1152–1159. [CrossRef] [PubMed]
25. Thorpe, D.E.; Niles, A.; Richardson, J.; Turner, J.; Tych, M. Enhancing Function, Fitness, and Participation in Adolescents with Cerebral Palsy. *Pediatr. Phys. Ther.* **2006**, *18*, 81–82. [CrossRef]
26. Lakes, K.D.; Sharp, K.; Grant-Beuttler, M.; Neville, R.; Haddad, F.; Sunico, R.; Ho, D.; Schneider, M.; Sawitz, S.; Paulsen, J.; et al. A Six Week Therapeutic Ballet Intervention Improved Gait and Inhibitory Control in Children with Cerebral Palsy—A Pilot Study. *Front. Public Health* **2019**, *7*, 137. [CrossRef] [PubMed]
27. Ryan, J.M.; Cassidy, E.E.; Noorduyn, S.G.; O'Connell, N.E. Exercise Interventions for Cerebral Palsy. *Cochrane Database Syst. Rev.* **2017**, *6*, CD011660. [CrossRef] [PubMed]
28. Verschuren, O.; Peterson, M.D.; Balemans, A.C.; Hurvitz, E.A. Exercise and Physical Activity Recommendations for People with Cerebral Palsy. *Dev. Med. Child Neurol.* **2016**, *58*, 798–808. [CrossRef]
29. Gaskin, C.J.; Imms, C.R.; Dagley, G.; Msall, M.E.; Reddihough, D. Successfully Negotiating Life Challenges: Learnings from Adults with Cerebral Palsy. *Qual. Health Res.* **2021**, *31*, 2176–2193. [CrossRef]
30. Ryan, R.M.; Deci, E.L. Self-Determination Theory and the Facilitation of Intrinsic Motivation, Social Development, and Well-Being. *Am. Psychol.* **2000**, *55*, 68–78. [CrossRef]
31. Ryan, R.M.; Deci, E.L. Intrinsic and Extrinsic Motivation From a Self-Determination Theory Perspective: Definitions, Theory, Practices, and Future Directions. *Contemp. Educ. Psychol.* **2020**, *61*, 101860. [CrossRef]
32. Teixeira, P.J.; Carraça, E.V.; Markland, D.; Silva, M.N.; Ryan, R.M. Exercise, Physical Activity, and Self-Determination Theory: A Systematic Review. *Int. J. Behav. Nutr. Phys. Act.* **2012**, *9*, 78. [CrossRef]
33. Flannery, M. Self-Determination Theory: Intrinsic Motivation and Behavioral Change. *Oncol. Nurs. Forum.* **2017**, *44*, 155–156. [CrossRef]
34. Duff, S.V.; Quinn, L. Motor Learning and Skill Acquisition. In *Functional Movement Development across the Life Span*, 2nd ed.; Cech, D., Martin, S., Eds.; WB. SaundersAspen Pub: Rockville, MD, USA, 2002; pp. 86–117.
35. Gentile, A.M. A Working Model of Skill Acquisition with Application to Teaching. *Quest* **1972**, *17*, 3–23. [CrossRef]
36. Gentile, A.M. Skill Acquisition: Action, Movement, and Neuromotor Processes. In *Movement Science: Foundations for Physical Therapy*, 2nd ed.; Carr, J.H., Shepherd, R.D., Eds.; Aspen Pub: Rockville, MD, USA, 2000; pp. 111–187.
37. Muratori, L.M.; Lamberg, E.M.; Quinn, L.; Duff, S.V. Applying Principles of Motor Learning and Control to Upper Extremity Rehabilitation. *J. Hand Ther.* **2013**, *26*, 94–102; quiz 103. [CrossRef]
38. Shumway-Cook, A.; Woollacott, M.; Rachwani, J.; Santamaria, V. *Motor Control: Translating Research into Clinical Practice*, 6th ed.; Wolters Kluwer: Philadelphia, PA, USA, 2023.
39. Sidaway, B.; Bates, J.; Occhiogrosso, B.; Schlagenhaufer, J.; Wilkes, D. Interaction of Feedback Frequency and Task Difficulty in Children's Motor Skill Learning. *Phys. Ther.* **2012**, *92*, 948–957. [CrossRef]
40. Winstein, C.J.; Pohl, P.S.; Lewthwaite, R. Effects of Physical Guidance and Knowledge of Results on Motor Learning: Support for the Guidance Hypothesis. *Res. Q. Exerc. Sport* **1994**, *65*, 316–323. [CrossRef]
41. Berridge, K.C. The Debate Over Dopamine's Role in Reward: The Case for Incentive Salience. *Psychopharmacology (Berl)* **2007**, *191*, 391–431. [CrossRef]
42. Ewell, L.A.; Leutgeb, S. Replay to Remember: A Boost from Dopamine. *Nat. Neurosci.* **2014**, *17*, 1629–1631. [CrossRef]
43. Ayres, A.J. *Sensory Integration and Learning Disorders*; Western Psychological Services: Los Angeles, CA, USA, 1972.
44. Gibson, J.J. The Theory of Affordances. In *Perceiving, Acting, and Knowing: Toward an Ecological Psychology*; Shaw, R., Bransford, J., Eds.; Erlbaum: Mahwah, NJ, USA, 1977; pp. 67–82.
45. Lauruschkus, K.; Nordmark, E.; Hallström, I. Parents' Experiences of Participation in Physical Activities for Children with Cerebral Palsy—Protecting and Pushing towards Independence. *Disabil. Rehabil.* **2017**, *39*, 771–778. [CrossRef]
46. Curran, T.; Wexler, L. School-Based Positive Youth Development: A Systematic Review of the Literature. *J. Sch. Health* **2017**, *87*, 71–80. [CrossRef]
47. Pritchard, L.; Phelan, S.; McKillop, A.; Andersen, J. Child, Parent, and Clinician Experiences with a Child-Driven Goal Setting Approach in Paediatric Rehabilitation. *Disabil. Rehabil.* **2022**, *44*, 1042–1049. [CrossRef]
48. Kimbel, J.D.; Duff, S.V.; Friel, K.M.; Grant-Beuttler, M.; Sukal Moulton, T.; Moreau, N. Incentives to Participate in Fitness Programming: Insights from Youth and Parents. *Qualtrics Survey* **2020**.
49. Fu, W.; Li, R.; Zhang, Y.; Huang, K. Parenting Stress and Parenting Efficacy of Parents Having Children with Disabilities in China: The Role of Social Support. *Int. J. Environ. Res. Public Health* **2023**, *20*, 2133. [CrossRef] [PubMed]
50. Sakwape, K.; Machailo, R.; Koen, M.P. Exploring role strain and experiences of caregivers of children living with disabilities. *Nurs. Open* **2023**, *10*, 2886–2894. [CrossRef]
51. McIntyre, L.L. Family-Based Practices to Promote Well-Being. *Am. J. Intellect. Dev. Disabil.* **2020**, *125*, 349–352. [CrossRef] [PubMed]
52. Clark, F.; Azen, S.P.; Zemke, R. Occupational Therapy for Independent Living Adults: A Randomized Controlled Trial. *JAMA* **1997**, *278*, 1321–1326. [CrossRef]

53. Hill, V.A.; Vickrey, B.G.; Cheng, E.M.; Valle, N.P.; Ayala-Rivera, M.; Moreno, L.; Munoz, C.; Dombish, H.; Espinosa, A.; Wang, D.; et al. A Pilot Trial of a Lifestyle Intervention for Stroke Survivors: Design of Healthy Eating and Lifestyle after Stroke (HEALS). *J. Stroke Cerebrovasc. Dis.* **2017**, *26*, 2806–2813. [CrossRef]
54. Jackson, J.; Carlson, M.; Mandel, D.; Zemke, R.; Clark, F. Occupation in Lifestyle Redesign®: The Well Elderly Study Occupational Therapy Program. *Am. J. Occup. Ther.* **1998**, *52*, 326–336. [CrossRef]
55. Pyatak, E.A.; Carandang, K.; Rice Collins, C.; Carlson, M. Optimizing Occupations, Habits, and Routines for Health and Well-Being with Lifestyle Redesign®: A Synthesis and Scoping Review. *Am. J. Occup. Ther.* **2022**, *76*, 7605205050. [CrossRef]
56. Slaman, J.; Roebroeck, M.; Dallmijer, A.; Twisk, J.; Stam, H.; Van Den Berg-Emons, R.; Learn 2 Move Research Group. Can a Lifestyle intervention Improve Physical Behavior in Adolescents and Young Adults with Spastic Cerebral Palsy? A Randomized Controlled Trial. *Dev. Med. Child Neurol.* **2015**, *57*, 159–166. [CrossRef]
57. Slaman, J.; Roebroeck, M.; van der Slot, W.; Twisk, J.; Wensink, A.; Stam, H.; van den Berg-Emons, R.; Learn 2 Move Research Group. Can a Lifestyle intervention Improve Physical Fitness in Adolescents and Young Adults with Spastic Cerebral Palsy? A Randomized Controlled Trial. *Arch. Phys. Med. Rehabil.* **2014**, *95*, 1646–1655. [CrossRef]
58. Law, M.; Baptiste, S.; McColl, M.; Opzoomer, A.; Polatajko, H.; Pollock, N. The Canadian Occupational Performance Measure: An Outcome Measure for Occupational Therapy. *Can. J. Occup. Ther.* **1990**, *57*, 82–87. [CrossRef]
59. Law, M.; Anaby, D.; Imms, C.; Teplicky, R.; Turner, L. Improving the Participation of Youth with Physical Disabilities in Community Activities: An Interrupted Time Series Design. *Aust. Occup. Ther. J.* **2015**, *62*, 105–115. [CrossRef]
60. Hay, J.A.; Hawes, R.; Faught, B.E. Evaluation of a Screening Instrument for Developmental Coordination Disorder. *J. Adolesc. Health* **2004**, *34*, 308–313. [CrossRef]
61. Grant-Beuttler, M.; Jennings, J.; McCauley, C.; Dulay, R.; Grossnickle, K.; Kill, K.; Hay, J. Development of an Electronic Version of the Children's Self-Perceptions of Adequacy in and Predilection for Physical Activity Scale. *Pediatr. Exerc. Sci.* **2017**, *29*, 153–160. [CrossRef]
62. Rollnick, S.; Miller, W.R.; Butler, C.C. Motivational Interviewing in Health Care: Helping Patients Change Behavior. *Am. J. Pharm. Educ.* **2009**, *73*, 127.
63. Rubak, S.; Sandbaek, A.; Lauritzen, T.; Christensen, B. Motivational Interviewing: A Systematic Review and Meta-analysis. *Br. J. Gen. Pract.* **2005**, *55*, 305–312.
64. Schwellnus, H.; King, G.; Baldwin, P.; Keenan, S.; Hartman, L.R. A Solution-Focused Coaching Intervention with Children and Youth with Cerebral Palsy to Achieve Participation-Oriented Goals. *Phys. Occup. Ther. Pediatr.* **2020**, *40*, 423–440. [CrossRef]
65. De Shazer, S.; Berg, I.K.; Lipchik, E.; Nunnally, E.; Molnar, A.; Gingerich, W.; Weiner-Davis, M. Brief Therapy: Focused Solution Development. *Fam. Process* **1986**, *25*, 207–221. [CrossRef]
66. Trepper, T.S.; Dolan, Y.; McCollum, E.E.; Nelson, T. Steve de Shazer and the Future of Solution-Focused Therapy. *J. Marital. Fam. Ther.* **2006**, *32*, 133–139. [CrossRef]
67. Moreau, N.G. Muscle Performance in Children and Youth with Cerebral Palsy: Implications for Resistance Training. In *Cerebral Palsy*, 2nd ed.; Miller, F., Bachrach, S., Lennon, N., O'Neil, M., Eds.; Springer: Cham, Switzerland, 2020; pp. 1–12. [CrossRef]
68. Moreau, N.G.; Falvo, M.J.; Damiano, D.L. Rapid Force Generation is Impaired in Cerebral Palsy and is Related to Decreased Muscle Size and Functional Mobility. *Gait Posture* **2012**, *35*, 154–158. [CrossRef]
69. Lewthwaite, R.; Chiviacowsky, S.; Drews, R.; Wulf, G. Choose to Move: The Motivational Impact of Autonomy Support on Motor Learning. *Psychon. Bull. Rev.* **2015**, *22*, 1383–1388. [CrossRef] [PubMed]
70. Darrah, J.; Wessel, J.; Nearingburg, P.; O'Connor, M. Evaluation of a Community Fitness Program for Adolescents with Cerebral Palsy. *Pediatr. Phys. Ther.* **1999**, *11*, 18–23. [CrossRef]

Disclaimer/Publisher's Note: The statements, opinions and data contained in all publications are solely those of the individual author(s) and contributor(s) and not of MDPI and/or the editor(s). MDPI and/or the editor(s) disclaim responsibility for any injury to people or property resulting from any ideas, methods, instructions or products referred to in the content.

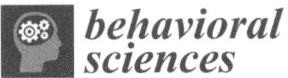

Article

Evidence for Using ACQUIRE Therapy in the Clinical Application of Intensive Therapy: A Framework to Guide Therapeutic Interactions

Stephanie C. DeLuca [1,2,3,*], Mary Rebekah Trucks [1], Dorian Wallace [1] and Sharon Landesman Ramey [1]

1. The Fralin Biomedical Research Institute's Neuromotor Clinic, Roanoke, VA 24016, USA; mrebekah@vtc.vt.edu (M.R.T.); wdorian6@vtc.vt.edu (D.W.); slramey@vt.edu (S.L.R.)
2. The School of Neuroscience, Virginia Tech, Blacksburg, VA 24061, USA
3. The Department of Pediatrics, Virginia Tech Carilion School of Medicine, Roanoke, VA 24016, USA
* Correspondence: stephdeluca@vt.edu; Tel.: +1-540-526-2098

Abstract: Intensive therapies have become increasingly popular for children with hemiparesis in the last two decades and are specifically recommended because of high levels of scientific evidence associated with them, including multiple randomized controlled trials and systematic reviews. Common features of most intensive therapies that have documented efficacy include: high dosages of therapy hours; active engagement of the child; individualized goal-directed activities; and the systematic application of operant conditioning techniques to elicit and progress skills with an emphasis on success-oriented play. However, the scientific protocols have not resulted in guiding principles designed to aid clinicians with understanding the complexity of applying these principles to a heterogeneous clinical population, nor have we gathered sufficient clinical data using intensive therapies to justify their widespread clinical use beyond hemiparesis. We define a framework for describing moment-by-moment therapeutic interactions that we have used to train therapists across multiple clinical trials in implementing intensive therapy protocols. We also document outcomes from the use of this framework during intensive therapies provided clinically to children (7 months–20 years) from a wide array of diagnoses that present with motor impairments, including hemiparesis and quadriparesis. Results indicate that children from a wide array of diagnostic categories demonstrated functional improvements.

Keywords: cerebral palsy; traumatic brain injury; hemispherectomy; hemiparesis; quadriparesis; intensive therapy; ACQUIRE therapy; pediatric constraint-induced movement therapy; hand arm bimanual therapy

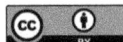

1. Introduction

Historically, pediatric rehabilitation has been eclectic in therapy delivery models in large part because of the need for individualized services in clinical models of care where the treated children have a wide range of diagnoses as well as variations in functional abilities and severity levels associated with their disability [1]. In this regard, the past few decades in pediatric rehabilitation have seen the development of many evidence-based therapeutic approaches based on five common constructs [2–10]:

1. Treatment delivery via an intensive therapeutic burst (i.e., many hours each day on multiple consecutive days per week across multiple weeks);
2. Goal-directed activities with componental parts of therapy activities progressing toward increased movement, function, and skill;
3. Active engagement of the child's current sensory-motor skills throughout all therapy sessions;

4. Activity selection guided by the child's interest with therapeutic modification to accomplish movement, function, and skill goals during playful, success-oriented interactions; and
5. Use of operant conditioning techniques, where positive reinforcement is provided to teach skills via variations in the contingencies of reinforcement to successively shape the child's skills toward a targeted goal.

The most documented of these constructs has been the concept of therapy being delivered in high dosages or in intensive therapeutic bursts of treatment where many hours of therapy are administered multiple days a week (often daily) within a time period that is limited to a few weeks. Two of the most well-known high-dosage therapies were designed specifically for hemiparetic cerebral palsy [2–10]. Pediatric constraint-induced movement therapy (PCIMT) and hand arm bimanual therapy (HABIT) are now routinely recommended as treatment approaches for children with hemiparesis to improve motor and functional skills [5,7,8,10,11]. Recent guidelines even recommend that these approaches begin in infancy [11] despite the fact that there is substantial evidence of the use in infancy being more limited [12]. These intensive high-dosage therapies have been the subject of numerous clinical trials and numerous systematic reviews serving as the basis for these recommendations, and high-dosage intensive therapies are now becoming commercially available. Despite these advances, these approaches are far from the clinical norm as the standard of care for children with disabilities, even for children with the specified diagnosis of hemiparesis. Rather, they are limitedly available for families that specifically seek these services.

There are many reasons for the limited dissemination of these therapeutic approaches and why they are not considered standard of care. These include limited coverage by third party payers for such services and the ability of the healthcare system to adequately provide these services within the current institutionalized models of care. However, there is another issue that is rarely addressed. Are therapists adequately prepared and trained to deliver intensive models of therapy? Intensive therapy models and distributed practice models both have a goal of increasing motor skills, but almost by definition they must approach the process of learning and teaching motor skills differently. Pediatric therapists who see children once or twice a week, usually for under an hour, must quickly identify a limited focus area at each visit and primarily educate parents and caregivers to focus on that one area to promote learning. Next, with multiple days between visits, they must rely on parental reports to understand reactions, levels of learning that promote gains or losses in motor skills, and then once again quickly decide on either the same or different focus area for the new visit. This model provides difficult decision points for therapists when children rarely have a singular need.

In contrast, most, if not all, high-dosage intensive therapies that have high-quality evidence to support their use stem from scientific investigations that were built, at least in part, on learning theories [13–15]. Protocols were built to include sufficient time where direct observations of child responses and reaction to those responses could be implemented across multiple repetitions. Furthermore, these protocols were built on the concept that the promotion of motor skills occurred within multi-contextual developmental domains that were interacting, and that those interactions were also a reflection of complex neurological pathways. This concept means that skill development is built across domains simultaneously (e.g., motor skills depend to a certain degree on cognitive skills and vice versa) and all of them need to be considered in the learning process, once again requiring time for a therapist to consider these cross-domain impacts. Above all, these scientifically investigated protocols were built on learning principles to guide therapeutic decision-making.

For example, decades of learning the literature has detailed the variations in reinforcement schedules needed to promote learning across differing ages [16,17]. A reinforcement that is delayed by a second for an infant negates the learning potential in that moment, whereas for a child of 3 or 4 years of age, the schedule of reinforcement has a broader time span to promote the desired learning [18–20]. Similarly, the scaffolding or progression of skill in operant conditioning must be progressed at certain levels of proficiency. Progression before 70–80% proficiency at a given level or even waiting until a child is completely proficient at a given level can stop or alter the progression of learning. These concepts were built on observations of children who were typically developing, but they have been robust in the promotion of learning across diagnostic categories and learning styles [13,14,16,21–24]. They were a primary and integral part of the early protocols and scientific investigations into intensive therapies. However, unlike the concept of high-dosage, they have been less built into the therapeutic lexicon and dissemination of high-dosage intensive therapies. They are also not routinely taught via therapy curriculums, causing many therapists to be ill-equipped at providing a high-dosage therapy clinically that maintains the levels of efficacy seen in clinical trials.

We sought to address this as we began to try to disseminate our research protocols and use of intensive therapies. The ACQUIRE framework as seen in Figure 1 represents a complex and reciprocal interplay between the child and the therapist that is under constant evolution because of the many different variables impacting therapeutic interactions. It was designed to inform and assist therapists in the delivery of high-dosage intensive therapy in order to create high-quality densely packed therapy activities that involve needed repetitions and skill refinement to promote motor learning.

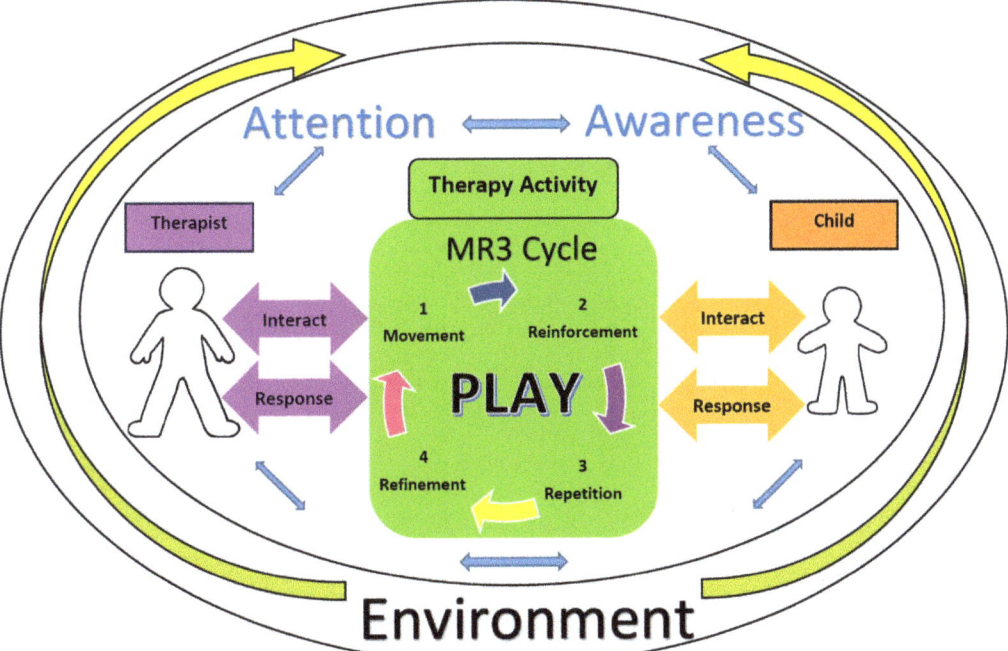

Figure 1. The ACQUIRE framework [8,13,14,25].

At the heart of the framework is a cyclical set of steps based on operant conditioning. We termed the central operant conditioning process as the MR3 Cycle: movement, reinforcement, repetition, and refinement [14]. This pattern guides the progression of learning by scaffolding supports and demands toward a targeted motoric and functional outcome or learning goal. As stated above, a key component of this process is to allow the sufficient repetition of tasks (via massed practice) to promote proficiency, combined with an understanding of when and how tasks might be refined and progressed by providing appropriate types, levels, and schedules of reinforcement. Refinement and progression are key. Massed practice alone does not move learning toward a target. The model also seeks to define the therapeutic environment in a manner to help the therapist understand the many components that overtly and subtly impact learning and the progression of skill. For example, a request for a movement that is above a child's skill level may result in a failed attempt at a movement, or it may also result in the child not responding at all. In both instances, a therapist must evaluate and react to the child and the demands of the task appropriately to promote learning. A parent entering the room may distract a child from a movement attempt where they were previously successful, making them unsuccessful secondary to the distraction. The therapist must recognize the basis of this failed attempt and respond to re-direct the child's attention. The process is quite complex. The collective and individualized attention, awareness, perception, and understanding of the task for both the therapist and the child are almost in a constant state of flux, creating unique demands on the therapy process; demands which therapists must be prepared to guide.

Figure 2 shows the complex decision-making process involved in that guidance. The process starts with a choice of an appropriate task. Remember that all tasks are dependent on multiple developmental domains, and thus many complexities must be considered. The choice of task must be motivating and meet a child's current ability levels. For example, if a parent has a goal that a child uses a paretic arm in dressing, but that child does not yet reach with their paretic arm, a choice for a task might be only to reach forward with the paretic arm toward a motivating toy. At first, that reach may even be untargeted. The therapist requests the child to reach for the toy with playful engagement, while providing cues and instructions to the child. The cues and instructions need to be specific and should include a modeling of the task. After modeling, if the child's attempt is not successful, the therapist may include hand-over-hand facilitation to help the child to complete the task in order to reinforce their attempts and allow a feeling of success. With each task request, the therapist must then allow sufficient time for a child to respond. This is key within a therapeutic context because not only does a task stem from multiple developmental domains, but a child's limitations may also be linked to many developmental domains (e.g., planning and processing limitations). Then, as shown in Figure 2, there are three possible child responses: a child successfully completes the requested task, the child is unsuccessful at completing the task, or the child does not respond. The MR3 operant conditioning cycle dictates that the therapist must respond, but the response is dependent on many constructs that a therapist needs to immediately evaluate. In the above example, if the child reaches forward and performs this on a sufficient number of occasions, the therapist may progress the skill by adding a reaching target (e.g., a large lever on a toy). As progression continues across hundreds of repetitions of reaching, the therapist may increase the complexity of having an open hand or to reach in different directional planes. Demands of a task can even be increased by changing how the request is made. A therapist may proceed from pairing a verbal and tactile request to merely a verbal request. All of this is relatively child-dependent and context-dependent because at each point in the process, the therapist must consider the many components impacting the child's learning. The ACQUIRE framework is meant to provide organization for many of the constructs to be considered.

We have now used this therapeutic process to train many therapists across two therapeutic research clinics, multiple clinical trials, and in the training of doctoral candidates in therapy professions. The clinical trials primarily focused on training therapists to complete intensive therapies where dosage levels and differing constraint types were used, including a bimanual approach involving no constraint. In our research clinics, we collected data gathered as practice-based evidence using the ACQUIRE therapy model while providing high-dosage clinical services across many different diagnostic categories, thus addressing another need in the dissemination of high-dosage intensive therapy models and their use across heterogenic clinical populations. We present that data below.

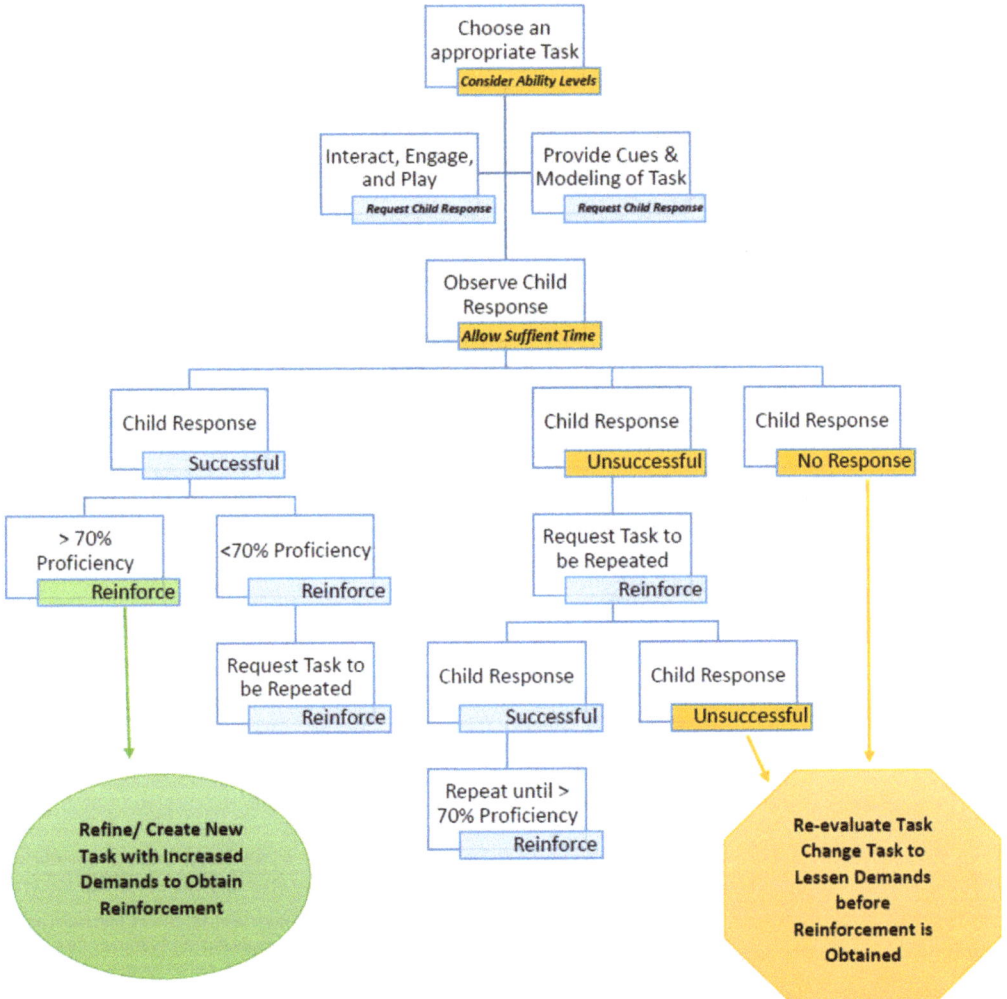

Figure 2. Therapeutic activity decision tree.

2. Materials and Methods

2.1. Participants/Clients

The sample is a convenience clinical sample collected across two research clinics at two different universities. The clinics were not operated concurrently. Children were brought to each of the clinics by caregivers to specifically receive intensive therapy services based on the ACQUIRE model of therapy. Families often sought services after interaction with other families via online support services. Children ranged in diagnoses, but were pre-screened by clinic personnel to ensure that there were no concerns about the children participating in intensive therapy. All levels of severity were included as long as the child was deemed medically stable, meaning that there were no existing movement/range of motion or behavioral requirements necessary for a child to receive services. While some children were quadriparetic, all children had some level of asymmetric functioning. Ethical approvals were obtained for all data collection at both clinics. All participants signed informed consent forms, permitting data during clinic-based services to be collected, analyzed, and published. The sample presented represents a subset of all clinical data collected at the two clinics. Some clinical data were unavailable for analyses because they have not yet been entered into the current database. The clinics did provide some children multiple epochs of intensive therapy if requested, but data from children who received additional epochs of treatment were not included. Children were also excluded if they did not finish the course of planned intervention (e.g., because of illness).

2.2. Intervention

ACQUIRE therapy was delivered between 4–6 h each weekday for 4 consecutive weeks, creating intensive therapy epochs of 80–120 therapy hours. Variations in dosage occurred for a variety of reasons, but most often was a function of parental requests or limitations in clinical coverage. A full arm constraint was used for children with hemiparesis via a PCIMT model called ACQUIREc therapy [13,14]. ACQUIREc Therapy is a specific form of ACQUIRE Therapy. Both the clinics were initially started to deliver this manualized PCIMT approach that served as the basis for our further development of the ACQUIRE framework. The basis for therapy for children with quadriparesis was ACQUIRE therapy, in which a constraint may or may not have been used, depending on the child's motor involvement, levels of asymmetry, and individual goals of the child and family.

2.3. Assessments

A battery of qualitative and clinical (quantitative) assessments were completed within 2 days prior to and after completion of ACQUIRE therapy. Quantitative data presented in this paper include the Emerging Behaviors Scale (EBS) [14], the Assisting Hand Assessment (AHA) [26], and the Pediatric Motor Activity log (PMAL) [14]. All assessments were primarily designed to examine asymmetric functioning of the upper extremities. The EBS is a count of 30 possible arm and hand skills. The AHA is a measure designed to examine bilateral performance of an assisting hand, and the PMAL is a parental report measure of 22 arm and hand skills where the parent reports how well and how often the child uses the more paretic arm and hand across a 5-point Likert scale, where 0 indicates no ability and no use of the more paretic arm and hand items where parents rate the functioning of the more paretic arm and hand across two scales that range between 0–5. The 'how often' scale provides an ordinal level ranking of how frequently children use the more paretic arm and hand and the 'how well' scale provides an ordinal level ranking of the quality of skills of the more paretic arm and hand.

2.4. Data Analysis

Descriptive statistics were prepared for sample characteristics and all quantitative data. Data between pre- and post-treatment were examined with repeated measures analysis of variance (ANOVA). Change scores were generated to compare between diagnostic categories and to compare outcomes between children with hemi- and quadriparesis. Analyses fused counts of the 30 potential behaviors for the EBS, logit scores for the AHA, and averages for PMAL 'how often' and 'how well' scales. Descriptive data were reported by parents.

3. Results

3.1. Participants/Clients

Participants/clients data are based on 139 children between 7 months to 20 years of age (mean = 62.1, S.D. = 53.41). There were 61 females and 78 males representing 44 and 56% of the sample, respectively. Ethnic or racial categories were not routinely recorded by the clinic, but retrospective examination of data indicated that about 10% of the sample represented children from racial and ethnic categories other than white or Caucasian. Table 1 presents the numbers of children by diagnostic categories compared across those with hemiparesis versus quadriparesis. ACQUIRE therapy was delivered for 6 h each weekday for 4 consecutive weeks for 118 of these children, making a dosage of 120 h of therapy. For four children, scheduling issues with their families caused three weeks to be delivered instead of four weeks at 6 h per day, resulting in a total dosage of 90 h. Four of twelve children's parents and therapists collaboratively decided to complete 4 h of therapy 5 days a week for 4 weeks, resulting in a total dosage of 80 h.

Table 1. Diagnostic categories by type of paresis.

	Hemiparesis	Quadriparesis
Cerebral Palsy (CP)	74	10
Cerebral Vascular Accident (CVA)	25	3
Arteriovenous Malformation (AVM)	1	0
Traumatic Brain Injury (TBI)	9	1
Hemispherectomy	4	0
Not Otherwise Specified Motor Delay	8	4
	121	18

3.2. The Emerging Behavior Scale

The EBS was the most consistent measure used across all children, and analysis included n = 121. Across all diagnostic categories and paresis types, children gained an average of 9.15 (S.D. = 5.98) new behaviors. Repeated measures ANOVA indicated a main effect of time between pre- to post-treatment with F = 23.51, $p < 0.001$. There were no significant differences found based on diagnosis or type of paresis. Table 2 shows mean change scores by diagnostic category and paresis type. Across all children with hemiparesis, the mean = 9.36 (S.D. = 6.03; n = 106), and across all children with quadriparesis, mean = 7.67 (S.D. = 5.51, n = 15). Results suggest that children with a variety of diagnoses that present with either hemi- or quadriparesis gained new unilateral skills.

Table 2. Mean Gain Scores (S.D.) by diagnostic categories.

Diagnosis		Emerging Behaviors Scale		Pediatric Motor Activity Log			
				Frequency of Use		Quality of Movement	
CP	Hemiparesis	9.71 (4.96)	n = 69	2.04 (1.14)	n = 45	1.50 (0.99)	n = 45
	Quadriparesis	7.56 (5.62)	n = 9	1.73 (0.68)	n = 6	1.47 (0.84)	n = 6
CVA	Hemiparesis	9.5 (9.29)	n = 20	2.18 (1.11)	n = 22	1.76 (1.05)	n = 22
	Quadriparesis	11.67 (6.43)	n = 3	2.39 (1.94)	n = 3	1.11 (0.96)	n = 3
TBI	Hemiparesis	7.86 (6.62)	n = 7	1.93 (0.97)	n = 8	1.55 (0.90)	n = 8
	Quadriparesis	5.00	n = 1	1.46	n = 1	1.42	n = 1
Hemispherectomy	Hemiparesis	9.00 (6.56)	n = 3	1.56 (0.91)	n = 4	2.00 (0.69)	n = 4
	Quadriparesis	N/A	n = 0	N/A	n = 0	N/A	n = 0
AVM	Hemiparesis	5.00	n = 1	2.63	n = 1	1.23	n = 1
	Quadriparesis	N/A	n = 0	N/A	n = 0	N/A	n = 0
Other	Hemiparesis	7.5 (1.80)	n = 6	1.78 (0.94)	n = 1	1.14 (0.71)	n = 1
	Quadriparesis	3.5 (0.71)	n = 2	N/A	n = 0	N/A	n = 0
			N = 121		N = 97		N = 97

3.3. The Pediatric Motor Activity Log

The PMAL was completed by 97 parents, of which 87 of the children presented with hemiparesis and 10 children presented with quadriparesis. Across all diagnostic categories and paresis types, parents rated their children as having increased amounts of use for the more paretic arm with a mean change = 2.17 (S.D. = 1.07), and they rated that their children's abilities with their more paretic arm and hands increased with a mean change = 1.54 (S.D. = 0.94). Repeated measures ANOVA, considering both the 'how often' and 'how well' scales indicated significant main effects of time between pre- to post-treatment. The 'how often' scale produced an F = 32.74, $p < 0.001$, and the 'how well' scale F = 17.58, $p < 0.001$. There were no significant differences found based on diagnosis or type of paresis. Table 2 shows mean changes for each scale by diagnostic category and paresis type. Across all children with hemiparesis, the mean = 2.03 (S.D. = 1.07; n = 87), and across all children with quadriparesis, mean = 1.91 (S.D. = 1.1, n = 10). Results demonstrate that parents reported changes in both the quality of their children's skills with the more paretic arm and hand, but reported even more changes in how frequently their children were using their more paretic arm and hand immediately after intensive therapy. Notably, this finding is true across diagnostic and paresis types (i.e., hemi- or quadriparetic).

3.4. The Assisting Hand Assessment

Data from the AHA were available for 26 children. All children were diagnosed with hemiparetic CP (n = 25) or stroke (n = 1). Three children were quadriparetic but highly asymmetrical. Across all diagnostic categories and paresis types, children gained an average of 11.19 (S.D. = 7.55) logit score points. Repeated measures ANOVA indicated no significant main effect of time between pre- to post-treatment, only a trend toward significance with F = 3.98, $p = 0.058$. There were no significant differences found based on diagnosis or type of paresis. Figure 3 demonstrates the pre- to post-changes by paresis type. Despite the fact that there was only a trend toward significance in this measure, as Figure 3 demonstrates, there were positive changes in all children. The lack of significance is likely related to the heterogeneity of the children and the fact that the measure was designed for measuring children with hemiparesis. As stated above, the children with quadriparesis that we chose to use the measure on in this clinical sample were extremely asymmetric. Results suggest that children with a variety of diagnoses that present with either hemi- or quadriparesis gained abilities to use their more paretic arm and hand in bimanual activities.

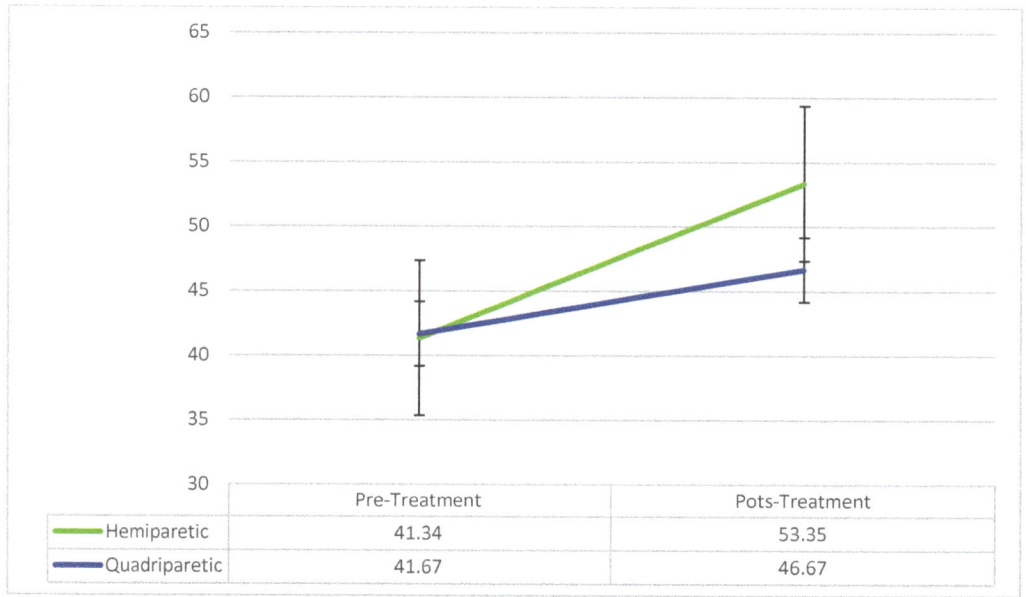

Figure 3. Pre- to post-treatment AHA logit scores.

4. Discussion

The usability of high-dosage intensive therapies in clinical settings is impacted by multiple issues. Two primary issues not adequately considered are, firstly, that clinical populations are usually highly heterogeneous, and secondly, that therapists are not adequately prepared to implement these high dosage therapeutic approaches. We sought to address both of these issues in this paper.

The ACQUIRE framework provides a more defined and detailed representation of the interactive therapeutic processes and provides specific constructs that impact learning during high-dosage intensive therapy. These concepts have a strong foundation in theories about learning, specifically operant conditioning, and should be seen as additive components to high-dosage therapies which have traditionally been defined more fundamentally in terms of frequency, intensity, and timing of therapy. Therapeutic encounters are complex, and the ACQUIRE framework and associated decision-making process seek to make therapeutic learning a collaborative and more definable interaction between the therapist and the child and must include sufficient time and opportunity for massed but refined processes to promote learning. In order to use high-dosage intensive therapies, therapists must be trained to understand these constructs. Concomitantly, high-dosage therapies and these processes allow therapists ample time to consider the whole child who is intermixing developmental domains almost on a continuous basis throughout development. We theorize that limited time constraints do not allow therapists to consider the interplay from both the therapeutic delivery side and the internal development side of the child, and that this is a major impediment for therapy delivery that routinely and systematically promotes the development of skills.

We have now used the ACQUIRE framework to train dozens of therapists and guide intensive therapy epochs for hundreds of children across many diagnoses. The data across etiologies presented in this paper begin to address the question about the use of high-dosage intensive therapy beyond merely hemiparesis. Across six diagnostic categories that included CP, CVA, TBI, AVM, hemispherectomy, and others (e.g., microcephaly, tumor resections), children consistently responded positively to receiving high-dosage intensive ACQUIRE therapy and gained movements and functional skills. The data in this paper were primarily focused on developing and measuring motor skills, primarily that of the upper extremity in children with multiple types of diagnoses. Importantly, children with varied diagnoses improved. In addition, we collapsed across levels of paralysis and comparing children with hemiparesis to children with quadriparesis, and both groups improved on the number of skills developed (e.g., the EBS) and by parental report (e.g., the PMAL). Magnitudes of change favored children with hemiparesis but all responded positively.

There are limitations to the data we present. First and foremost, we present data collected for clinical purposes and to internally understand if the intensive therapy services we were providing were indeed producing positive changes. Both of the clinics were initially designed to provide our manualized version of pediatric constraint-induced movement therapy, ACQUIRE Therapy [14], and we have published numerous clinical trials [26–29] based on this protocol, but our assessment and expanded treatment protocols were built on this legacy by incorporating all the components of that protocol outside the constraint with children who had bilateral paresis. Our routinely used measurements of change are limited for this reason. We often saw changes and parents reported changes in other motor areas (e.g., gross motor skills) and developmental domains (e.g., language) not routinely tested. We further recognize that children in this sample received a minimum of 80 h of therapy within a four-week period. While this meets recommendations made within the literature [3], it is well above the current standard of practice and perhaps more importantly what is routinely covered by third party reimbursement. This is a major factor that prevents many children from receiving intensive therapy. While our data cannot adequately address the health disparities associated with this fact, it is incumbent upon us to recognize it as a limitation.

5. Conclusions

The field of pediatric rehabilitation, or at least therapists on a provider level, appear to be increasing the amount of therapeutic services provided to children in traditional settings [25–29]. Perhaps this change, in part, is due to the overall increase in pediatric therapy services, driven mostly by demand of caregivers. There also appears to be an increase in the number of facilities providing intensive pediatric therapy services, again likely driven by caregiver demand. While the increase in intensity is necessary, our experience with providing intensive services for children with neuromotor impairments, both in research and clinic settings, has led us to a greater understanding of the multiple necessary components that exist for the effective and efficacious delivery of high-quality intensive therapies that excel beyond merely the component of dosage. Dosage is a highly recognized and needed component [3,25], but it is not the only essential component for intensive therapies to be delivered in a manner that maximizes efficacy. The ACQUIRE framework and therapy delivery are meant to guide the necessary interactions between the therapist and the child in order maximize intensive therapy services for both the therapeutic delivery side provided by the therapist and on the developmental side for the child. As the field makes further investments into pediatric rehabilitation to utilize high-dosage therapies, we need to better establish how we prepare therapists to deliver these therapeutic efforts.

The next steps are always difficult when considering how to translate research findings into practice. Defining these intensive therapies in terms of frequency, density, and dosage was a major addition to the pediatric rehabilitation field driven by research, but it has led to an eclectic mix of therapies with varying levels of results. The next steps include a greater standardization of guiding methodologies and decision-making processes used to deliver intensive therapies.

Author Contributions: Conceptualization of all materials and ideas in the manuscript included all authors. M.R.T. and D.W. were responsible for implementing the ACQUIRE Therapy model with many of the participants. S.L.R. and S.C.D. directed and oversaw all data collection involved with the participants. S.C.D. conducted all data and prepared the original draft of the manuscript. Further writing, review and editing were conducted by all authors. Visualizations were drafted by S.C.D., M.R.T. and D.W. Funding acquisition was developed by S.L.R. and S.C.D. All authors have read and agreed to the published version of the manuscript.

Funding: This research received no external funding, but involves data based on a clinical service. The authors are funded for other projects that supported the refinement of the ACQUIRE therapy model in addition to the clinical services based on the use of ACQUIRE therapy. These included the CHAMP study funded by NIH grant R01HD068345, the Baby CHAMP study funded by NIH grant R01HD074574, and the National Pediatric Rehabilitation Resource Center grant P2CHD101912. All grants were awarded by the Eunice Kennedy Shriver National Institute of Child Health and Human Development, National Center for Medical Rehabilitation Research, National Institutes of Health.

Institutional Review Board Statement: The use of clinical data was conducted in accordance with the Declaration of Helsinki, and approved by the Institutional Review Board of Virginia Tech protocol numbers 13-196 and 13-093 with dates of approval continuous since 2013. Protocol 13-196 was originally approved on 9 August 2013 and the most recent approval was 11 January 2023, and protocol 13-093 was originally approved on 13 February 2013 and the most recent approval was 22 January 2023.

Informed Consent Statement: Written informed consent (parental permission) for the use of all clinical data was obtained from each child's guardian(s).

Data Availability Statement: Data collected were collected for clinical purposes and therefore individual data are not available for distribution or public use.

Acknowledgments: The authors wish to acknowledge the families and children who graciously allowed us to learn from them. We would also like to thank the Fralin Biomedical Research Institute at Virginia Tech Carilion, Virginia Tech and the Sparks Clinic at the University of Alabama at Birmingham for the support of our research clinics at these institutions.

Conflicts of Interest: The authors declare no conflict of interest.

References

1. Barry, M. Evidence-based practice in pediatric physical therapy. *Phys. Ther.* **2001**, *9*, 39–51.
2. Jackman, M.; Sakzewski, L.; Morgan, C.; Boyd, R.N.; Brennan, S.E.; Langdon, K.; Toovey, R.A.M.; Greaves, S.; Thorley, M.; Novak, I. Interventions to improve physical function for children and young people with cerebral palsy: International clinical practice guideline. *Dev. Med. Child Neurol.* **2021**, *64*, 536–549. [CrossRef] [PubMed]
3. Jackman, M.; Lannin, N.; Galea, C.; Sakzewski, L.; Miller, L.; Novak, I. What is the threshold dose of upper limb training for children with cerebral palsy to improve function? A systematic review. *Aust. Occup. Ther. J.* **2020**, *67*, 269–280. [CrossRef] [PubMed]
4. Hoare, B.; Wallen, M.A.; Thorley, M.N.; Jackman, M.L.; Carey, L.M.; Imms, C. Constraint-induced movement therapy in children with unilateral cerebral palsy. *Cochrane Database Syst. Rev.* **2019**, *4*, CD004149. [CrossRef]
5. Novak, I.; McIntyre, S.; Morgan, C.; Campbell, L.; Dark, L.; Morton, N.; Stumbles, E.; Wilson, S.-A.; Goldsmith, S. A systematic review of interventions for children with cerebral palsy: State of the evidence. *Dev. Med. Child Neurol.* **2013**, *55*, 885–910. [CrossRef] [PubMed]
6. Novak, I.; Honan, I. Effectiveness of paediatric occupational therapy for children with disabilities: A systematic review. *Aust. Occup. Ther. J.* **2019**, *66*, 258–273. [CrossRef]
7. Ramey, S.L.; DeLuca, S.C. Pediatric CIMT: History and definition. In *Handbook of Pediatric Constraint-Induced Movement Therapy (CIMT): A Guide for Occupational Therapy and Health Care Clinicians, Researchers, and Educators*; Ramey, S.L., Coker-Bolt, P., DeLuca, S.C., Eds.; AOTA Press: Bethesda, MD, USA, 2013; pp. 19–40.
8. Ramey, S.L.; DeLuca, S.C.; Coker-Bolt, P. Operationalizing pediatric CIMT: Guidelines for transforming basic principles and scientific evidence into clinical practice for individual children. In *Handbook of Pediatric Constraint-Induced Movement Therapy (CIMT): A Guide for Occupational Therapy and Health Care Clinicians, Researchers, and Educators*; Ramey, S.L., Coker-Bolt, P., DeLuca, S.C., Eds.; AOTA Press: Bethesda, MD, USA, 2013; pp. 115–128.
9. Hoare, B.; Eliasson, A.C. Evidence to practice commentary: Upper limb constraint in infants: Important perspectives on measurement and the potential for activity-dependent withdrawal of corticospinal projections. *Phys. Occup. Ther. Pediatr.* **2014**, *34*, 22–25. [CrossRef]
10. Eliasson, A.C.; Krumlinde-Sundholm, L.; Gordon, A.M.; Feys, H.; Klingels, K.; Aarts, P.B.M.; Rameckers, E.; Autti-Rämö, I.; Hoare, B. Guidelines for future research in Constraint-Induced Movement Therapy for children with unilateral cerebral palsy: An expert consensus. *Dev. Med. Child Neurol.* **2014**, *56*, 125–137. [CrossRef]
11. Morgan, C.; Fetters, L.; Adde, L.; Badawi, N.; Bancale, A.; Boyd, R.N.; Chorna, O.; Cioni, G.; Damiano, D.L.; Darrah, J.; et al. Early Intervention for Children Aged 0 to 2 Years with or at high risk of cerebral palsy: International clinical practice guideline based on systematic reviews. *JAMA Pediatr.* **2021**, *175*, 846–858. [CrossRef]
12. Baker, A.P.; Niles, N.P.; Kysh, L.M.; Sargent, B.P. Effect of motor intervention for infants and toddlers with cerebral palsy: A systematic review and meta-analysis. *Pediatr. Phys. Ther.* **2022**, *34*, 297–307. [CrossRef]
13. DeLuca, S.C.; Ramey, S.L.; Trucks, M.R.; Lutenbacher, R.; Wallace, D.A. The ACQUIREc protocol: What we have learned from a decade of delivering a signature form of Pediatric CIMT. In *Handbook of Pediatric Constraint-Induced Movement Therapy: A Guide for Occupational Therapy and Health Care Clinicians, Researchers, and Educators*; Ramey, S.L., Coker-Bolt, P., DeLuca, S.C., Eds.; AOTA Press: Bethesda, MD, USA, 2013; pp. 129–147.
14. DeLuca, S.C.; Echols, K.; Ramey, S.L. *ACQUIREc Therapy: A Training Manual for Effective Application of Pediatric Constraint-Induced Movement Therapy*; Mindnurture: Karnal, India, 2007.
15. Gordon, A.M.; Hung, Y.-C.; Brandao, M.; Ferre, C.L.; Kuo, H.-C.; Friel, K.; Petra, E.; Chinnan, A.; Charles, J.R. Bimanual training and constraint-induced movement therapy in children with hemiplegic cerebral palsy: A randomized trial. *Neurorehabilit. Neural Repair* **2011**, *25*, 692–702. [CrossRef] [PubMed]
16. Reynolds, G.S. *A Primer of Operant Conditioning*, Rev. ed.; Scott, Foresman: Northbrook, IL, USA, 1975; p. 155.
17. Kelleher, R.T.; Gollub, L.R. A review of positive conditioned reinforcement. *J. Exp. Anal. Behav.* **1962**, *5* (Suppl. S4), 543–597. [CrossRef] [PubMed]
18. Ramey, C.T.; Hieger, L.; Klisz, D. Synchronous reinforcement of vocal responses in failure-to-thrive infants. *Child Dev.* **1972**, *43*, 1449–1455. [CrossRef] [PubMed]
19. Ramey, C.T.; Ourth, L.L. Delayed reinforcement and vocalization rates of infants. *Child Dev.* **1971**, *42*, 291–297. [CrossRef] [PubMed]
20. Ramey, C.T.; Watson, J.S. Nonsocial reinforcement of infants' vocalizations. *Dev. Psychol.* **1972**, *6*, 538. [CrossRef]
21. Skinner, B.F. Contingencies of reinforcement in the design of a culture. *Syst. Res. Behav. Sci.* **1966**, *11*, 159–166. [CrossRef]
22. Skinner, B.F. *The Technology of Teaching*; Appleton-Century-Crofts: Coopersburg, PA, USA, 1968.
23. Skinner, B.F. What is the experimental analysis of behavior? *J. Exp. Anal. Behav.* **1966**, *9*, 213–218. [CrossRef]
24. Hoare, B.; Greaves, S. Unimanual versus bimanual therapy in children with unilateral cerebral palsy: Same, same, but different. *J. Pediatr. Rehabilitation Med.* **2017**, *10*, 47–59. [CrossRef]
25. Ramey, S.L.; DeLuca, S.C.; Stevenson, R.D.; Conaway, M.; Darragh, A.R.; Lo, W.; CHAMP. Constraint-Induced Movement Therapy for cerebral palsy: A Randomized Trial. *Pediatrics* **2021**, *148*, e2020033878. [CrossRef]

26. Krumlinde-Sundholm, L.; Holmefur, M.; Kottorp, A.; Eliasson, A.C. The Assisting Hand Assessment: Current evidence of validity, reliability, and responsiveness to change. *Dev. Med. Child Neurol.* **2007**, *49*, 259–264. [CrossRef] [PubMed]
27. Ramey, S.L.; DeLuca, S.; Stevenson, R.D.; Case-Smith, J.; Darragh, A.; Conaway, M. Children with Hemiparesis Arm and Movement Project (CHAMP): Protocol for a multisite comparative efficacy trial of paediatric constraint-induced movement therapy (CIMT) testing effects of dosage and type of constraint for children with hemiparetic cerebral palsy. *BMJ Open* **2019**, *9*, e023285. [CrossRef]
28. Taub, E.; Ramey, S.L.; DeLuca, S.; Echols, K. Efficacy of Constraint-Induced Movement Therapy for children with cerebral palsy with asymmetric motor impairment. *Pediatrics* **2004**, *113*, 305–312. [CrossRef] [PubMed]
29. DeLuca, S.C.; Case-Smith, J.; Stevenson, R.; Ramey, S.L. Constraint-induced movement therapy (CIMT) for young children with cerebral palsy: Effects of therapeutic dosage. *J. Pediatr. Rehabil. Med.* **2012**, *5*, 133–142. [CrossRef] [PubMed]

Disclaimer/Publisher's Note: The statements, opinions and data contained in all publications are solely those of the individual author(s) and contributor(s) and not of MDPI and/or the editor(s). MDPI and/or the editor(s) disclaim responsibility for any injury to people or property resulting from any ideas, methods, instructions or products referred to in the content.

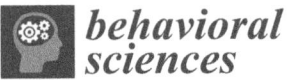

Article

Powered Mobility Device Use and Developmental Change of Young Children with Cerebral Palsy

Samuel W. Logan [1,*], Bethany M. Sloane [1], Lisa K. Kenyon [2] and Heather A. Feldner [3]

1. College of Health, Oregon State University, Corvallis, OR 97331, USA; sloaneb@oregonstate.edu
2. Department of Physical Therapy, Grand Valley State University, Grand Rapids, MI 49504, USA; kenyonli@gvsu.edu
3. Department of Rehabilitation Medicine, University of Washington, Seattle, WA 98195, USA; hfeldner@uw.edu
* Correspondence: sam.logan@oregonstate.edu

Abstract: Mobility is a fundamental human right and is supported by the United Nations and the ON Time Mobility framework. The purpose of this study was to understand the effect of a powered mobility intervention on developmental changes of children with cerebral palsy (CP). This study was a randomized, crossover clinical trial involving 24 children (12–36 months) diagnosed with CP or with high probability of future CP diagnosis based on birth history and current developmental status. Children received the Explorer Mini and a modified ride-on car in randomized order, each for 8 weeks. The Bayley Scales of Infant and Toddler Development—4th Edition was administered at baseline, mid-study, and end-of-study. Raw change scores were used for analysis. Total minutes of use per device was categorized as low or high use for analysis based on caregiver-reported driving diaries. Explorer Mini: The high use group exhibited significantly greater positive change scores compared to the low use group on receptive communication, expressive communication, and gross motor subscales ($p < 0.05$). Modified ride-on car: No significant differences between low and high use groups. Regardless of device, low use was associated with no significant developmental change and high use was associated with positive developmental changes. Mobility access is critical to maximize the development of children with CP and may be augmented by using powered mobility devices. Results may have implications for the development of evidence-based guidelines on dosage for powered mobility use.

Keywords: cerebral palsy; disability; mobility; technology

1. Introduction

Mobility is a fundamental human right [1,2]. The United Nations supports this position of mobility equity as outlined in the Conventions on the Rights of Persons with Disabilities and the Rights of Children [3,4]. The ON Time Mobility framework further outlines children's right to explore the environment, develop social relationships, and serve as active participants in co-creating experiences in their daily lives [2]. Mobility access is critical to maximize the development of children with neuromotor disabilities, including cerebral palsy (CP). Mobility may include traditional motor skill intervention as well as use of powered mobility devices such as motorized wheelchairs, modified ride-on cars, and the Explorer Mini, a mobility device designed specifically for toddlers.

Young children with CP demonstrate positive outcomes in mobility, development, and participation following a powered mobility intervention with a motorized wheelchair [5–7]. For example, young children with CP who used powered mobility devices exhibited increased mobility skills and independence [5,6,8,9], parent perceptions of social skills [6,10], receptive communication and self-care skills [7], sleep–wake patterns [10], and participation [11]. Children as young as 7 months old who have a range of motor abilities, including complex disabilities, have demonstrated successful engagement with powered mobility [7,12].

Despite these positive outcomes, there remain challenges to widespread adoption of powered mobility use, including child-related reasons such as perceived readiness based on age [13], cognitive, physical, or behavioral factors [14], and family or environment-related reasons such as lack of support, ability to transport the device, and home environment [14]. Another challenge includes caregiver perceptions that powered mobility use will interfere with their child's motor development [11]. However, results of a randomized controlled trial suggest no significant differences in fine or gross motor skill between a powered mobility intervention group and a control group [7]. The ON Time Mobility framework does not provide readiness criteria for children to meet prior to consideration of powered mobility use but rather embraces a mobility rights perspective to advocate for multimodal access to mobility in many forms based on each child's complex needs and environmental conditions [2]. Current recommendations indicate that powered mobility may be considered for children with disabilities as a means to explore mobility at ages and stages similar to their peers without disabilities, regardless of whether this is temporary, concurrent with gross motor skill intervention or as an anticipated long-term mobility solution [15].

Modified ride-on cars are an additional powered mobility option for young children with CP. Modified ride-on car use in young children with disabilities, including CP, is a feasible powered mobility option in home, hospital, and school settings and has been associated with positive activity and participation outcomes [16]. Modified ride-on cars include adaptation of commercially available, off-the-shelf, battery-operated toy cars. Modified ride-on cars can be adapted through installation of a large and easy to press activation switch on the steering wheel and customized seating support created from low-cost and readily available materials. The adapted switch usually includes an "all-or-nothing" activation mechanism where, once a child presses the switch, the car is turned on to its maximum speed until the switch is released, though, in some cases, potentiometers are also integrated to provide families with the ability to adjust speed. The total cost is about $200 for a modified ride-on car and modification supplies [17,18]. The do-it-yourself movement of modifying ride-on cars highlights a systemic gap in commercially available mobility technology for pediatric populations.

The Explorer Mini is a Food and Drug Administration cleared 510k medical device for young children 12–36 months old and was commercially released in March 2020. The Explorer Mini is activated with a midline joystick that provides proportional speed control. Other features include its zero-degree turning radius, five speed options, and the ability to be used in either a seated or standing position. A recent study of the Explorer Mini included 33 children 6–35 months old, 12 of which were diagnosed with CP. Results established initial feasibility for young children to successfully use the joystick for mobility and the observation that they appeared to enjoy the experience during a single driving session [19].

The current study extends previous work in three ways. First, this study addresses the potential effect of low and high device use on developmental outcomes in young children diagnosed with CP or with a high probability of future CP diagnosis. Previous intervention studies have examined powered mobility use and the onset of mobility skills [8,9] or generally reported use and developmental change without an interpretation of potential dosage effects [7]. Similarly, modified ride-on car use is highly variable, and, often, low adherence to use recommendations have been reported [16]. There are no studies with the Explorer Mini that report device use beyond a single driving session. Further, Permobil, manufacturer of the Explorer Mini, recently released "A Guideline for Introducing Powered Mobility to Infants and Toddlers." [20]. The guideline acknowledges there are no specific recommendations for dosage of powered mobility use based on a lack of available evidence and the individually variable needs and abilities of many young drivers. Thus, the current study may have implications for the development of evidence-based guidelines for powered mobility use.

Second, this study examines children's individual pathways from device use to developmental outcomes. Previous powered mobility intervention studies have used single-subject and case series designs to provide rich descriptions of behavior and developmental change [16,21]. However, the current study extends this work by using a unique approach of examining a larger sample size to synthesize individual-level data into larger trends that have the potential to impact clinical practice.

Third, our study aims, design, and interpretation of results are grounded in dynamic systems theory (DST) [22]. Regardless of device type, powered mobility intervention research is typically not grounded in theoretical frameworks of motor development. There are three key principles of DST: complexity, continuity in time, and dynamic stability. These principles interact to encourage an individual's path toward a developmental cascade of change over time [22]. Complexity relates to the synergistic and interconnectedness of multiple systems that interact together and are influenced by the convergence of individual, task, and environmental constraints that influence behaviors. In the context of DST, constraints do not refer to limitations or restrictions but are the holistic context of how multiple systems interact to facilitate behaviors. We recognize that child development is complex and may be influenced by children's Gross Motor Function Classification System (GMFCS) level (individual constraint) and the use of the Explorer Mini and modified ride-on car (task constraints) in different family, home, neighborhood, and community spaces that present varying real-world situations of powered mobility use (environmental constraints). Continuity in time recognizes that change in functioning is dependent on the past, which influences the path toward future levels of functioning. Our study acknowledges continuity through examining children's individual pathways of developmental change, thereby recognizing that each child is likely to experience their own unique trajectory dependent upon their previous developmental past. Dynamic stability regards behaviors as stable and flexible to varying degrees, depending upon the behavior and state of the system at a given point in time. Our study embraces that dynamic stability of developmental change may be influenced by the frequency of powered mobility device use between assessments of developmental domains.

The purpose of this study was to examine the effect of powered mobility use on the developmental changes of young children (12–36 months) diagnosed with CP or with a high likelihood of future CP diagnosis following separate 8-week use periods for the Explorer Mini and modified ride-on car. Children between 12 and 36 months of age were the focus of this study because early childhood is a critical developmental time and provision of powered mobility is not standard of practice at this age [13,14] despite previous positive research findings [7–10,12,16]. Therefore, the overall objective was to understand the effect of a powered mobility intervention on developmental changes. In the United States, there was no commercially available powered mobility device for children under 3 years of age until the Explorer Mini was released in 2020. Prior to the Explorer Mini, modified ride-on cars were popularized as a do-it-yourself powered mobility option for young children. Both devices were chosen for the current study because of their use for children 12–36 months as a powered mobility device for this population. In addition, there are cost and access differences between the devices. The Explorer Mini costs $2944 and requires a physician's prescription for access. In contrast, a modified ride-on car costs $200–$400 and requires minimal technical skills for access. These factors contributed to the use of a randomized, crossover study design that included children using each device during an intervention period.

There were two aims of the current study. Aim 1: Compare the relationship between device use frequency (low and high use) of each device to change scores of Bayley-4 subscales (e.g., cognitive, receptive communication, expressive communication, fine motor, and gross motor). H1: *We hypothesized that change scores across all Bayley-4 subscales would be higher for the high use group compared to the low use group for both devices.* Aim 2: Describe children's individual pathways of developmental change on Bayley-4 subscales considering device use and GMFCS levels. H2: *We hypothesized that high use would be associated with positive developmental changes for both devices.* H3: *We also hypothesized that low use would be associated with no developmental changes.* H4: *Lastly, we hypothesized that children classified* at GMFCS Levels I, II, and III would exhibit more pathways to positive developmental change compared to children classified at GMFCS Levels IV and V.

2. Materials and Method

This study was a randomized, crossover, multi-site clinical trial, and children received the Explorer Mini or a modified ride-on car in a randomized order, each for 8 weeks. There was no wash out period between devices since both devices are intended to support self-initiated mobility. This study is part of a larger study. Please see [23] for a published protocol with full methodological details.

2.1. Participants

Recruitment of potential participants was conducted through local physical, occupational, and early intervention agencies and clinics at each site (Washington, Oregon, and Michigan). Twenty-four children between 12 and 36 months of age diagnosed with CP or with high probability of future CP diagnosis based on birth history or current developmental status were included in this study. A high probability of future CP diagnosis was confirmed through caregiver report based on birth history or current developmental status, demonstrated delays of the onset of mobility, and receipt of therapeutic services. One family did not return the caregiver-reported driving diary about device use and were excluded from analysis, resulting in a final sample of 23 children for the current study. See Table 1 for demographic information.

Table 1. Demographic information for participants and individual device use data.

			Device Use (Mins)	
ID	Age	GMFCS Level	Explorer Mini	Modified Ride-On Car
2	17 months	V	182	203
3	2 years	II	435	95
4	19 months	V	374	370
5	18 months	V	1185	526
6	2 years and 4 months	II	980	923
7	21 months	III	165	15
8	2 years and 5 months	III	563	48
10	15 months	V	505	86
11	17 months	II	177	99
12	15 months	IV	335	0
13	2 years and 6 months	V	35	60
14	12 months	IV	330	200
15	2 years and 5 months	III	1270	547
16	21 months	I	17	92
17	2 years and 7 months	V	165	30
18	20 months	V	206	0
19	2 years and 5 months	IV	613	0
20	23 months	IV	613	529
21	23 months	V	217	571
22	16 months	IV	1105	119
23	2 years 8 months	V	823	96
24	12 months	II	1110	230
25	18 months	II	547	165

2.2. Description of Devices

Explorer Mini. The Explorer Mini is commercially available and Food and Drug Administration cleared 510k medical device intended for use of children 12–36 months of age. The Explorer Mini includes a rechargeable, 12-volt battery, maximum speed of 1.5 mph, a 0-inch turning radius, five speed options, can be driven in sitting or standing positions, 35 lbs. weight limit, and is activated and steered through an omni-directional and proportional controlled joystick. See Figure 1.

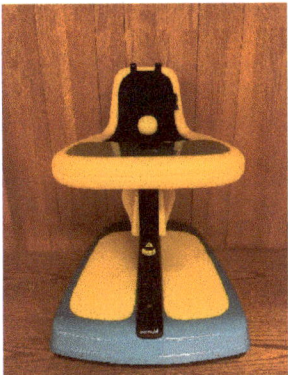

Figure 1. Photograph of the Explorer Mini.

Modified ride-on car. The Fisher Price Cars 3 Lil' Lightning McQueen is commercially available and intended for use of children 12–36 months. The McQueen includes a rechargeable, 6-volt battery, maximum speed of 2 mph, a 37.5 inch turning radius, one speed option, can be used in the sitting position only, 40 lbs. weight limit, steered via a handheld steering wheel, and activated through an all-or-nothing switch pressed via a finger or thumb located on the steering wheel. Modifications included (a) replacing the small switch with an all-or-nothing adapted switch that is large (5-inch diameter), easy to press, and installed on the steering wheel, (b) the addition of a potentiometer to allow for variable speed control, and (c) customized and individual seating support based on each child's positioning needs. See Figure 2.

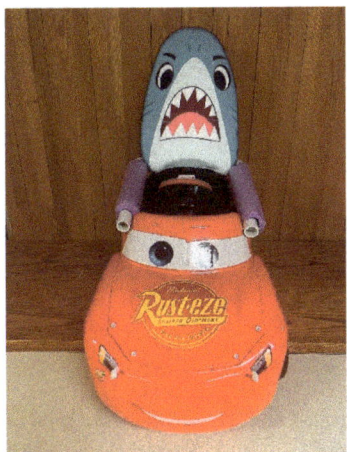

Figure 2. Photograph of the modified ride-on car.

2.3. Dependent Variables

Device use. Caregivers reported device use as minutes per driving session in a caregiver-reported driving diary. Several modified ride-on car studies recommended to families at least 20–30 min per day for 5 days per week of device use; however, actual device use is often low and highly variable [16]. Families in the current study were encouraged to incorporate the devices into their everyday routines and participated in two standardized check-in periods per device to encourage driving and identify/remove potential driving barriers; however, they were not provided specified device use recommendations. We created definitions of low and high use based on our research, clinical experience, and previous literature [16,24]. Low use was defined as 480 min or less across an 8-week period. This is equivalent to an average of 20 min per day for 3 days per week (i.e., 1 h per week or less, which is similar to dosage of early intervention services) [24]. High use was defined as 481 min or more across an 8-week period. Low and high use groups were used for data analysis.

2.4. Bayley Scales of Infant and Toddler Development—4th Edition (Bayley-4) [25]

The Bayley-4 is a norm-referenced standardized measure that was validated with a sample of children mostly without disabilities. Scaled and raw scores may be used to identify change over time, but scaled scores must be used to compare a child's performance to their age-matched peers. However, in a heterogenous sample of children with disabilities, even in the presence of significant change in raw scores, scaled scores may remain steady or decline/decrease due to the inherent comparison against age-matched peers. Raw scores were used to calculate change scores for each subscale between each period of device use because of the sample and relatively short intervals between assessment (8 weeks). Raw scores and change scores more accurately reflect the presence or absence of change in our participants who served as their own controls, which considers our population (i.e., CP) heterogeneity. Further, caregivers reported that 14 of the 23 children (~61%) functioned at GMFCS Levels IV or V. These children are expected to develop at a decreased rate compared to other GMFCS levels, or compared to children with typical development who were the basis for the norm referenced scaled and standard scores in the Bayley-4 manual.

The Bayley-4 was administered at T0 (prior to any device use), T1 (after 8 weeks of first device use), and T2 (after 8 weeks of second device use) and included assessment of the cognitive, receptive communication, expressive communication, fine motor, and gross motor subscales. Change scores were calculated by subtracting the raw score at one time point from the raw score at another timepoint for each individual child. The percentage of change was calculated by dividing the change score by the raw score at first timepoint $\times 100$. For example, a raw score of 57 at T0 and 70 at T1 would result in a change score of 13 (70−57), which represents 23% positive change ($13/57 = 0.2280 \times 100 = 23\%$). The magnitude of the percentage of change was defined as follows: stable (+/−9% or less), small change (+/−10–19%), moderate change (+/−20–29%), or large change (+/−30% or more). We used a conservative approach informed by our collective research and clinical experience to define magnitudes of percentage of change. The context of social validity, including the importance of the treatment effect, guided the classification of magnitudes [26,27]. Similar to a previous powered mobility study, the lowest level of change determined as meaningful was defined as at least 10% because this level of change may inform intervention planning [28].

2.5. Data Analysis

Aim 1: Compare the relationship between device use frequency (low and high use) of each device to change scores of Bayley-4 subscales. Non-parametric tests were used due to small sample size of groups and the violation of the assumption of normality (Shapiro–Wilk test; $p < 0.05$) for the receptive communication and gross motor change scores. The Mann–Whitney U test was used to compare two independent groups (low vs high use) on Bayley-4 change scores. Separate tests were conducted across Bayley-4 subscales (cognitive, receptive communication, expressive communication, fine motor, and gross motor) and across devices (Explorer Mini; modified ride-on car).

Aim 2: Describe children's individual pathways of developmental change on Bayley-4 subscales considering device use and GMFCS levels. Visual analysis was used to narratively describe trends through a series of figures. Figures are presented that include children's individual pathways of percentage change (stable, small, moderate, large) across Bayley-4 subscales (cognitive, receptive communication, expressive communication, fine motor, and gross motor), devices (Explorer Mini; modified ride-on car), use levels (low use; high use), and GMFCS Levels (I–III; IV–V).

3. Results

Aim 1: See Table 2 for descriptive information about device use. **Explorer Mini.** Expressive communication change scores of the high use group (Mdn = 4) were higher than those of the low use group (Mdn = 1.5). A Mann–Whitney U test indicated that this difference was statistically significant, $U(N_{high\ use} = 11, N_{low\ use} = 12) = 32.00, z = -2.1, p = 0.037$. Receptive communication change scores of the high use group (Mdn = 4) were higher than those of the low use group (Mdn = 0). A Mann–Whitney U test indicated that this difference was statistically significant, $U(N_{high\ use} = 11, N_{low\ use} = 12) = 15.50, z = -3.1, p < 0.001$. Gross motor change scores of the high use group (Mdn = 5) were higher than those of the low use group (Mdn = −0.5). A Mann–Whitney U test indicated that this difference was statistically significant, $U(N_{high\ use} = 11, N_{low\ use} = 12) = 32.00, z = -2.1, p = 0.037$. **Modified ride-on car.** No significant differences in change scores resulted between low and high use groups.

Table 2. Summary information about device use.

	Explorer Mini		Modified Ride-On Car	
	Minutes of Use		Minutes of Use	
	Low Use (*n* = 12)	High Use (*n* = 11)	Low Use (*n* = 18)	High Use (*n* = 5)
Min	17	505	0	526
Max	435	1270	370	923
Median	193.8	823	93.5	538
Mean	219.8	846.7	106.4	631.3
Standard Deviation	128	290.6	96.9	194.7

Aim 2: A narrative description is provided for children's individual pathways of developmental change on Bayley-4 subscale scores. See Figures 3–7.

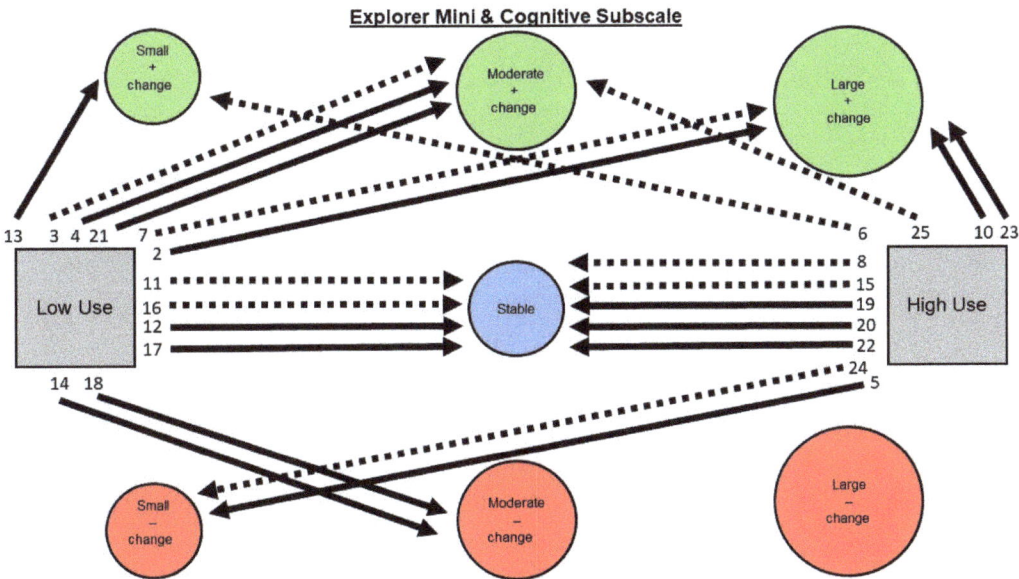

Figure 3. *Cont.*

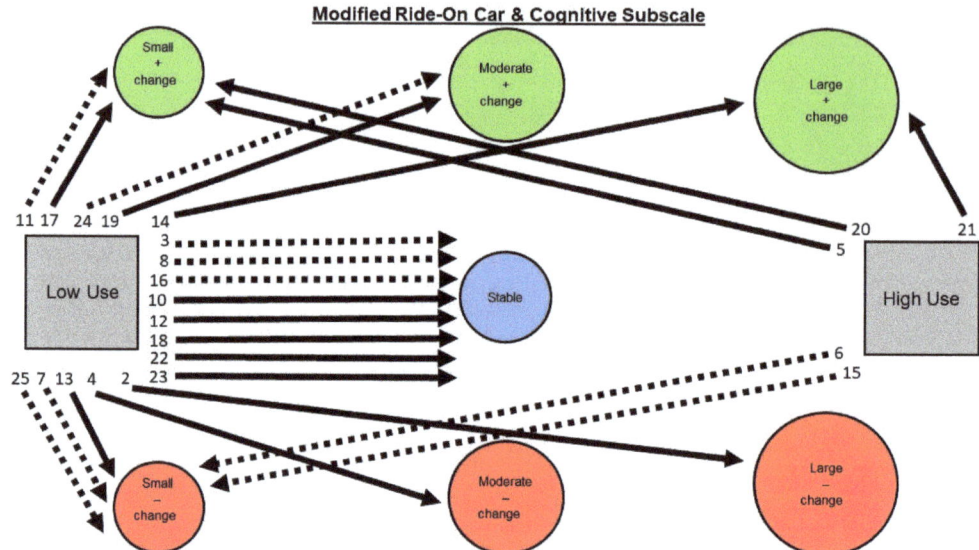

Figure 3. Pathways for each child from Explorer Mini (**top**) and modified ride-on car (**bottom**) low and high use groups to developmental change on the cognitive subscale of the Bayley-4. Low use was defined as 480 min or less across an 8-week period. High use was defined as 481 min or more across an 8-week period. The magnitude of the percentage of change for Bayley-4 subscales was defined as follows: stable (+/−9% or less), small change (+/−10–19%), moderate change (+/−20–29%), or large change (+/−30% or more). The #s indicate participant ID. Bolded lines represent children GMFCS Levels IV or V. Dashed lines represent children GMFCS Levels I, II, or III.

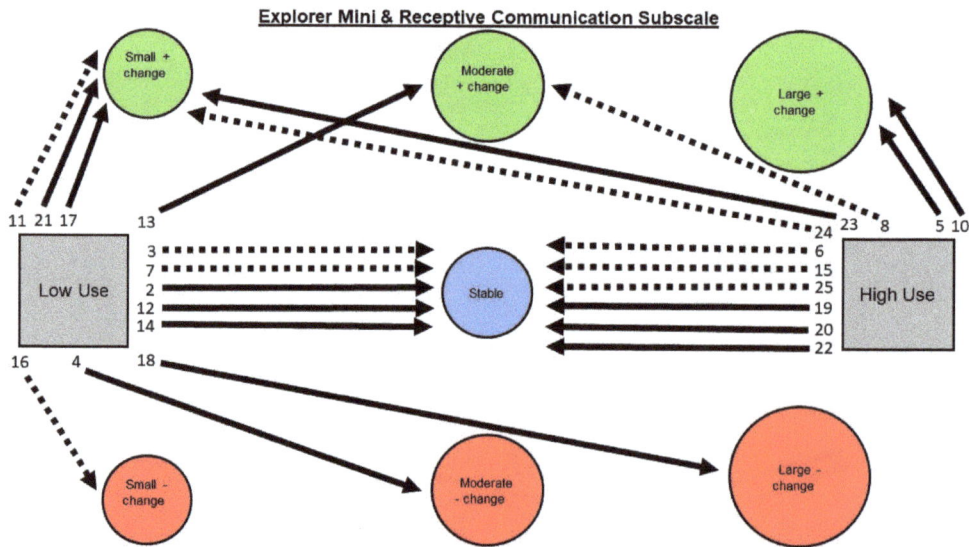

Figure 4. *Cont.*

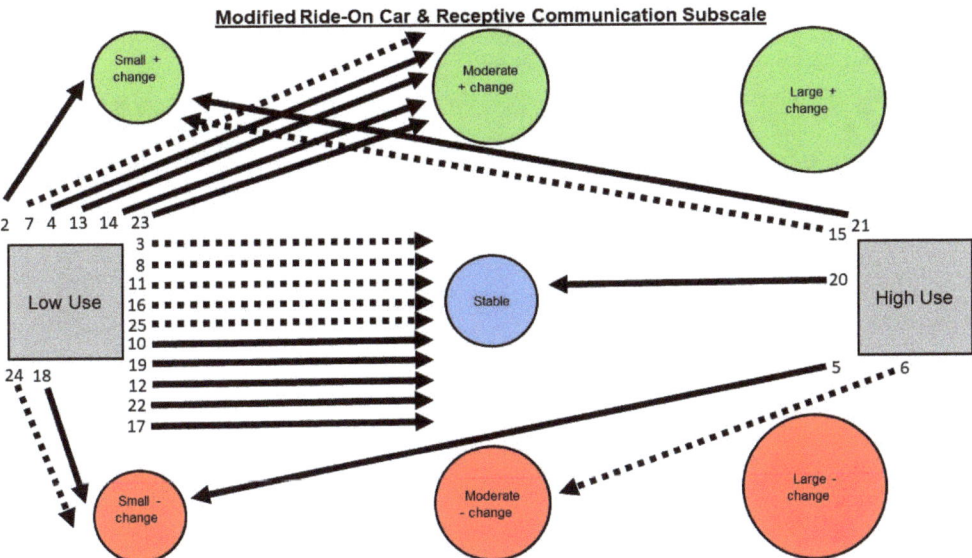

Figure 4. Pathways for each child from Explorer Mini (**top**) and modified ride-on car (**bottom**) low and high use groups to developmental change on the receptive communication subscale of the Bayley-4.

Cognitive subscale. Explorer Mini: Low use (n = 12; 52%). Children exhibited five of seven possible individual pathways from low use to developmental change. The most common pathway was low use to positive change (n = 6; 50%), including small (n = 1), moderate (n = 3), and large (n = 2). The next most common pathway was low use to stable (n = 4; 33%). The least common pathway was low use to negative change (n = 2; 17%), including small (n = 0), moderate (n = 2), and large (n = 0). Children with GMFCS I–III and IV–V appeared to show similar patterns. **High use (n = 11; 48%).** Children exhibited five of seven possible individual pathways from high use to developmental change. The most common pathway was high use to stable (n = 5; 46%). The next most common pathway was high use to positive change (n = 4; 36%), including small (n = 1), moderate (n = 1), and large (n = 2). The least common pathway was high use to negative change (n = 2; 18%), including small (n = 2). Children with GMFCS I–III and IV–V appeared to show similar patterns.

Modified ride-on car: Low use (n = 18; 78%). Children exhibited seven of seven possible individual pathways from low use to developmental change. The most common pathway was low use to stable (n = 8; 44%). The remaining two pathways were equal in commonality, including low use to negative change (n = 5; 28%), including small (n = 3), moderate (n = 1), and large (n = 1); and positive change (n = 5; 28%), including small (n = 2), moderate (n = 2), and large (n = 1). Children with GMFCS I–III and IV–V appeared to show similar patterns. **High use (n = 5; 22%).** Children exhibited three of seven possible individual pathways from high use to developmental change. The most common pathway was high use to positive change (n = 3; 60%), including small (n = 2) and large (n = 1). The next most common pathway was high use to negative change (n = 2; 40%), including small (n = 2). The least common pathway was high use to stable (n = 0; 0%). Children with GFMCS I–III all showed negative change while all children with GMFCS IV–V showed positive change.

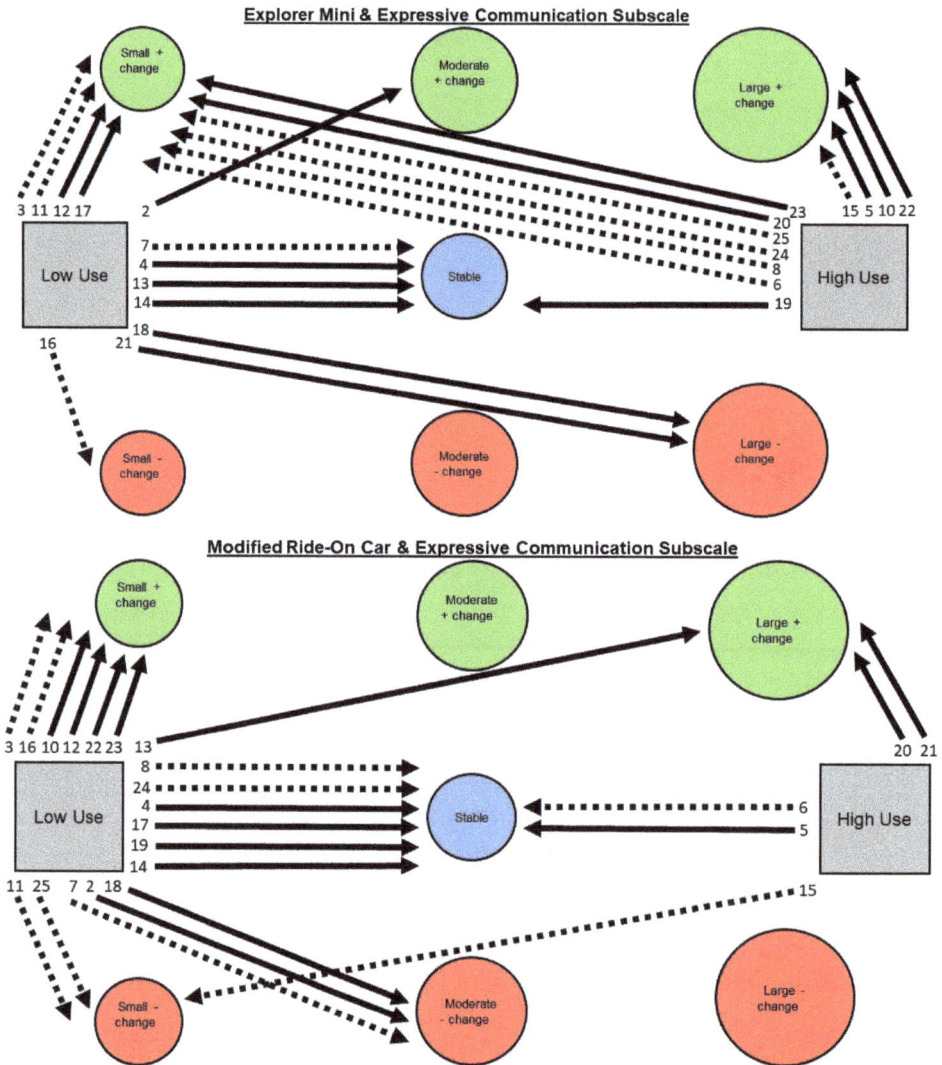

Figure 5. Pathways for each child from Explorer Mini (**top**) and modified ride-on car (**bottom**) low and high use groups to developmental change on the expressive communication subscale of the Bayley-4.

Receptive subscale. Explorer Mini: Low use (*n* = 12; 52%). Children exhibited six of seven possible individual pathways from low use to developmental change. The most common pathway was low use to stable (*n* = 5; 42%). The next most common pathway was low use to positive change (*n* = 4; 33%), including small (*n* = 3) and moderate (*n* = 1). The least common pathway was low use to negative change (*n* = 3; 25%), including small (*n* = 1), moderate (*n* = 1), and large (*n* = 1). Children with GMFCS I–III and IV–V appeared to show similar patterns. **High use (*n* = 11; 48%).** Children exhibited four of seven possible individual pathways from high use to developmental change. The most common pathway was high use to stable (*n* = 6; 66%). The next most common pathway was high use to positive change (*n* = 5; 46%), including small (*n* = 2), moderate (*n* = 1), and large (*n* = 2).

The least common pathway was high use to negative change (*n* = 0; 0%). Children with GMFCS I–III and IV–V appeared to show similar patterns.

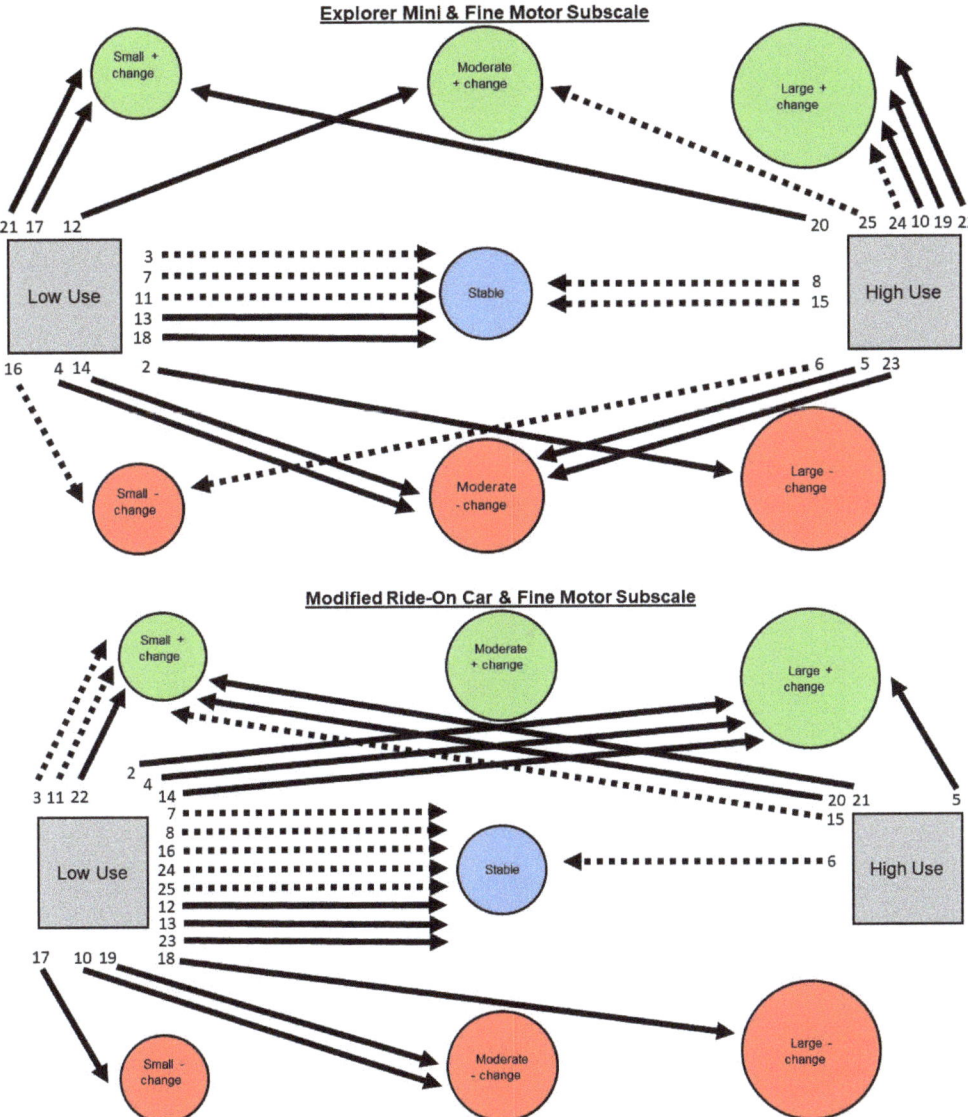

Figure 6. Pathways for each child from Explorer Mini (**top**) and modified ride-on car (**bottom**) low and high use groups to developmental change on the fine motor subscale of the Bayley-4.

Modified ride-on car: Low use (*n* = 18; 78%). Children exhibited four of seven possible individual pathways from low use to developmental change. The most common pathway was low use to stable (*n* = 10; 56%). The next most common pathway was low use to positive change (*n* = 6; 33%), including small (*n* = 1) and moderate (*n* = 5). The least common pathway was low use to negative change (*n* = 2; 11%), including small (*n* = 2). Children with GMFCS IV–V appeared to show more positive changes compared to GMFCS I–III. **High use (*n* = 5; 22%).** Children exhibited four of seven possible individual pathways from high use to developmental change. There were two most common pathways: high use to positive change (*n* = 2; 40%), including small (*n* = 2); and high use to negative change (*n* = 2; 40%), including small (*n* = 1) and moderate (*n* = 1). The least common pathway was high use to stable (*n* = 1; 20%). Children with GMFCS I–III and IV–V appeared to show similar patterns.

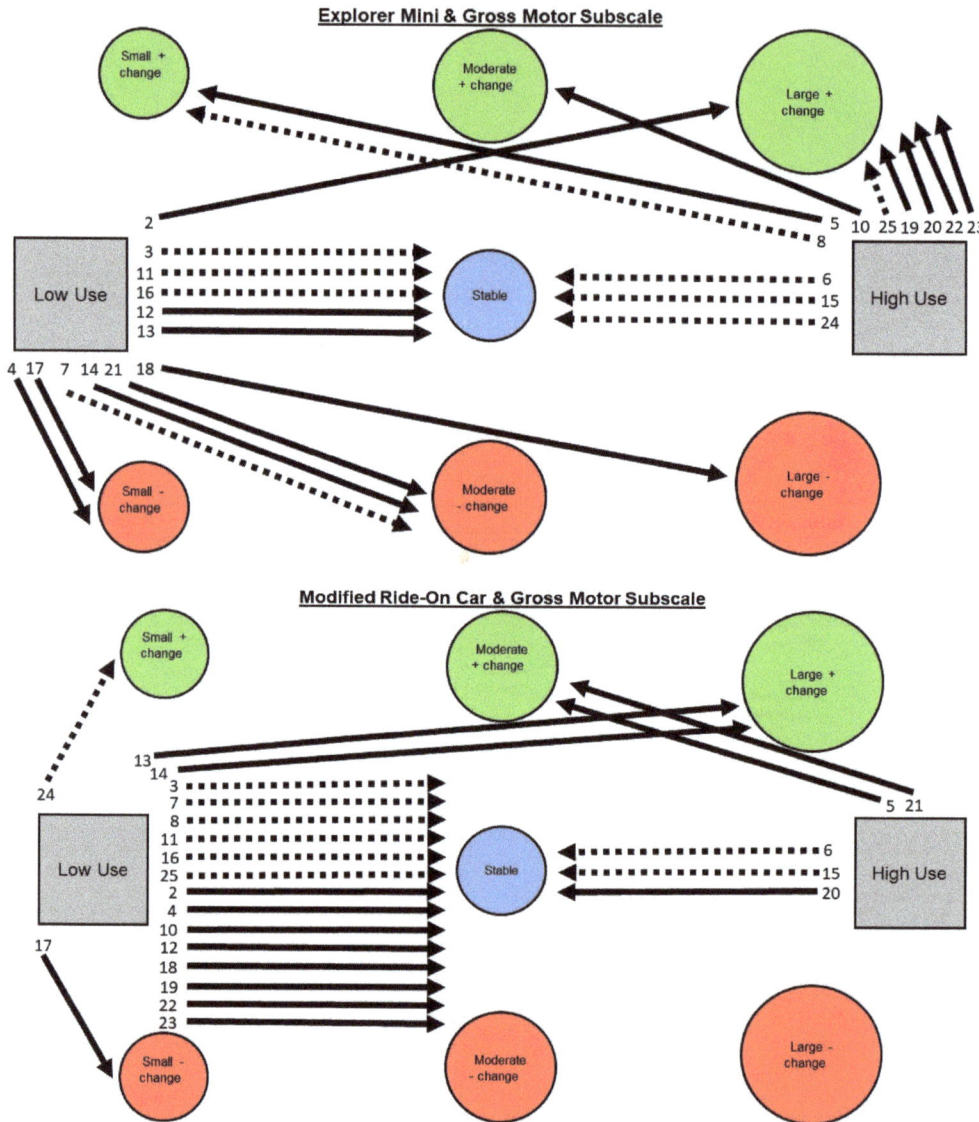

Figure 7. Pathways for each child from Explorer Mini (**top**) and modified ride-on car (**bottom**) low and high use groups to developmental change on the gross motor subscale of the Bayley-4.

Expressive subscale. Explorer Mini: Low use (*n* = 12; 52%). Children exhibited five of seven possible individual pathways from low use to developmental change. The most common pathway was low use to positive change (*n* = 5; 42%), including small (*n* = 4) and moderate (*n* = 1). The next most common pathway was low use to stable (*n* = 4; 33%). The least common pathway was low use to negative change (*n* = 3; 25%), including small (*n* = 1) and large (*n* = 2). Children with GMFCS I–III and IV–V appeared to show similar patterns. **High use (*n* = 11; 48%).** Children exhibited three of seven possible individual pathways from high use to developmental change. The most common pathway was high use to positive change (*n* = 10; 91%), including small (*n* = 6) and large (*n* = 4). The next most common pathway was high use to stable (*n* = 1; 9%). The least common pathway was high use to negative change (*n* = 0; 0%). Children with GMFCS I–III and IV–V appeared to show similar patterns.

Modified ride-on car: Low use (*n* = 18; 78%). Children exhibited five of seven possible individual pathways from low use to developmental change. The most common pathway was low use to positive change (*n* = 7; 39%), including small (*n* = 6) and large (*n* = 1). The next most common pathway was low use to stable (*n* = 6; 33%). The least common pathway was low use to negative change (*n* = 5; 28%), including small (*n* = 2) and moderate (*n* = 3). Children with GMFCS I–III and IV–V appeared to show similar patterns. **High use (*n* = 5; 22%).** Children exhibited three of seven possible individual pathways from high use to developmental change. There were two most common pathways: high use to positive change (*n* = 2; 40%), including large (*n* = 2); and high use to stable (*n* = 2; 40%). The least common pathway was from high use to negative change, including small (*n* = 1; 20%). Children with GMFCS I–III and IV–V appeared to show similar patterns.

Fine motor subscale. Explorer Mini: Low use (*n* = 12; 52%). Children exhibited six of seven possible individual pathways from low use to developmental change. The most common pathway was low use to stable (*n* = 5; 42%). The next most common pathway was low use to negative change (*n* = 4; 33%), including small (*n* = 1), moderate (*n* = 2), and large (*n* = 1). The least common pathway was low use to positive change (*n* = 3; 25%), including small (*n* = 2) and moderate (*n* = 1). Children with GMFCS IV–V showed positive, stable, and negative change, while children with GMFCS I–III showed only stable or negative change. **High use (*n* = 11; 48%).** Children exhibited six of seven possible individual pathways from high use to developmental change. The most common pathway was high use to positive change (*n* = 6; 55%), including small (*n* = 1), moderate (*n* = 1), and large (*n* = 4). The next most common pathway was high use to negative change (*n* = 3; 27%), including small (*n* = 1) and moderate (*n* = 2). The least common pathway was high use to stable (*n* = 2; 18%). Children with GMFCS I–III and IV–V appeared to show similar patterns.

Modified ride-on car: Low use (*n* = 18; 78%). Children exhibited six of seven possible individual pathways from low use to developmental change. The most common pathway was low use to stable (*n* = 8; 44%). The next most common pathway was low use to positive change (*n* = 6; 33%), including small (*n* = 3) and large (*n* = 3). The least common pathway was low use to negative change (*n* = 4; 22%), including small (*n* = 1), moderate (*n* = 2), and large (*n* = 1). Children with GMFCS IV–V showed positive, stable, and negative change, while children with GMFCS I–III showed only stable or positive change. **High use (*n* = 5; 22%).** Children exhibited 3 of 7 possible individual pathways from high use to developmental change. The most common pathway was high use to positive change (*n* = 4; 80%), including small (*n* = 3) and large (*n* = 1). The next most common pathway was high use to stable (*n* = 1; 20%). The least common pathway was from high use to negative change (*n* = 0; 0%). Children with GMFCS I–III and IV–V appeared to show similar patterns.

Gross motor subscale. Explorer Mini: Low use (*n* = 12; 52%). Children exhibited five of seven possible individual pathways from low use to developmental change. The most common pathway was low use to negative change (*n* = 6; 50%), including small (*n* = 2), moderate (*n* = 3), and large (*n* = 1). The next most common pathway was low use to stable (*n* = 5; 42%). The least common pathway was low use to positive change (*n* = 1; 8%), including large (*n* = 1). Children with GMFCS I–III showed stable pathways compared to children with GMFCS IV–V, who tended to show negative changes. **High use (*n* = 11; 48%).** Children exhibited 4 of 7 possible individual pathways from high use to developmental change. The most common pathway was high use to positive change (*n* = 8; 73%), including small (*n* = 2), moderate (*n* = 1), and large (*n* = 5). The next most common pathway was high use to stable (*n* = 3; 27%). The least common pathway was high use to negative change (*n* = 0; 0%). Children with GMFCS IV–V always showed positive change, while children with GFMCS I–III showed stable pathways and positive change.

Modified ride-on car: Low use (*n* = 18; 78%). Children exhibited four of seven possible individual pathways from low use to developmental change. The most common pathway was low use to stable (*n* = 14; 78%). The next most common pathway was low use to positive change (*n* = 3; 17%), including small (*n* = 1) and large (*n* = 2). The least common pathway was low use to negative change (*n* = 1; 6%), including small (*n* = 1). Children with GMFCS I–III and IV–V appeared to show similar patterns. **High use (*n* = 5; 22%).** Children exhibited two of seven possible individual pathways from high use to developmental change. The most common pathway was high use to stable (*n* = 3; 60%). The next most common pathway was high use to positive change (*n* = 2; 40%), including moderate (*n* = 2). The least common pathway was from high use to negative change (*n* = 0; 0%). Children with GMFCS IV–V showed stable pathways and positive change, while children with GMFCS I–III showed only stable pathways.

Summary of individual pathways across all Bayley-4 domains. See Table 3. Regardless of device, the most common pathway for low use was to stable (*n* = 69; 46%) and for high use to positive change (*n* = 46; 57.5%).

Table 3. Frequency and percentages of paths from low and high use to developmental change for each device on the Bayley-4 (all subscales).

Explorer Mini					
Low Use (*n* = 12; 60 paths)			High Use (*n* = 11; 55 paths)		
(+) Change	Stable	(−) Change	(+) Change	Stable	(−) Change
19 (32%)	**23 (38%)**	18 (30%)	**33 (60%)**	17 (31%)	5 (9%)
Modified Ride-On Car					
Low Use (*n* = 18; 90 paths)			High Use (*n* = 5; 25 paths)		
(+) Change	Stable	(−) Change	(+) Change	Stable	(−) Change
27 (30%)	**46 (51%)**	17 (19%)	**13 (52%)**	7 (28%)	5 (20%)

Explorer Mini: Low use (*n* = 12; 52%). There were 60 pathways recorded from low use to developmental change (positive, stable, negative). The most common pathway was low use to stable (*n* = 23; 38%). **High use (*n* = 11).** There were 55 pathways recorded from high use to developmental change (positive, stable, negative). The most common pathway was high use to positive change (*n* = 33; 60%).

Modified ride-on car: Low use (*n* = 18). There were 90 pathways recorded from low use to developmental change (positive, stable, negative). The most common pathway was low use to stable (*n* = 46; 51%). **High use (*n* = 5).** There were 25 pathways recorded from high use to developmental change (positive, stable, negative). The most common pathway was high use to positive change (*n* = 13; 52%).

4. Discussion

The purpose of this study was to examine the effect of powered mobility use on the developmental changes of young children diagnosed with CP or with a high likelihood of future CP diagnosis. Our first hypothesis was partially supported and stated that change scores across all Bayley-4 subscales would be higher for the high use group compared to the low use group for both devices. Findings indicate that high use of the Explorer Mini resulted in significantly greater change scores compared to low use on receptive communication, expressive communication, and gross motor domains. There were no significant differences between low use and high use of a modified ride-on car.

One potential explanation for our findings is that children's high use of the Explorer Mini may have contributed to new exploratory experiences that resulted in increased, varied, and novel social interactions with caregivers, siblings, and/or others in the environment, which, in turn, facilitated changes in receptive communication and expressive communication. The powered mobility experiences may have motivated children to be more active and mobile outside of the device, contributing to advanced gross motor skills. A substantially higher percentage of children were in the high use group for the Explorer Mini (48%) compared to the modified ride-on car (22%). Further, there was a low percentage of children who were in the high use group for both devices (17%). These results are consistent with previous work that indicates variable duration and frequency of device use during an intervention period [16] that is likely due to several perceived barriers related to the caregiver, child, device, and environment [29,30]. Our study protocol attempted to address these issues through providing families with two standardized check ins during each 8-week period of device use. These check ins included time for the caregiver to ask questions and discuss perceived barriers, and for the research team to provide activity suggestions and facilitating strategies to encourage both device use and children's learning. Future research is warranted to understand the exploratory experiences of young children during powered mobility device use to determine if and how these experiences contribute to developmental change, including communication skills.

Another potential explanation is the caregivers' and children's device preferences. There were 11 families in the high use group of the Explorer Mini. Based on our qualitative data, 8 out of 11 families indicated that both caregiver and child preferred the Explorer Mini compared to the modified ride-on car. It is possible the preference for the Explorer Mini both in quantitative (i.e., use) and qualitative ways influenced the frequency, quality, and type of opportunities children were provided to use the device that contributed to the observed developmental changes.

Lastly, a potential explanation for the findings is related to the functional difference in how the Explorer Mini and modified ride-on car are operated and used to navigate the environment. The Explorer Mini uses a joystick for activation of omni-directional steering, while the modified ride-on car uses an all-or-nothing and single switch for activation that is separate from steering control. In combination with high use, the joystick navigation of the Explorer Mini may have resulted in different mobility experiences that can at least partially explain the findings. To our knowledge, there are no research studies that directly compares children's driving experiences of powered mobility devices that are activated through a single switch versus a joystick within home and community settings, and further research is warranted.

Our second and third hypotheses were supported and stated that, through visual analysis of individual pathways, high use would be associated with positive developmental changes and that low use would be associated with no developmental changes for both devices. The most common pathway from high use was to positive change for the Explorer Mini (60% of pathways) and modified ride-on car (53% of pathways). The most common pathway from low use was to no developmental change (i.e., stable) for the Explorer Mini (38% of pathways) and modified ride-on car (51% of pathways). Despite the common pathways, it is clear that this is not a hard and fast rule, and there are several factors that influence a child's developmental trajectory that align with dynamic systems theory. Bi-directional interactions amongst individual (children's previous developmental history and current GMFCS level), task (device preference and use), and environmental (settings of device use) constraints likely contributed in different ways to development change for each child in the current study. These results align with a classic study in motor development where researchers examined individual pathways in the development of the fundamental motor skill of throwing [31]. They found common pathways, yet there was variability in how the trunk, humerus, and forearm actions coordinate to produce throwing across trials and time. Analyses of different groups are important in research studies, but there is also value in examining individual data to understand the underlying patterns of change.

Our fourth hypothesis was not supported; it stated that, through visual analysis of individual pathways, children classified at GMFCS Levels I, II, and III would exhibit more pathways to positive developmental change compared to children classified at GMFCS

Levels IV and V. On the cognitive subscale, all children at GMFCS Levels I, II, and III showed negative change while all children at GMFCS Levels IV and V showed positive change following modified ride-on car use. On the gross motor subscale, a mix of stable pathways and positive change were demonstrated across GMFCS levels and devices. There were no discernable trends on the receptive communication, expressive communication, and fine motor subscales. These findings were not dependent on high use of devices since there was a similar breakdown of children in the high use group for each device at GMFCS Levels I, II, III and GMFCS Levels IV and IV (45% and 55% respectively for high use of the Explorer Mini; 40% and 60% respectively for high use of a modified ride-on car). These results have important research and clinical applications. Children at GMFCS Levels IV and V are often excluded from powered mobility research trials due to safety and readiness concerns related to limited head, trunk, and limb control. Often, an inclusion or exclusion criteria is related to a child's ability to sit with support as a requirement for study enrollment [19,32]. Our results clearly demonstrate that children at GMFCS Levels IV and V should be included in powered mobility research trials. In the current study, children at GMFCS Levels IV and V demonstrated the most frequent amount of positive change for certain Bayley-4 domains, further highlighting the clinical applicability of powered mobility intervention in this population.

It is important to acknowledge the limitations of the current study. First, our study is statistically powered for its primary aims [23]. However, the study is not statistically powered to examine differences amongst several subgroups such as device use (i.e., high, low), device type (i.e., Explorer Mini, modified ride-on car), and GMFCS Levels (i.e., I, II, II and IV, V). Nonetheless, this study is part of the largest powered mobility clinical trial to date, and the examination of individual pathways of developmental change provides new knowledge. Second, the current study included children from 12 to 36 months of age at the time of enrollment. Although this is a common age range of powered mobility research studies [7,16], it is important to note that any observed effects may have been influenced by an interaction of age, experience, and functional mobility. Third, the classification of low and high use of devices was based on caregiver-reported driving diaries. A recent study compared modified ride-on car use measured through objective tracking or caregiver diaries [32]. There were no significant differences between objective tracking and diaries on average session duration or total driving time. The authors noted that over- or under-reporting of use through diaries may have occurred, but researchers can reasonably expect that caregiver diaries accurately represent their child's device use. The objective tracking used in previous work involves directly integrating hardware components into the electrical system of the modified ride-on car [32]. These components are not compatible with the Explorer Mini. There is a need for further sensor development and integration with powered mobility devices to understand how they are used in home and community spaces. This type of technology is readily available on traditional power chairs for adults, but this remains a salient need in the pediatric population. Fourth, in-depth information about other factors that may have contributed to the observed changes in the current study were not systematically measured and controlled for in analyses, such as the frequency, duration, and specific activities of other therapies received, interactions between caregivers and children during device use, participation in other play-based experiences, or any number of environmental circumstances such as the size and type of house or surrounding built environment of the neighborhood and community. Fifth, differences between the use amounts, device characteristics, and family preferences of devices makes it difficult to draw conclusions about specific factors that may have contributed to the observed developmental changes. Our results suggest more work is needed with separate groups assigned to each device and a standardized dosage to further understand effects of a powered mobility intervention. Lastly, Bayley-4 standard scores are not available for young children with CP across each GMFCS level. Therefore, it is unknown whether the magnitude of our observed changes in raw scores are expected for this population; however, it is unlikely, given the short time of 8 weeks between assessments. In addition, we used change scores relative to each child, so they served as their own control. Results of the current study should be interpreted with caution and may not be generalizable to all young children with CP.

5. Conclusions

In conclusion, mobility is a fundamental human right [1]. This is a position supported by the United Nations and the ON Time Mobility framework [2–4]. The multimodal principle of this framework advocates for children to have a range of technology options for mobility depending upon what works best for them based on an interaction of their individual and environmental constraints. Powered mobility is one mobility option for young children with CP. The results of the current study indicate the potential for positive developmental change following high use of a powered mobility device, and they recognize the variability of individual differences in children's developmental trajectories and potentially differing responses to intervention.

Author Contributions: Conceptualization, S.W.L., L.K.K. and H.A.F.; data curation, S.W.L., B.M.S., L.K.K. and H.A.F.; funding acquisition, S.W.L., L.K.K. and H.A.F.; methodology, S.W.L., L.K.K. and H.A.F.; project administration, H.A.F.; visualization, H.A.F.; writing—original draft, S.W.L.; writing—review and editing, B.M.S., L.K.K. and H.A.F. All authors have read and agreed to the published version of the manuscript.

Funding: This study was funded by the American Academy for Cerebral Palsy and Developmental Medicine and the National Pediatric Rehabilitation Resource Center (C PROGRESS) through the National Institute of Child Health and Human Development (NICHD) (P2CHD101912).

Institutional Review Board Statement: This study was conducted according to the guidelines of the Declaration of Helsinki and approved by the Institutional Review Board of the University of Washington (protocol # STUDY00011386; date of approval: 1 December 2020).

Informed Consent Statement: Informed consent was obtained from all participants involved in the study.

Data Availability Statement: De-identified individual participant data, including score report data from participation and developmental measures and device use reports, will be made available to other researchers and reported on clinicaltrials.gov per NIH funding requirements and will be made available 6 months following publication of study results. This study has been registered with the US National Library of Medicine Clinical Trial Registry under the National Clinical Trial (NCT) identified number NCT04684576 (Protocol Version 1) on 24 December 2020.

Acknowledgments: Permobil, the manufacturer of the Explorer Mini, loaned 6 of the 12 Explorer Minis needed to complete the study. The funding agencies and equipment manufacturer have no role in the design of the study, data analysis, interpretation, or preparation of scientific manuscripts or presentations. We thank Dinah Schultz for her assistance with creating and revising the figures.

Conflicts of Interest: The authors declare no conflict of interest.

References

1. Feldner, H.A.; Logan, S.W.; Galloway, J.C. Why the time is right for a radical paradigm shift in early powered mobility: The role of powered mobility technology devices, policy and stakeholders. *Disabil. Rehabil. Assist. Technol.* **2016**, *11*, 89–102. [CrossRef]
2. Sabet, A.; Feldner, H.A.; Tucker, J.; Logan, S.W.; Galloway, J.C. ON TIME mobility: Advocating for mobility as a human right. *Pediatr. Phys. Ther.* **2022**, *34*, 546–550. [CrossRef] [PubMed]
3. United Nations. Convocation on the Rights of Persons with Disabilities. 2006. Available online: https://www.un.org/development/desa/disabilities/convention-on-the-rights-of-persons-with-disabilities.html (accessed on 21 July 2021).
4. United Nations Convention on the Rights of the Child. United Nations Office of High Commissioner. Updated November 2002. Available online: https://www.ohchr.org/en/professionalinterest/pages/crc.aspx (accessed on 21 July 2021).
5. Bottos, M.; Bolcati, C.; Sciuto, L.; Ruggeri, C.; Feliciangeli, A. Powered wheelchairs and independence in young children with tetraplegia. *Dev. Med. Child Neurol.* **2001**, *43*, 769–777. [CrossRef] [PubMed]
6. Guerette, P.; Furumasu, J.; Tefft, D. The positive effects of early powered mobility on children's psychosocial and play skills. *Assist. Technol.* **2013**, *25*, 39–48. [CrossRef] [PubMed]
7. Jones, M.A.; McEwen, I.R.; Neas, B.R. Effects of powered wheelchairs on the development and function of young children with severe motor impairments. *Pediatr. Phys. Ther.* **2012**, *24*, 131–140. [CrossRef] [PubMed]

8. Butler, C.; Okamoto, G.; McKay, T. Motorized wheelchair driving by disabled children. *Arch. Phys. Med. Rehabil.* **1984**, *65*, 95–97.
9. Ragonesi, C.B.; Galloway, J.C. Short-term, early intensive power mobility training: Case report of an infant at risk for cerebral palsy. *Pediatr. Phys. Ther.* **2012**, *24*, 141–148. [CrossRef] [PubMed]
10. Tefft, D.; Guerette, P.; Furumasu, J. The impact of early powered mobility on parental stress, negative emotions, and family social interactions. *Phys. Occup. Ther. Pediatr.* **2011**, *31*, 4–15. [CrossRef]
11. Wiart, L.; Darrah, J.; Hollis, V.; Cook, A.; May, L. Mothers' perceptions of their children's use of powered mobility. *Phys. Occup. Ther. Pediatr.* **2004**, *24*, 3–21. [CrossRef]
12. Lynch, A.; Ryu, J.-C.; Agrawal, S.; Galloway, J.C. Power mobility training for a 7-month-old infant with spina bifida. *Pediatr. Phys. Ther.* **2009**, *21*, 362–368. [CrossRef]
13. Kenyon, L.K.; Jones, M.; Breaux, B.; Tsotsoros, J.; Gardner, T.; Livingstone, R. American and Canadian therapists' perspectives of age and cognitive skills for paediatric power mobility: A qualitative study. *Disabil. Rehabil. Assist. Technol.* **2020**, *15*, 692–700. [CrossRef]
14. Kenyon, L.K.; Schmitt, J.; Otieno, S.; Cohen, L. Providing paediatric power wheelchairs in the USA then and now: A survey of providers. *Disabil. Rehabil. Assist. Technol.* **2020**, *15*, 708–717. [CrossRef]
15. Rosen, L.; Plummer, T.; Sabet, A.; Lange, M.L.; Livingstone, R. RESNA position on the application of power mobility devices for pediatric users. *Assist. Technol.* **2023**, *2*, 14–22. [CrossRef] [PubMed]
16. Hospodar, C.M.; Feldner, H.A.; Logan, S.W. Active mobility, active participation: A systematic review of modified ride-on car use by children with disabilities. *Disabil. Rehabil. Assist. Technol.* **2021**, epub ahead of print. [CrossRef] [PubMed]
17. Huang, H.-H.; Galloway, J.C. Modified ride-on toy cars for early power mobility: A technical report. *Pediatr. Phys. Ther.* **2012**, *24*, 149–154. [CrossRef] [PubMed]
18. Logan, S.W.; Feldner, H.A.; Bogart, K.R.; Goodwin, B.; Ross, S.M.; Catena, M.A.; Whitesell, A.A.; Sefton, Z.J.; Smart, W.D.; Galloway, J.C. Toy-based technologies for children with disabilities simultaneously supporting self-directed mobility, participation, and function: A tech report. *Front. Robot AI* **2017**, *4*, 1–10. [CrossRef]
19. Plummer, T.; Logan, S.W.; Morress, C. Explorer Mini: Infants' initial experience with a novel pediatric powered mobility device. *Phys. Occup. Ther. Pediatr.* **2020**, *41*, 192–208. [CrossRef]
20. Feldner, H.A.; Plummer, T.; Hendry, A. A Guideline for Introducing Powered Mobility to Infants and Toddlers. 2022. Available online: https://permobilwebcdn.azureedge.net/media/stwou5go/a-guideline-for-introducing-powered-mobility-to-infants-and-toddlers_v0122.pdf (accessed on 10 February 2023).
21. Livingstone, R.; Field, D. Systematic review of power mobility outcomes for infants, children and adolescents with mobility limitations. *Clin. Rehabil.* **2014**, *28*, 954–964. [CrossRef]
22. Thelen, E. Dynamic systems theory and the complexity of change. *Psych. Dialog.* **2005**, *15*, 255–283. [CrossRef]
23. Feldner, H.; Logan, S.W.; Kenyon, L.K. In the driver's seat: A randomized, crossover clinical trial protocol comparing home and community use of the Permobil Explorer Mini and a modified ride-on car by children with cerebral palsy. *Phys. Ther.* **2022**, *102*, pzac062. [CrossRef]
24. An, M.; Dusing, S.C.; Harbourne, R.T.; Sheridan, S.M. What really works in intervention? Using fidelity measures to support optimal outcomes. *Phys. Ther.* **2020**, *100*, 757–765. [CrossRef] [PubMed]
25. Bayley, N.; Aylward, G.P. *Bayley Scales of Infant and Toddler Development*, 4th ed.; BAYLEY-4; Pearson: Bloomington, MN, USA, 2019.
26. Portney, L.G. *Foundations of Clinical Research: Applications to Evidence-Based Practice*; FA Davis: Philadelphia, PA, USA, 2020.
27. Wolf, M.M. Social validity: The case for subjective measurement or how applied behavior analysis is finding its heart. *J. Appl. Behav. Anal.* **1978**, *11*, 203–214. [CrossRef] [PubMed]
28. Logan, S.W.; Feldner, H.A.; Lobo, M.A.; Winden, H.N.; MacDonald, M.; Galloway, J.C. Power-up: Exploration and play in a novel modified ride-on car for standing. *Pediatr. Phys. Ther.* **2017**, *29*, 30–37. [CrossRef] [PubMed]
29. Logan, S.W.; Feldner, H.A.; Bogart, K.R.; Catena, M.A.; Hospodar, C.M.; Raja Vora, J.; Smart, W.D.; Massey, W.V. Perceived barriers before and after a 3-month period of modified ride-on car use. *Pediatr. Phys. Ther.* **2020**, *32*, 243–248. [CrossRef] [PubMed]
30. Logan, S.W.; Feldner, H.A.; Bogart, K.R.; Catena, M.A.; Hospodar, C.M.; Raja Vora, J.; Smart, W.D.; Massey, W.V. Perceived barriers of modified ride-on car use of young children with disabilities: A content analysis. *Pediatr. Phys. Ther.* **2020**, *32*, 129–135. [CrossRef]
31. Langendorfer, S.J.; Roberton, M.A. Individual pathways in the development of forceful throwing. *Res. Q. Exerc. Sport* **2002**, *73*, 245–256. [CrossRef]
32. Logan, S.W.; Hospodar, C.M.; Bogart, K.R.; Catena, M.A.; Feldner, H.A.; Fitzgerald, J.; Schaffer, S.; Sloane, B.; Phelps, B.; Phelps, J.; et al. Real world tracking of modified ride-on car usage in young children with disabilities. *J. Mot. Learn. Dev.* **2019**, *7*, 336–353. [CrossRef]

Disclaimer/Publisher's Note: The statements, opinions and data contained in all publications are solely those of the individual author(s) and contributor(s) and not of MDPI and/or the editor(s). MDPI and/or the editor(s) disclaim responsibility for any injury to people or property resulting from any ideas, methods, instructions or products referred to in the content.

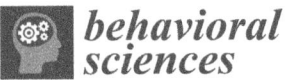

behavioral sciences

Article

Task-Related Differences in End-Point Kinematics in School-Age Children with Typical Development

Julia Mazzarella [1,*], Daniel Richie [2], Ajit M. W. Chaudhari [1,2], Eloisa Tudella [3], Colleen K. Spees [4] and Jill C. Heathcock [1]

1. Division of Physical Therapy, School of Health and Rehabilitation Sciences, College of Medicine, The Ohio State University, Columbus, OH 43210, USA; jill.heathcock@osumc.edu (J.C.H.)
2. Department of Biomedical Engineering, College of Engineering, The Ohio State University, Columbus, OH 43210, USA
3. Department of Physical Therapy, Federal University of São Carlos, São Carlos 13565-905, SP, Brazil
4. Division of Medical Dietetics, School of Health and Rehabilitation Sciences, College of Medicine, The Ohio State University, Columbus, OH 43210, USA
* Correspondence: julia.mazzarella@mso.umt.edu

Abstract: Understanding whether and how children with typical development adapt their reaches for different functional tasks could inform a more targeted design of rehabilitation interventions to improve upper extremity function in children with motor disabilities. This prospective study compares timing and coordination of a reach-to-drink, reach-to-eat, and a bilateral reaching task in typically developing school-aged children. Average speed, straightness, and smoothness of hand movements were measured in a convenience sample of 71 children, mean age 8.77 ± 0.48 years. Linear mixed models for repeated measures compared the variables by task, phases of the reach, task x phase interactions, and dominant versus non-dominant hands. There were significant main effects for task and phase, significant task x phase interactions ($p < 0.05$), and a significant difference between the dominant and non-dominant hand for straightness. Hand movements were fastest and smoothest for the reach-to-eat task, and least straight for the bilateral reaching task. Hand movements were also straighter in the object transport phases than the prehension and withdrawal phases. These results indicate that children with typical development change their timing and coordination of reach based on the task they are performing. These results can inform the design of rehabilitation interventions targeting arm and hand function.

Keywords: upper extremity; technology; pediatric; functional reach; assessment

Citation: Mazzarella, J.; Richie, D.; Chaudhari, A.M.W.; Tudella, E.; Spees, C.K.; Heathcock, J.C. Task-Related Differences in End-Point Kinematics in School-Age Children with Typical Development. *Behav. Sci.* **2023**, *13*, 528. https://doi.org/10.3390/bs13070528

Academic Editor: Scott D. Lane

Received: 31 May 2023
Revised: 19 June 2023
Accepted: 20 June 2023
Published: 23 June 2023

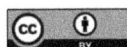

Copyright: © 2023 by the authors. Licensee MDPI, Basel, Switzerland. This article is an open access article distributed under the terms and conditions of the Creative Commons Attribution (CC BY) license (https://creativecommons.org/licenses/by/4.0/).

1. Introduction

Functional reach is essential for children to complete tasks like feeding, self-care, school participation, and leisure activities. Intentional reach is essential for driving other areas of development, such as cognitive and fine motor, in young children. Intentional reach-to-grasp skills emerge between 4–6 months of age in typical development as infants begin reaching for toys [1,2] and reach adult-like performance by 8–11 years [3–5]. Reaching and grasping are challenging skills for many children with motor disabilities, such as cerebral palsy (CP), and often a major focus of rehabilitation. The most common measures of functional upper extremity use in this population apply clinical observation and subjective scoring of performance, which have limitations in precision and rater bias [6,7]. Kinematic variables collected using three-dimensional (3D) motion capture offer an objective and quantitative measurement of upper extremity movements in early child development [3,8–16] such as reach and grasp. Timing and coordination of reach and grasp in infants and children are well-documented in the literature [3,5,9,14,16–20].

When quantifying upper extremity movement, a reach is typically defined as a movement towards an object, ending when the hand contacts the object. Straightness and smoothness are variables that quantify the coordination of a reach [17]. Straightness describes the trajectory of the hand, with a straighter movement following a shorter trajectory from the start- to end-point of the movement. Smoothness describes the shape of the velocity profile of the hand, with fewer peaks in the velocity profile indicating a smoother movement. A volitional reach in a healthy adult typically presents with a single velocity peak and a near-straight trajectory with a single, shallow curve [18]. Speed of the reach is calculated to measure timing of the reach movement and both average velocity and peak velocity are frequently used. Speed of a reach increases with maturity [3].

In the past decade, a few studies have applied 3D kinematics to objectively measure reach in a functional task, such as reaching for food to eat or a cup to drink [17,19–21]. Butler et al. [17,20] published the Reach and Grasp Cycle, a protocol developed to objectively measure upper extremity movement during a functional reach-to-drink task. Butler et al. [17,20] and Machado et al. [19] have applied this protocol in samples of children with typical development and children with cerebral palsy with upper extremity motor impairments. Hung et al. [21] used a similar reach-grasp-eat task, which involved reaching to eat a cracker, to evaluate functional upper extremity movement in children with CP. These studies provide detailed information about reach and grasp during discrete functional tasks in populations of children with typical development and CP. They did not compare differences in reach kinematics with the type of task and use of the dominant versus non-dominant upper extremity. Previous research in adults has investigated differences in kinematics when reaching for different objects; however, these did not include functional, multi-phase reaching tasks [22–24]. This study aims to fill the gap in understanding about how children with typical development change their reaches for different functional tasks. This will inform more precise treatment planning for the improvement of functional upper extremity use and coordination in children with motor impairments.

We adapted the set-up, procedure, and movement sequence from the Reach and Grasp Cycle [20] to three different tasks: a reach-to-drink, reach-to-eat, and a bilateral reach. Our purpose was to measure kinematics of functional reach in typically developing school-aged children when performing various everyday tasks to identify differences in spatiotemporal characteristics of reach. We measured straightness, smoothness, and average speed of hand movement for each phase of the Reach and Grasp Cycle. We hypothesized that there would be significant differences in all three kinematic variables by type of task, phases of the Reach and Grasp Cycle, and between the dominant and non-dominant hands for unilateral tasks. Specifically, we expected the initial reach (prehension) to be less straight, less smooth, and slower than the other 3 phases. We expected movements in the first 3 phases to be straighter, smoother, and slower in the reach-to-drink task compared to the other two tasks. We also expected movements to be less straight, less smooth, and slower in the bilateral reach, due to the bilateral coordination aspect. Last, we expected movements with the dominant hand to be straighter, smoother, and faster than with the non-dominant hand.

2. Materials and Methods

2.1. Participants

Participants were 71 typically developing children (38 male, 33 female), 7–10 years old (mean 8.77 ± 0.48), with 10 left-hand dominant and 61 right-hand dominant, as determined by the child's preferred writing hand. Participants were a convenience sample of children recruited from low-resource neighborhoods in Central Ohio, USA. Children were excluded if they were unable to follow instructions given in English, or if they had a motor impairment that prevented them from being able to perform the reach and grasp tasks. Given the exploratory nature of this investigation, the sample size was determined based on recommendations for normative datasets in pediatric populations [25].

This study was approved by the Institutional Review Board at The Ohio State University (2017B0110). Parents or legal guardians provided informed consent, and all child participants provided verbal assent.

2.2. Procedure

Participants were assessed at the Pediatric and Rehabilitation (PEARL) Laboratory at The Ohio State University. Retroreflective markers (8 mm) were placed on the children on their sternum, bilateral acromia, lateral epicondyles, radial and ulnar styloid processes, and heads of the third metacarpals. Markers were also placed on the 4 corners of the table, the back of the chair, and the objects that the children were reaching for (Figure 1). Children were seated at the table with the chair positioned so that their hips, knees, and ankles were flexed to 90°. The objects for which children were reaching (a 5.6 cm diameter cup of water, a 4.6 cm diameter Ritz cracker, or a 21.6 cm diameter ball) were positioned in front of the child at 75% of their arm's length away, consistent with the set-up from Butler et al. and Machado et al. [19,20]. This position was marked with tape on the table for each participant. The participants began with their hands resting on the table, shoulders neutral, elbows flexed to 90°, and wrists neutral. The resting hand placement was marked on the table with hand-shaped outlines, within which the children placed their hands. For the reach-to-drink and reach-to-eat tasks, children were instructed: "With your [left/right] hand, reach for the [object], pick up the [object], take a [drink/bite], return the [object] to the marked position on the table, and return your hand to the start position. Do this twice." For the bilateral task, the children were instructed: "Reach for the ball with both hands, pick it up, touch it to your chin, return the ball to the marked position, and return your hands to the start position. Do this twice." Participants were allowed one practice trial per hand with each object. Two repetitions were recorded for each condition with a 10-camera VICON Motion Capture system at 120 Hz and filtered with a low-pass Butterworth filter at 4 Hz.

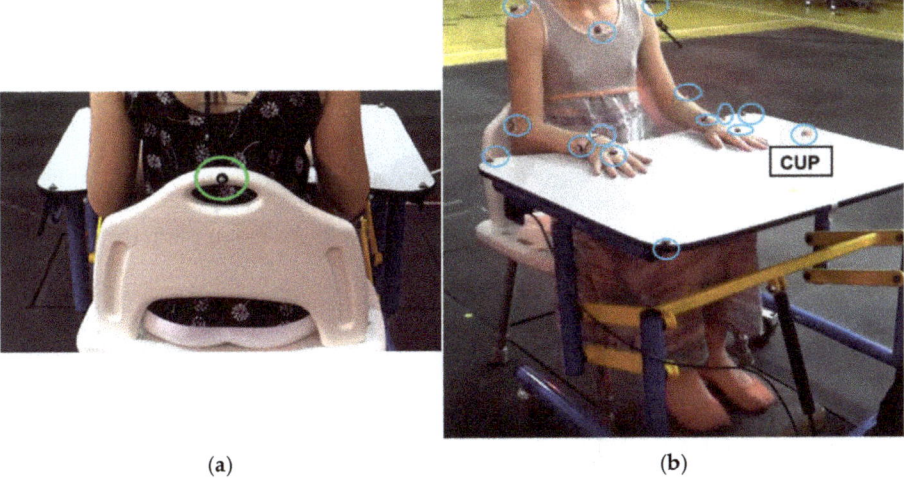

(a)   (b)

Figure 1. Marker placement and child positioning; (**a**) view from behind; (**b**) view from front.

2.3. Data Analysis

Phases of the movement (Figure 2) were visually identified and marked as events in the Vicon recordings. The task was divided into the following 4 phases of movement, based on the Reach and Grasp Cycle created by Butler et al. [20]:

1. Prehension: The movement begins with the hand(s) in the marked start position and ends when the hand(s) contact the object.
2. Transport 1: The movement begins with the hand(s) lifting the object from the table and ends with the object contacting the mouth or chin.
3. Transport 2: The movement begins with the object leaving the mouth or chin and ends with the object contacting the table at its marked position.

4. Withdrawal: The movement begins with the hand(s) releasing the object and ends with the hands contacting the marked start position on the table.

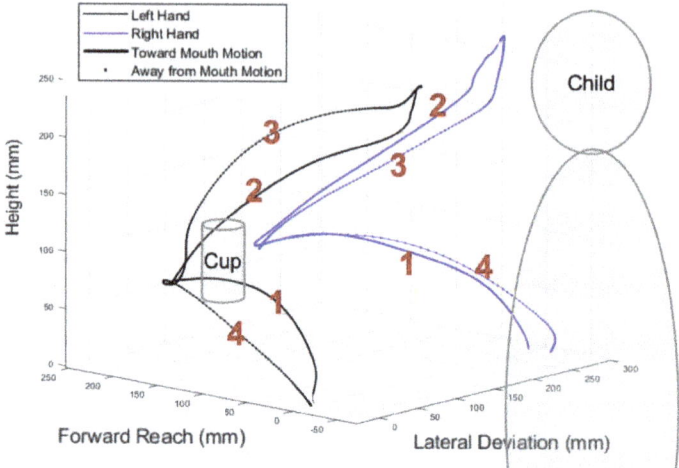

Figure 2. Four phases of the reaching task: (1) Prehension; (2) Transport 1; (3) Transport 2; (4) Withdrawal.

A custom MATLAB script was used to calculate spatial and temporal variables of reach for each phase of the Reach and Grasp Cycle. The variables were calculated based on the hand position, which was defined as the center point between the markers on the 3rd metacarpal, ulnar styloid process, and radial styloid process. The spatial and temporal variables were defined as:

- Straightness (ratio): ratio of the hand path length (total path the hand travels) to the movement length (difference between start- and end-points of the movement), with a value closer to one indicating a straighter movement.
- Smoothness (count): measured as the number of velocity peaks in a movement, with fewer velocity peaks indicating a smoother movement.
- Average speed (mm/s): calculated at each position of the marker using a 4-point central difference numerical differentiation.

A generalized linear mixed model for repeated measures for Gaussian distributions was applied using the SAS GLIMMIX procedure to compare each kinematic variable by task, phase, task x phase interactions, and dominant versus non-dominant hand for unilateral tasks (reach-to-drink and reach-to-eat). The model was created using a restricted maximum likelihood estimation technique, and the Kenward–Roger degrees of freedom method and fixed effects standard error adjustment. The alpha level was set to $\alpha = 0.05$. This model was chosen because it accounts for correlations between dependent variables, as well as a response that is not normally distributed. This is the case for straightness ratio and smoothness, for which values can only be >1. Least squared means were calculated for post hoc testing of task x phase interactions. The Bonferroni correction was applied for post hoc comparisons, setting $\alpha = 0.0005$.

3. Results

Means and standard deviation for kinematic variables of interest by task, type, and phase were calculated (Table 1).

Table 1. Mean and standard deviation of straightness ratio, smoothness, and average speed of hand movement by task type and phase.

Task Type	Phase	Variable	Mean	Std. Deviation
Bilateral	Prehension	Straightness Ratio	1.18	0.109
		Smoothness	1.70	3.59
		Speed (mm/s)	465	125
	Transport 1	Straightness Ratio	1.06	0.049
		Smoothness	1.75	2.68
		Speed (mm/s)	467	113
	Transport 2	Straightness Ratio	1.10	0.0528
		Smoothness	1.97	3.44
		Speed (mm/s)	450	99.9
	Withdrawal	Straightness Ratio	1.25	0.150
		Smoothness	1.43	1.31
		Speed (mm/s)	407	114
Reach-to-eat	Prehension	Straightness Ratio	1.11	0.0792
		Smoothness	1.10	0.357
		Speed (mm/s)	460	104
	Transport 1	Straightness Ratio	1.04	0.0294
		Smoothness	1.14	0.415
		Speed (mm/s)	514	116
	Transport 2	Straightness Ratio	1.05	0.0799
		Smoothness	1.11	0.345
		Speed (mm/s)	514	105
	Withdrawal	Straightness Ratio	1.28	0.171
		Smoothness	1.18	0.435
		Speed (mm/s)	423	121
Reach-to-drink	Prehension	Straightness Ratio	1.10	0.0692
		Smoothness	1.19	0.852
		Speed (mm/s)	429	93.6
	Transport 1	Straightness Ratio	1.02	0.0174
		Smoothness	1.34	1.70
		Speed (mm/s)	420	87.4
	Transport 2	Straightness Ratio	1.03	0.0185
		Smoothness	1.48	2.07
		Speed (mm/s)	389	76.3
	Withdrawal	Straightness Ratio	1.21	0.175
		Smoothness	1.33	0.807
		Speed (mm/s)	399	128

3.1. Straightness Ratio

There were significant main effects of straightness ratio for type of task ($F(2) = 107.26$, $p < 0.0001$), phase of task ($F(3) = 801.98$, $p < 0.0001$), type x phase interaction ($F(6) = 12.59$, $p < 0.0001$), and hand dominance ($F(1) = 13.05$, $p = 0.0003$), with straighter movement on the dominant side (Table 2; Figure 3a). Post hoc analysis revealed significant differences ($p < 0.0005$) for all comparisons, except: the prehension, transport 1, and transport 2 phases between the reach-to-drink versus the reach-to-eat tasks; the transport 1 and withdrawal phases between the bilateral versus reach-to-eat tasks; and within the reach-to-drink and reach-to-eat tasks, the transport 1 versus transport 2 phases; these comparisons showed no significant differences (Table 3).

Table 2. Main effects for least squares means.

Effect	Num DF	Straightness Ratio			Smoothness			Speed		
		Den DF	F	p-Value	Den DF	F	p-Value	Den DF	F	p-Value
Task	2	3124	107.26	<0.0001 *	3122	21.06	<0.0001 *	3112	176.31	<0.0001 *
Phase	3	3113	801.98	<0.0001 *	3114	2.26	0.0798	3109	64.87	<0.0001 *
Task x Phase	6	3111	12.59	<0.0001 *	3113	1.68	0.1230	3109	25.38	<0.0001 *
Hand	1	3124	13.05	0.0003	3122	1.03	0.3107	3112	0.18	0.6674

* Significant effect.

Table 3. Differences of task x phase least squares means.

Task	Phase	Task	Phase	Straightness Ratio		Smoothness		Speed	
				t Value	p-Value	t Value	p-Value	t Value	p-Value
Ball	1	Ball	2	14.88	<0.0001 *	−0.31	0.7596	−0.33	0.7386
Ball	1	Ball	3	10.06	<0.0001 *	−2.02	0.0438	2.11	0.0352
Ball	1	Ball	4	−9.02	<0.0001 *	1.55	0.1208	8.13	<0.0001 *
Ball	2	Ball	3	−4.75	<0.0001 *	−1.69	0.0902	2.42	0.0158
Ball	2	Ball	4	−23.44	<0.0001 *	1.84	0.0664	8.39	<0.0001 *
Ball	3	Ball	4	−18.73	<0.0001 *	3.50	0.0005 *	6.00	<0.0001 *
Cracker	1	Cracker	2	9.71	<0.0001 *	−0.25	0.8026	−7.60	<0.0001 *
Cracker	1	Cracker	3	7.84	<0.0001 *	−0.04	0.9664	−7.63	<0.0001 *
Cracker	1	Cracker	4	−19.94	<0.0001 *	−0.76	0.4476	4.82	<0.0001 *
Cracker	2	Cracker	3	−1.86	0.0626	0.21	0.8365	−0.03	0.9773
Cracker	2	Cracker	4	−29.31	<0.0001 *	−0.51	0.6102	12.22	<0.0001 *
Cracker	3	Cracker	4	−27.47	<0.0001 *	−0.71	0.4757	12.25	<0.0001 *
Cup	1	Cup	2	10.72	<0.0001 *	−1.04	0.2992	1.17	0.2426
Cup	1	Cup	3	9.78	<0.0001 *	−1.96	0.0499	5.52	<0.0001 *
Cup	1	Cup	4	−13.65	<0.0001 *	−0.92	0.3589	3.74	0.0002 *
Cup	2	Cup	3	−0.93	0.3546	−0.92	0.3585	4.33	<0.0001 *
Cup	2	Cup	4	−24.13	<0.0001 *	0.11	0.9129	2.57	0.0102
Cup	3	Cup	4	−23.21	<0.0001 *	1.02	0.3085	−1.71	0.0868
Ball	1	Cracker	1	8.41	<0.0001 *	3.40	0.0007	0.68	0.4961
Ball	1	Cup	1	9.75	<0.0001 *	2.78	0.0054	5.06	<0.0001 *
Cracker	1	Cup	1	1.29	0.1987	−0.62	0.5331	4.33	<0.0001 *
Ball	2	Cracker	2	3.41	0.0007	3.39	0.0007	−6.60	<0.0001 *
Ball	2	Cup	2	5.62	<0.0001 *	2.00	0.0452	6.47	<0.0001 *
Cracker	2	Cup	2	2.17	0.0301	−1.39	0.1641	13.00	<0.0001 *
Ball	3	Cracker	3	6.22	<0.0001 *	5.26	<0.0001 *	−9.01	<0.0001 *
Ball	3	Cup	3	9.40	<0.0001 *	2.77	0.0057	8.39	<0.0001 *
Cracker	3	Cup	3	3.12	0.0018	−2.51	0.0121	17.33	<0.0001 *
Ball	4	Cracker	4	−2.91	0.0037	0.99	0.3226	−2.46	0.0139
Ball	4	Cup	4	4.76	<0.0001 *	0.25	0.8019	0.58	0.5595
Cracker	4	Cup	4	7.65	<0.0001 *	−0.74	0.4569	3.05	0.0023

* Significant effect.

3.2. Smoothness

There was a significant main effect of smoothness for type of task ($F(2) = 21.06$, $p < 0.0001$). Main effects for phase, type x phase interaction, and dominant versus non-dominant hand were not significant (Table 2; Figure 3b). Post hoc analysis revealed that the reaching movements for the bilateral task were significantly less smooth than in the reach-to-eat task for transport 2 ($p < 0.0005$). The reaching movement for transport 2 was also significantly less smooth than withdrawal for the bilateral task ($p = 0.0005$). All other comparisons were not significantly different (Table 3).

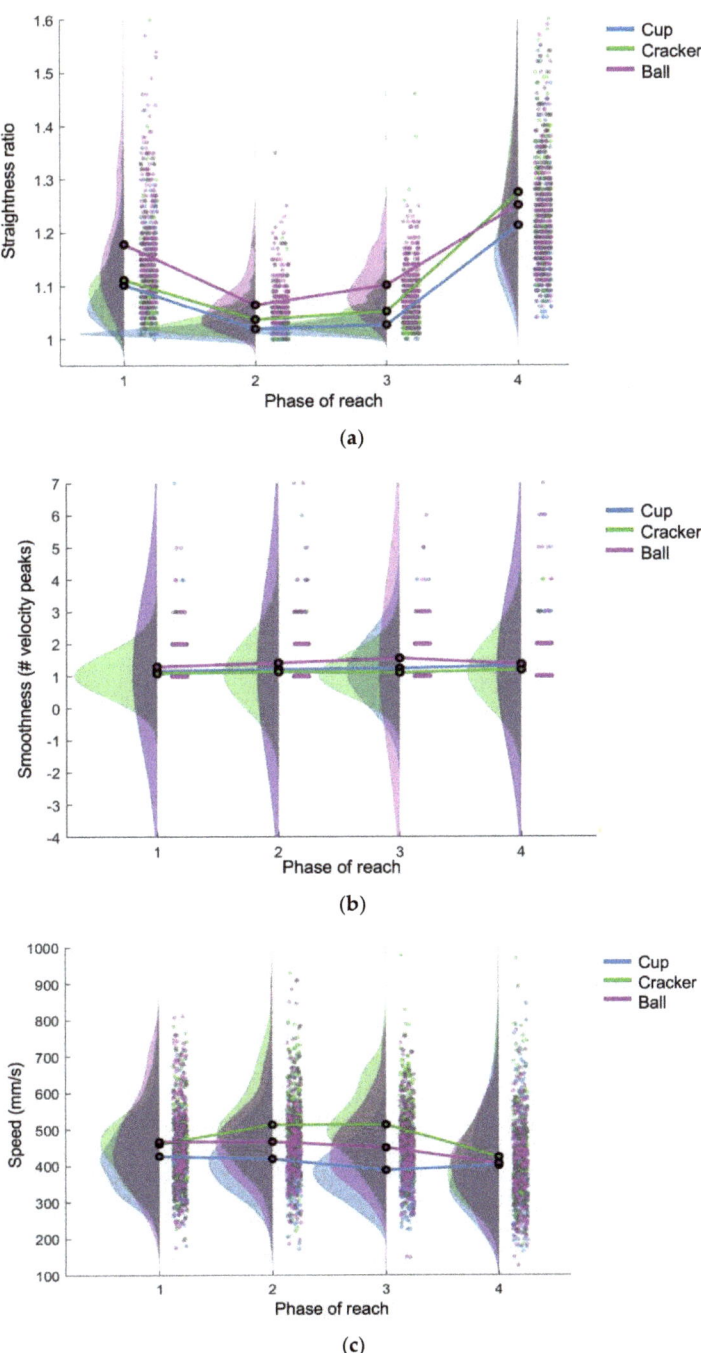

Figure 3. Raincloud plot by task and phase of straightness ratio (**a**), smoothness (**b**), and speed (**c**) [26].

3.3. Speed

There were significant main effects of speed for type of task ($F(2) = 176.31, p < 0.0001$), phase of task ($F(3) = 64.87, p < 0.0001$), and type x phase interaction ($F(6) = 25.38, p < 0.0001$), but not for dominant versus non-dominant hand (Table 2; Figure 3c). Post hoc testing revealed the following phase differences within each task: reaching movements in the prehension phase were faster than transport 2 and withdrawal, and reaching movements in the transport 1 phase were faster than transport 2; for the reach-to-eat task, reaching movements were faster in the prehension phase than the three other phases, and withdrawal was slower than all three other phases; reaching movements in the bilateral reach were significantly slower in the withdrawal phase than all other phases (Table 3). The following differences between tasks by phase were also found: for prehension and transport 1, reach movement was faster in both the bilateral and reach-to-eat tasks versus the reach-to-drink task; reaching movement in the reach-to-eat task was also significantly faster than the bilateral task for both transport phases.

4. Discussion

The objective of this study was to evaluate the coordination and timing of reaching movements in typically developing school-aged children when performing functional reaching tasks, applying the Reach and Grasp Cycle [20]. We were able to measure the straightness, smoothness, and speed of reaching movements of 71 children performing three different tasks: reach-to-drink, reach-to-eat, and a bilateral reach. The results from this study support our main hypothesis, indicating that reaching movement varies significantly based on the task being performed, even when the individual is following the same reaching pattern of the Reach and Grasp Cycle [20]. Support for our specific hypotheses was mixed. The prehension movement was slower and straighter than the two transport phases, as predicted, but not the withdrawal phase. Additionally, there was no significant difference in smoothness between the phases. This might have been due to a ceiling effect, as the mean was close to 1 for all phases. As we expected, bilateral movements were less straight than the other two tasks. The bilateral movements were also slower than the reach-to-eat movements, but not reach-to-drink, providing partial support for that hypothesis. Last, the dominant hand did move significantly straighter than the non-dominant hand, but not smoother nor faster. These results highlight the complex interplay of task and object characteristics that impact the timing and coordination of reaching behaviors in children. Since most of the research on the impacts of varying task and object constraints on reach kinematics has focused on an adult population, we will compare and contrast our results with those.

Research in adults has demonstrated changes in reaching behaviors with different task constraints. For example, when adults reach for an empty cup of water, their movements are significantly faster than reaches toward a full cup of water [24,27]. It is not yet known if these effects are the same in a pediatric population. In support of our hypotheses, some of the results in this study were consistent with these findings, such as: reaches were faster in the prehension and transport 1 phases for the reach-to-eat and bilateral tasks than for the reach-to-drink task. This is likely due to greater constraints on the reach-to-drink task, with the need for precision to keep the water in the cup. Consistent with this theory, movements in the two transport phases were straightest for the reach-to-drink task, although only significantly different from the bilateral task. This type of task requires feedback motor control to maintain a straight movement to keep the water from spilling out of the cup [23], meaning that the sensory systems are providing real-time feedback on the position of the cup, water, hand, etc., which the motor system then uses to guide the movement of the upper extremity to complete the task successfully. The children likely slowed their speed in the reach-to-drink task to allow time for this sensory processing to occur.

Changes in object size also affects reach speed in adults performing a reach and grasp task, with slower reaches toward smaller objects [23,28]. In contrast, children in this study had the fastest reaching speeds in the reach-to-eat task, even though the cracker was the smallest of the three objects. In this instance, there are likely other factors that had greater influence on reach behavior than object size. One factor might be that reaching for a cup full of water requires more precision and visuomotor feedback than reaching for a small object, as described previously. An additional factor could be motivation to complete the task. Motivation and reward can impact movement speed, amplitude, and variability in multiple types of movement tasks in adults [22,29–31]. In the present study, it is possible that the children found the reward of eating a cracker to be more motivating than drinking water or touching a ball to their chin. This would be consistent with previous research, which indicated that reaching movements were faster and less variable for tasks that offered a reward, compared to tasks with no reward [22,29].

The differences between phases of the Reach and Grasp Cycle in this study were partially consistent with our hypotheses and might indicate that familiarity with specific movements has a strong influence on timing and coordination of the reach. For example, reaches were fastest and straightest in the object transport phases, which is consistent with previous research and our predictions [17,32]. It is possible that these movements, or at least transport 1, can be completed using primarily feedforward control, which is much faster than feedback control [33]. Feedforward motor control relies on stored motor representations, which are created over many repetitions of a motor task, rather than from processing of sensory information in real time. Children bring objects to and from their mouth many times a day; however, the position of the object they are reaching for is variable, and thus the prehension phase requires more feedback control to accomplish. We had also hypothesized that movements would be faster and straighter in the withdrawal phase compared to the prehension phase, which was not supported by our results. It is possible that in the context of this study procedure, participants needed to use feedback control for the withdrawal phase as well, because there was a marked position on which they needed to place their hands. Overall, it is clear that there is a complex interplay of task and object characteristics that impact timing and coordination of reaching behaviors in children via motor control mechanisms.

Last, we found that the dominant hand movements were significantly straighter than the non-dominant hand movements, as we expected. Contrary to our hypothesis, and contrary to studies in adults, we found no differences in speed or smoothness of movement between the dominant and non-dominant hands [34,35]. Given the age and typical development of the participants (7–12 years old), we would expect them to demonstrate a strong hand preference, and our result partially supported this [36]. It is possible that this procedure is not sensitive enough to detect the difference in speed and smoothness between the dominant and non-dominant hands in typical development; however, Butler et al. have shown that it can detect differences between typical and motor-impaired movement [17]. Future investigations should determine the magnitude of difference required to detect a meaningful change for each of these kinematic variables in the Reach and Grasp Cycle. This would help determine whether measuring kinematics of functional reaching tasks could be used to detect clinically important improvements with rehabilitation.

5. Conclusions

Kinematic measurement of coordination and timing of reaching movement in functional reaching tasks is a promising objective, quantitative measure of upper extremity function in a pediatric population, as it can provide detailed information about movement timing and coordination. Results from this study provide insight into how task familiarity, constraints, and motivation might impact the coordination and timing of reach in typically developing children, and the role that motor control systems might play in those differences. This information could be used to further refine clinical rehabilitation approaches for pediatric populations with upper extremity motor impairment. Application to clinical practice could include: (1) routinely using kinematics as an outcome measure to track progress; (2) using information about timing and coordination and task constraints to target improvements in skills that are inherent to participation in daily life activities. Some examples of precise treatment planning based on the results of this study would be to choose larger target objects or more motivating tasks to train increased reach speed, and to use tasks that require feedback control, such as transporting a cup of water, to train straightness and smoothness. Future research could further investigate the impact of specific task characteristics on kinematics in a reach and grasp task in children. An important next step would be to determine a minimal clinically important difference for average speed, smoothness, and straightness of hand movement in the Reach and Grasp Cycle. In the future, data could be used as a normative comparison for age-matched children with motor disability to measure improvements in everyday reaching function with targeted upper extremity therapy interventions.

Author Contributions: Conceptualization, J.M., J.C.H. and E.T.; methodology, J.M., J.C.H., A.M.W.C., E.T. and D.R.; software, D.R.; validation, J.M., D.R. and A.M.W.C.; formal analysis, J.M. and D.R.; investigation, J.M.; resources, C.K.S. and A.M.W.C.; data curation, J.M., C.K.S. and D.R.; writing—original draft preparation, J.M.; writing—review and editing, J.C.H., D.R., A.M.W.C., C.K.S. and E.T.; visualization, J.M.; supervision, J.C.H., A.M.W.C., E.T. and C.K.S.; project administration, J.M. and C.K.S.; funding acquisition, C.K.S. All authors have read and agreed to the published version of the manuscript.

Funding: This research was funded by United States Department of Agriculture, grant number 2017-68001-26353; the Foundation for Physical Therapy Research Combined Promotion of Doctoral Studies II-New Investigator Fellowship Initiative; the Eunice Kennedy Shriver National Institute of Child Health and Human Development award number 5F30HD104379-02; and C-PROGRESS award number P2CHD101912-04.

Institutional Review Board Statement: The study was conducted in accordance with the Declaration of Helsinki, and approved by the Institutional Review Board of The Ohio State University (protocol code 2017B0110, approved 6 July 2017).

Informed Consent Statement: Informed consent was obtained from all subjects involved in the study. Written informed consent has been obtained from the patient(s) to publish this paper.

Data Availability Statement: The data presented in this study are available on request from the corresponding author.

Acknowledgments: Additional contributions: Gardenia Barbosa, Rachel Bican, Kim Scott, and Thais Cabral for their contributions to protocol design and data collection.

Conflicts of Interest: The authors declare no conflict of interest. The funders had no role in the design of the study; in the collection, analyses, or interpretation of data; in the writing of the manuscript; or in the decision to publish the results.

References

1. Coluccini, M.; Maini, E.S.; Martelloni, C.; Sgandurra, G.; Cioni, G. Kinematic characterization of functional reach to grasp in normal and in motor disabled children. *Gait Posture* **2007**, *25*, 493–501. [CrossRef] [PubMed]
2. Thelen, E.; Corbetta, D.; Spencer, J.P. Development of reaching during the first year: Role of movement speed. *J. Exp. Psychol. Hum. Percept. Perform.* **1996**, *22*, 1059–1076. [CrossRef] [PubMed]
3. Simon-Martinez, C.; dos Santos, G.L.; Jaspers, E.; Vanderschueren, R.; Mailleux, L.; Klingels, K.; Ortibus, E.; Desloovere, K.; Feys, H. Age-related changes in upper limb motion during typical development. *PLoS ONE* **2018**, *13*, e0198524. [CrossRef] [PubMed]
4. Schneiberg, S.; Sveistrup, H.; McFadyen, B.; McKinley, P.; Levin, M.F. The development of coordination for reach-to-grasp movements in children. *Exp. Brain Res.* **2002**, *146*, 142–154. [CrossRef] [PubMed]
5. Gilliaux, M.; Dierckx, F.; Vanden Berghe, L.; Lejeune, T.M.; Sapin, J.; Dehez, B.; Stoquart, G.; Detrembleur, C. Age Effects on Upper Limb Kinematics Assessed by the REAplan Robot in Healthy School-Aged Children. *Ann. Biomed. Eng.* **2015**, *43*, 1123–1131. [CrossRef]
6. DeMatteo, C.; Law, M.; Russell, D.; Pollock, N.; Rosenbaum, P.; Walter, S. *QUEST: Quality of Upper Extremity Skills Test*; McMaster University, CanChild Centre for Childhood Disability Research: Hamilton, ON, Canada, 1992.
7. Krumlinde-Sundholm, L.; Eliasson, A.C. Development of the assisting hand assessment: A Rasch-built measure intended for children with unilateral upper limb impairments. *Scand. J. Occup. Ther.* **2003**, *10*, 16–26. [CrossRef]
8. Chen, C.-Y.; Tafone, S.; Lo, W.; Heathcock, J.C. Perinatal stroke causes abnormal trajectory and laterality in reaching during early infancy. *Res. Dev. Disabil.* **2015**, *38*, 301–308. [CrossRef]

9. Bhat, A.N.; Galloway, J.C. Toy-oriented changes during early arm movements: Hand kinematics. *Infant Behav. Dev.* **2006**, *29*, 358–372. [CrossRef]
10. Corbetta, D.; Thelen, E. Lateral Biases and Fluctuations in Infants' Spontaneous Arm Movements and Reaching. *Dev. Psychobiol.* **1999**, *34*, 237–255. [CrossRef]
11. Rachwani, J.; Santamaria, V.; Saavedra, S.L.; Wood, S.; Porter, F.; Woollacott, M.H. Segmental trunk control acquisition and reaching in typically developing infants. *Exp. Brain Res.* **2013**, *228*, 131–139. [CrossRef]
12. Nelson, E.L.; Konidaris, G.D.; Berthier, N.E. Hand preference status and reach kinematics in infants. *Infant Behav. Dev.* **2014**, *37*, 615–623. [CrossRef]
13. Marchi, V.; Belmonti, V.; Cecchi, F.; Coluccini, M.; Ghirri, P.; Grassi, A.; Sabatini, A.M.; Guzzetta, A. Movement analysis in early infancy: Towards a motion biomarker of age. *Early Hum. Dev.* **2020**, *142*, 104942. [CrossRef]
14. Lynch, A.; Lee, H.M.; Bhat, A.; Galloway, J.C. No stable arm preference during the pre-reaching period: A comparison of right and left hand kinematics with and without a toy present. *Dev. Psychobiol.* **2008**, *50*, 390–398. [CrossRef] [PubMed]
15. Karch, D.; Kim, K.; Wochner, K.; Pietz, J.; Dickhaus, H.; Philippi, H. Quantification of the segmental kinematics of spontaneous infant movements. *J. Biomech.* **2008**, *41*, 2860–2867. [CrossRef]
16. Lee, M.; Ranganathan, R.; Newell, K.M. Changes in Object-Oriented Arm Movements that Precede the Transition to Goal-Directed Reaching in Infancy. *Dev. Psychobiol.* **2011**, *53*, 685–693. [CrossRef] [PubMed]
17. Butler, E.E.; Ladd, A.L.; LaMont, L.E.; Rose, J. Temporal-spatial parameters of the upper limb during a Reach & Grasp Cycle for children. *Gait Posture* **2010**, *32*, 301–306. [CrossRef] [PubMed]
18. Morasso, P. Spatial Control of Arm Movements. *Exp. Brain Res.* **1981**, *42*, 223–227. [CrossRef]
19. Machado, L.R.; Heathcock, J.; Carvalho, R.P.; Pereira, N.D.; Tudella, E. Kinematic characteristics of arm and trunk when drinking from a glass in children with and without cerebral palsy. *Clin. Biomech.* **2019**, *63*, 201–206. [CrossRef]
20. Butler, E.E.; Ladd, A.L.; Louie, S.A.; LaMont, L.E.; Wong, W.; Rose, J. Three-dimensional kinematics of the upper limb during a Reach and Grasp Cycle for children. *Gait Posture* **2010**, *32*, 72–77. [CrossRef]
21. Hung, Y.-C.; Henderson, E.R.; Akbasheva, F.; Valte, L.; Ke, W.S.; Gordon, A.M. Planning and coordination of a reach-grasp-eat task in children with hemiplegia. *Res. Dev. Disabil.* **2012**, *33*, 1649–1657. [CrossRef] [PubMed]
22. Summerside, E.M.; Shadmehr, R.; Ahmed, A.A. Vigor of reaching movements: Reward discounts the cost of effort. *J. Neurophysiol.* **2018**, *119*, 2347–2357. [CrossRef] [PubMed]
23. Berthier, N.E.; Clifton, R.K.; Gullapalli, V.; McCall, D.D.; Robin, D.J. Visual Information and Object Size in the Control of Reaching. *J. Mot. Behav.* **1996**, *28*, 187–197. [CrossRef]
24. Flindall, J.W.; Doan, J.B.; Gonzalez, C.L.R. Manual asymmetries in the kinematics of a reach-to-grasp action. *Laterality Asymmetries Body Brain Cogn.* **2014**, *19*, 489–507. [CrossRef] [PubMed]
25. Bridges, A.J.; Holler, K.A. How Many is Enough? Determining Optimal Sample Sizes for Normative Studies in Pediatric Neuropsychology. *Child Neuropsychol.* **2007**, *13*, 528–538. [CrossRef] [PubMed]
26. Allen, M.; Poggiali, D.; Whitaker, K.; Marshall, T.R.; Kievit, R.A. Raincloud plots: A multi-platform tool for robust data visualization. *Wellcome Open Res.* **2019**, *4*, 63. [CrossRef] [PubMed]
27. Nelson, E.L.; Berthier, N.E.; Konidaris, G.D. Handedness and Reach-to-Place Kinematics in Adults: Left-Handers Are Not Reversed Right-Handers. *J. Mot. Behav.* **2018**, *50*, 381–391. [CrossRef]
28. Grosskopf, A.; Kuhtz-Buschbeck, J.P. Grasping with the left and right hand: A kinematic study. *Exp. Brain Res.* **2006**, *168*, 230–240. [CrossRef]
29. Bryden, P.J.; Roy, E.A. Preferential reaching across regions of hemispace in adults and children. *Dev. Psychobiol.* **2006**, *48*, 121–132. [CrossRef]
30. Steenbergen, B. Achieving Coordination in Prehension: Joint Freezing and Postural Contributions. *J. Mot. Behav.* **1995**, *27*, 333. [CrossRef]
31. Gentilucci, M. Object motor representation and reaching-grasping control. *Neuropsychologia* **2002**, *40*, 1139–1153. [CrossRef]
32. Mosberger, A.C.; De Clauser, L.; Kasper, H.; Schwab, M.E. Motivational state, reward value, and Pavlovian cues differentially affect skilled forelimb grasping in rats. *Learn. Mem.* **2016**, *23*, 289–302. [CrossRef] [PubMed]
33. Takikawa, Y.; Kawagoe, R.; Itoh, H.; Nakahara, H.; Hikosaka, O. Modulation of saccadic eye movements by predicted reward outcome. *Exp. Brain Res.* **2002**, *142*, 284–291. [CrossRef] [PubMed]
34. Mir, P.; Trender-Gerhard, I.; Edwards, M.J.; Schneider, S.A.; Bhatia, K.P.; Jahanshahi, M. Motivation and movement: The effect of monetary incentive on performance speed. *Exp. Brain Res.* **2011**, *209*, 551–559. [CrossRef] [PubMed]
35. Mackey, A.H.; Walt, S.E.; Stott, N.S. Deficits in upper-limb task performance in children with hemiplegic cerebral palsy as defined by 3-dimensional kinematics. *Arch. Phys. Med. Rehabil.* **2006**, *87*, 207–215. [CrossRef] [PubMed]
36. Seidler, R.D.; Noll, D.C.; Thiers, G. Feedforward and feedback processes in motor control. *Neuroimage* **2004**, *22*, 1775–1783. [CrossRef]

Disclaimer/Publisher's Note: The statements, opinions and data contained in all publications are solely those of the individual author(s) and contributor(s) and not of MDPI and/or the editor(s). MDPI and/or the editor(s) disclaim responsibility for any injury to people or property resulting from any ideas, methods, instructions or products referred to in the content.

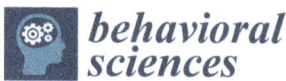

Article

Use of Goal Attainment Scaling to Measure Educational and Rehabilitation Improvements in Children with Multiple Disabilities

Kimberly Kascak [1,*], Everette Keller [2] and Cindy Dodds [3]

1 Office of Interprofessional Initiatives, Medical University of South Carolina, Charleston, SC 29425, USA
2 Department of Public Health Sciences, Medical University of South Carolina, Charleston, SC 29425, USA; kellerev@musc.edu
3 College of Health Professions, Medical University of South Carolina, Charleston, SC 29425, USA; doddscb@musc.edu
* Correspondence: kascak@musc.edu

Abstract: With a focus on children with multiple disabilities (CMD), the purpose of this quality improvement project was to elevate educational measurement and practices involving CMD. Using the goal attainment scaling (GAS) methodology, this project was conducted within a public charter school, Pattison's Academy for Comprehensive Education (PACE), focusing on 31 CMD and measuring student improvement and program effectiveness. For 2010–2011 and 2011–2012, improvements were demonstrated for the majority of CMD by meeting or exceeding their goals. Goal attainment scaling was able to capture improvement in educational and rehabilitation goals in the majority of CMD. Goal attainment scaling can provide an indication of a program's effectiveness. The use of GAS in CMD has potential to maximize participation across the school setting where all children in the United States commonly develop and learn skills as well as find meaning.

Keywords: children with multiple disabilities; goal attainment scaling; quality of life; individual education program

1. Introduction

The United Nations Convention on the Rights of Children states that "a child with mental or physical disabilities is entitled to enjoy a full and decent life, in conditions that ensure dignity, promote self-reliance and facilitate the child's active participation in the community [1]". Solutions to ensure that the rights of children with disabilities are upheld are multi-contextual, complicated, and often involve struggles between health care and rehabilitation as well as between health care and public-school systems that provide special education and related services (e.g., physical therapy (PT) and occupational therapy (OT)) in the least restrictive environment to ensure a free and appropriate education. Across childhood, school environments provide an essential participatory setting and context in which children develop and learn motor, self-care, social–emotional, and cognitive skills. This is not only true for typical children, but also and possibly more importantly, for children with disabilities, including those with multiple disabilities.

In the United States, the 7.2 million children with disabilities account for 15% of children enrolled in public school, and children with multiple disabilities (CMD) account for 2% of that total [2]. Descriptions and definitions for this 2% of children vary across educational and rehabilitation institutions. Through the Individuals with Disabilities Education Act (IDEA), the Department of Education defines CMD as those with concomitant impairments (such as intellectual disability–blindness or intellectual disability–orthopedic impairment) that in combination cause such severe educational needs that they cannot be accommodated in special education programs solely for one of the impairments [3]. In

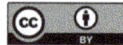

Citation: Kascak, K.; Keller, E.; Dodds, C. Use of Goal Attainment Scaling to Measure Educational and Rehabilitation Improvements in Children with Multiple Disabilities. *Behav. Sci.* **2023**, *13*, 625. https://doi.org/10.3390/bs13080625

Academic Editors: Stephanie C. DeLuca and Jill C. Heathcock

Received: 21 April 2023
Revised: 14 July 2023
Accepted: 21 July 2023
Published: 27 July 2023

Copyright: © 2023 by the authors. Licensee MDPI, Basel, Switzerland. This article is an open access article distributed under the terms and conditions of the Creative Commons Attribution (CC BY) license (https://creativecommons.org/licenses/by/4.0/).

the field of healthcare, children with medical complexity (CMC) are most similar to CMD. Berry and colleagues [4] defined CMC as a subset of children with special health care needs who have primary diagnoses that may be acquired or congenital. They also demonstrate multisystem impairments, resulting in considerable functional activity limitations (e.g., walking, dressing, talking) and participatory restrictions (e.g., school, community); experiencing frequent and extensive hospitalizations; and requiring multiple primary care, subspecialty care, and multi-disciplinary rehabilitation visits. Poly-pharmacology, medical equipment, and care coordination are commonplace. Because this project involves children within a school "setting", the term "children with multiple disabilities" (CMD) will be used in this paper.

The Individuals with Disabilities Education Act [3] is a federal law that ensures that children with disabilities (0–21 years) receive a free, appropriate public education in the least restrictive environment. To ensure the delivery of this education, each child served by special education has an Individualized Educational Program (IEP) that is a binding legal document. It is made up of present levels of performance based on evidence-based educational and rehabilitation assessments, special education services, related services (PT, OT, transportation, etc.), supplementary services, assistive technology (AT), and measurable annual goals. It is important to note that one single assessment cannot determine a child's educational placement and tests cannot be discriminatory (e.g., racial, cultural, gender). The facilitation of parental participation is strongly encouraged across the IEP process.

Children with multiple disabilities have multiple bodily and environment barriers, which can challenge comprehensive assessment, objective measurement, and overall functional achievement in life. To properly evaluate the present levels of CMD, the use of multiple assessments is necessary because of the heterogeneity within the population and individual nature of each CMD's ability. One conceptual framework that has been used to describe, measure, and guide assessment and treatment in individuals with disabilities, including CMD, is the International Classification of Functioning, Disability and Health (ICF) [5,6]. The ICF is a biosocial framework for communicating and describing health and disability. It is an interactive framework made up of the domains in body structure and function, activity, participation, and environmental and personal factors [5]. Best practice supports the use of evidence-based measurement tools to capture outcomes across that ICF. For CMD specifically, measurement across the ICF in combination with the assessment of their unique characteristics allows for ideal individualization. Because CMD have multiple system impairments, activity limitations, and participatory restrictions, multiple measurement tools are necessary to document individual abilities and goal areas while the ICF framework provides an excellent model for organizing and prioritizing goal areas and subsequent treatment strategies.

Many of the commonly used assessments target appropriate skills and functional activities for children with disabilities; however, they are not sensitive enough for the subtle and slower changes that may occur in CMD [7–10]. In addition, the majorities of these measures were not specifically developed with CMD in mind. As such, documenting change or responsiveness for change is often negligible for this population, which means improvement is either not objectively captured or there is a no perception of educational or rehabilitative improvement [9]. One measure that has been used to document change in children with disabilities within education and rehabilitation settings including school settings is goal attainment scaling (GAS) [11–13].

Goal attainment scaling provides an individualized and patient- and family-informed method toward achieving a desired outcome and its approach to individualization is well suited for inclusion within an IEP. Steenbeek and colleagues [14] compared positive findings from GASs, the Pediatric Evaluation of Disability Inventory (PEDI), and the Gross Motor Function Measure (GMFM)-66 of children with cerebral palsy (CP) across all Gross Motor Function Classification System levels and determined that 20% of items found within the GASs were not captured within the PEDI and GMFM-66. This suggests that GASs may better measure unique aspects of the patient and family experiences as compared with fixed-item patient-reported measures like the PEDI or GMFM [14–16]. In a systematic review including 52 pediatric rehabilitation studies, implications are that GAS can be effectively used across a variety of diagnoses and interventions and is reflective of meaningful change. REF Three of these studies were conducted in school environments, and eight studies involved children with CP at Gross Motor Function Classification System levels of IV and V (i.e., 111 out of 444 children), which is commonly reflective of CMD. None of the studies specifically addressed CMD or CMC. The aim of this project was to describe assessment to guide GAS development as well as the implementation and measurement/analyses of GAS integrated into the IEP of 31 CMD in a school setting.

2. Methods

2.1. Protections for Human Participants

Conducted within a public charter school for CMD, this project was considered a quality improvement with the goal of elevating educational measurement and practices involving CMD. Parents and legal guardians of participating children did consent to participation in the school that provided individualized assessment, goal creation and measurement, and associated interventional strategies. The Board of Directors approved the school's data collection processes and annually reviewed findings from annual outcome data collection. It should be noted that 50% of the board members were employees of an academic medical center and other healthcare facilities, which supported their clear understanding and oversight concerning the consent process.

2.2. Project Site and Participants

Pattison's Academy for Comprehensive Education (PACE) is a public charter school with a mission to improve the quality of life (QOL) for children with multiple disabilities by providing the high-quality integration of education and rehabilitation. It was considered a separate school by the Department of Education that served only CMD. The school was conceptualized and implemented based on the market testing of the non-profit Pattison's Academy, which hosted 5-week summer camps for CMD. One underlying principle of the summer camp was to actively engage the sensory and motor abilities of children to encourage optimal participation across the camp day with the goal of each child being physically engaged for 180 min across the 6-h day [17]. This 180-min expectation was translated to PACE upon its opening and often was reflected in goals.

Pattison's Academy for Comprehensive Education was made up of five classrooms with 6 to 7 CMD students. In total, 5 special education teachers, 7 educational assistants, 2 physical therapists, 2 occupational therapists, 1 speech and language pathologist, and 1 school administrator made up the faculty. The indoor and outdoor environment was fully accessible and a wide variety of assistive and adaptive equipment was available. The children attended school eight hours a day (8 a.m. to 3 p.m.) from mid-August to mid-June.

Thirty-one CMD between the ages of 4 and 16 years attended PACE in Charleston, South Carolina. Thirteen children were African American, seventeen were White, and one identified as Other. All children were non-Hispanic. Fifteen were male and sixteen were female. See Table 1 for additional demographic details.

Table 1. Demographics and Characteristics of the Participants (N = 31).

Demographic and Characteristics	# of Children [1]
DIAGNOSIS	
Cerebral palsy	17
Genetic health conditions	11
Traumatic brain injury	3

Table 1. Cont.

Demographic and Characteristics	# of Children [1]
CO-OCCURRING CONDITIONS	
Seizures	19
Cortical visual impairment	15
Tracheostomy	1
GENDER	
Male	15
Female	16
RACE and ETHNICITY	
Black/African American	13
White	17
Other	1
Not Hispanic/Latino	31
MOBILITY FUNCTION	
Wheelchair users propelled by caregiver	29
Wheelchair user self-propel	2
FEEDING FUNCTION	
Gastronomy or Jejunostomy tube	13
Gastronomy Tube/Oral	4
Oral	14
SELFCARE FUNCTION	
Maximum assistance	30
Moderate assistance	1
EXPRESSIVE and RECEPTIVE FUNCTION	
Maximum assistance	29
Moderate assistance	2

[1] One student only attended the 2010-11 school year and not the 2011-12 school year.

3. Outcomes

Goal attainment scaling was the primary outcome used by PACE to measure student improvement and program effectiveness. Goal attainment scaling is an objective goal writing approach that allows for individualization and should involve child and family input. The standardized process is well suited for measuring educational and rehabilitation capacity and performance across the ICF [5]. Goals using GAS methodology should also follow "SMART" criteria: specific (i.e., "who", "what", "when", "why", and "where"), measurable, attainable, relevant, and realistic within a temporal boundary [18,19]. Scalings are found to be more reliable and valid when developed in collaboration with families and educational and rehabilitation providers [11,12,19].

The normal distribution of a bell-shaped curve serves as the statistical foundation for GAS. Based on family interviewing and evidence-based educational and rehabilitation assessments, levels of performance that the child is expected to achieve are assigned values equally spaced across the five levels between -2 and 2 (i.e., $-2, -1, 0, 1, 2$). Across the expected levels of performance, only one specific variable, such as repetitions, duration, frequency, distance, assistance level, and steps across a task (task analysis) should be measured. The -2 and $+2$ values correspond to 2 standard deviations below and above the expected mean, respectively. Although, several acceptable options are available for defining

GAS scores [11,12,20]; this project defined −2 as the "current level of performance", which is the most common GAS methodology used. The −1, 0, 1, and 2 values are defined as progress toward the expected level of performance, expected level of performance, greater than the expected level of performance, and much greater than the expected level of performance. Goals should be designed to achieve the expected level of performance.

Scoring requires assigning a raw score between −2 and 2 to every individual GAS. For a group of GASs, raw scores are summed. Scaled and T-scores are derived from the GAS raw scores using the statistical formula or tables entitled *Conversion Key for Follow-Up Guides Having One Scored Scale* available in *Goal Attainment Scaling: Applications, Theory, and Measurement* [11] (p. 274) or the GOALed app [21]. The T-scores are the standardized statistic that allows within or between subject comparisons. T-scores are reflective of small sample sizes (n < 30) with unknown population standard deviations, which points to individuality [22]. The interpretation of T-scores can reflect an individual's single goal, an individual's groups of goals, a group's group of goals, or more broadly, an entire program's goals. Interpretations from collective groups and program goals are reflective of a program's effectiveness.

4. Procedures

As a public charter school serving children within the domain of special education, PACE required annual IEPs with measurable annual goals. Because GAS was a primary outcome of the school, goals formatted into the GASs were integrated into annual IEPs. To guide and support the development of IEP goals using the GAS methodology, four steps were carried out.

4.1. Step 1: Evidence-Based Assessment

4.1.1. Required Assessments: These Assessments Were Administered for All Enrolled Students Developmental Assessment for Individuals with Severe Disabilities

The Developmental Assessment for Individuals with Severe Disabilities (DASH) 2 [23] was the required annual educational and rehabilitation assessment that was administered to every student by the educational and rehabilitation faculty members. The DASH is a criterion-referenced assessment that measures skills across five scales (i.e., academic, sensory–motor, activities of daily living, language, and social–emotional) in children and adults who have severe physical and sensory disabilities.

Caregiver Priorities and Child Health Index of Life with Disabilities

With a mission to improve QOL for CMD, annually measuring QOL was important, so parents completed the Caregiver Priorities and Child Health Index of Life with Disabilities (CPCHILD) [24]. The CPCHILD has demonstrated validity and measures health-related QOL in non-ambulant children with severe developmental disabilities. It is composed of 37 questions across six domains: Personal Care/Activities of Daily Living; Positioning, Transferring and Mobility; Comfort and Emotions; Communication and Social Interaction; Health; and Overall Quality of Life. Scores are on a 5- or 6-point Likert scale with levels of assistance and intensity also documented. A higher score on the CPCHILD indicates a more enhanced HRQL.

Faces Pain Scale—Revised

Although 180-min of active participation for CMD has been found to be safe [17,25,26] and as such was implemented each school day, it was important to monitor pain severity and discomfort in the event that this intensity was problematic for some CMD. To measure pain severity, the validated 10-point metric Faces Pain Scale—Revised was used and reported by parents [27]. It displays gender-neutral faces in various degrees of pain. The "0" space on the scale displays a face with a neutral expression while the "most pain possible" face is described as the "10" space [28,29].

Pediatric Evaluation of Disability Inventory

The Pediatric Evaluation of Disability Inventory (PEDI) [30] is a valid measurement tool, which considers functional skills and caregiver assistance across the three domains of self-care, mobility, and social function. Self-care, mobility, and social function domains for both the functional skills and caregiver assistance sections were administered and scored by therapists (i.e., PT, OT, SLP) based on observations in the school setting. The use of this measure allowed for a more in-depth examination of the child's needs for caregiver assistance and overall functional abilities, which informed goals [31,32].

4.1.2. Commentary Assessments: These Assessments Were Completed When Appropriate for Individual Children

In addition to the required assessments, complementary assessments were administered according to each child's individual characteristics and needs of the educational and rehabilitation team. Because many of the CMD presented with cortical visual impairment (CVI) and had assistive technology needs, the Cortical Visual Impairment Range Assessment and Matching Assistive Technology to Child-Augmentative Communication Evaluations Simplified Assessment (MATCH-ACES) was also administered as needed. Findings from these assessments expanded descriptive data available on each child, which better guided goal development and intervention delivery.

Cortical Visual Impairment Range Assessment

The Cortical Visual Impairment Range Assessment (CVIRA) [33] is a reliable functional vision assessment designed to investigate the visual characteristics associated with CVI. It measures the degree of CVI severity on a 0–10 continuum where 0 represents no visual function and 10 represents near typical visual function [34,35].

Matching Assistive Technology to Child-Augmentative Communication Evaluations Simplified Assessment

The Matching Assistive Technology to Child-Augmentative Communication Evaluations Simplified Assessment (MATCH-ACES) [36] is an evidence-based comprehensive evaluative process that is child-centered and is used to identify the need for assistive technology in the educational setting. The administration of the MATCH-ACES was found to be an effective process for appropriately matching students with assistive technology (AT) in order to meet educational goals [36]. To ensure data obtained from each child were accurate and best reflected their abilities, no more than two assessments occurred in a day and the completion of all assessments occurred over 2 weeks at a minimum.

4.2. Step 2: Family Interview

As outcome measures were being administered, the educational and rehabilitation team also interviewed parents/legal guardians to identify and discuss skills and goals that were important to the child and family. These interviews were conducted at the school or in children's homes. Again, because PACE's mission was to impact QOL, a school-specific QOL questionnaire was developed that was derived from a QOL model created by Patrick and Chiang [37,38]. See Appendix A for this questionnaire. This questionnaire served as a script or guide for enhancing discussion between the family and school faculty. It was not required that each question had to be asked and answered, but it was essential that the information gathered was thorough and meaningful to families. This process ensured that created goals were collectively relevant for the home, community, and school environments. For example, one child's grandmother was interested in her grandchild learning to manage her drooling and the school team agreed this was a great idea. As such, a goal attainment scaling was created to address the skill. Similarly, the grandmother wanted the child to learn to operate a remote control for the home television channel selection and although this was not an appropriate school goal, we were able to incorporate switch access into a communication device and school socialization goal.

4.3. Step 3: ICF and GAS Development

Following the assessment and family interview phases, all findings were organized across the ICF framework. See Appendix B for an example involving a CMD. This summative document was instrumental in helping the team to organize and prioritize goals that would be incorporated into the IEP. From the ICF document, the interprofessional educational and rehabilitation team (i.e., School Principal, Director of Therapy, each student's special educator, physical therapist, occupational therapist, speech and language pathologist) could more easily prioritize and initially develop goals using GAS methodology. Goals for each student were developed across the categories of physical activity/adaptive physical education, gross and fine motor, language, feeding, cognition, self-care, academics, social and emotional, and transition. Goals were also written across the ICF framework. Once school team members reached a consensus on goals, goals were sent to families for review, revisions, and/or approval prior to the formal IEP meeting. Because of the high level of IEP pre-planning, oftentimes few, if any, changes were made to the goals areas, GASs, or actual IEP document at the final and formal IEP meeting. In cases where GASs were achieved during the school year, the team reconvened to create more advanced goals based on children's annual assessments. Parents again edited or approved the more advanced goals. Appendix C contains examples of a student's goal attainment scalings.

4.4. Step 4: Goal Measurement across the Year

Each child's GASs were measured weekly by educational and/or rehabilitation professionals using a specifically created data sheet that was modified from the Murdoch Center Data Sheet from the Murdoch Program Library [39]. See Appendix D for an example. Formal reporting to parents concerning GASs on the IEP data occurred every 9 weeks. If progress reporting indicated the mastery of a GAS with a score of 0 or above, then a more advanced GAS was established. The expected duration of GASs was 1 year, as it aligned with the annual development of IEPs. At the end of the year, raw scores were summed for each student's set of IEP/GAS goals. This summed raw score is similar to an overall grade point average for a regular education student taking courses in a variety of subjects (e.g., math, English, social studies). The summed raw scores were then translated into scaled and T-scores for each child. Collectively scoring GASs for all children in each classroom and the entire school allowed for T-score calculations for each classroom and the entire school to be generated. These T-scores were reflective of overall classroom and school effectiveness, which were used to inform improvements [11].

5. Results

For the 2010–2011 school year, 204 IEP GASs were created for 31 children with disabilities. The average number of goals per student was 6.58, ranging from 5 to 7 goals. Raw scores were converted to T-scores using tables provided in Kiresuk et al.'s book [11] (pp. 274–278). Student, classroom, and overall school scores are displayed in Table 2 and Figure 1. The scores in Table 2 reflect the T-score for each individual child, classroom, and school, having been adjusted for the number of goals a student had during that school year, as students with the same scaled score may have differing T-scores based on their individual number of goals. Based on summed T-scores, seven students demonstrated T-scores of 50 (50 to 71.11), indicating the meeting or exceeding of expectations. Twenty children demonstrated improvement beyond baseline, but below the expected values projected. Four CMD demonstrated no improvement from baseline. One classroom met expectations with a T-score of 50.4. A second classroom was close to meeting expectations with a T-score of 45.1. The remaining classrooms demonstrated improvement beyond baseline, approximating an increase of 1 standard deviation. Reflective of all student goals, the school effectiveness T-score was 35.74.

Table 2. Goal Attainment Scaling Scores across students for years 2010–2011 and 2011–2012.

	2010–2011 Number of Goals	Scaled Score	T-Score	Classroom T-Score	School T-Score	2011–2012 Number of Goals	Scaled Score	T-Score	Classroom T-Score	School T-Score	Bell Curve of Adjusted Scores Based on Number of Goals
CLASSROOM 1				50.396	35.74				32.65	29.45	
1	6	0.83	62.91			5	−1.2	31.91			
2	6	0.33	44.84			5	−1.2	31.91			
3	5	0.2	53.02			7	−0.86	36.45			
4	7	−2	18.28			5	−1.2	31.91			
5	7	0	50			7	−1.14	31.93			
6	7	−0.14	47.74			7	−0.14	47.74			

Table 2. *Cont.*

	2010–2011 Number of Goals	Scaled Score	T-Score	Classroom T-Score	School T-Score	2011–2012 Number of Goals	Scaled Score	T-Score	Classroom T-Score	School T-Score	Bell Curve of Adjusted Scores Based on Number of Goals
7	7	0	50			8	−0.88	35.94			
CLASSROOM 2				27.356					22.95		
8	7	−1.29	29.67			8	−0.88	35.94			
9	6	−0.67	39.67			7	−1.71	22.89			
10	8	−2	17.87			5	−1	34.92			
11	6	−1.17	31.93			7	−1.71	22.89			
12	8	−1.38	30.12			7	−1.57	25.15			

Table 2. Cont.

	2010–2011 Number of Goals	Scaled Score	T-Score	Classroom T-Score	School T-Score	2011–2012 Number of Goals	Scaled Score	T-Score	Classroom T-Score	School T-Score	Bell Curve of Adjusted Scores Based on Number of Goals
13	7	−1.29	29.67			8	−1.25	29.92			
CLASSROOM 3				30.413					20.15		
14	5	−0.8	37.94			6	−2	19.02			
15	6	−1.67	24.18			7	−1.57	25.15			
16	5	−0.6	40.95			6	−1.67	24.18			
17	7	−2	18.38			6	−2	19.02			
18	7	−0.29	45.48			6	−1.33	29.34			

Table 2. Cont.

	2010–2011 Number of Goals	Scaled Score	T-Score	Classroom T-Score	School T-Score	2011–2012 Number of Goals	Scaled Score	T-Score	Classroom T-Score	School T-Score	Bell Curve of Adjusted Scores Based on Number of Goals
19	8	−1.13	31.93			7	−1.57	25.15			
CLASSROOM 4				45.058					33.12		
20	7	−0.57	40.96			7	−1.71	22.89			
21	6	−1.33	29.34			6	−1.33	29.34			
22	8	0.25	54.02			5	−1	34.92			
23	5	1.4	71.11			4	1	64.51			
24		0	50				−2	30			

Table 2. *Cont.*

	2010–2011 Number of Goals	Scaled Score	T-Score	Classroom T-Score	School T-Score	2011–2012 Number of Goals	Scaled Score	T-Score	Classroom T-Score	School T-Score	Bell Curve of Adjusted Scores Based on Number of Goals
25	8	−0.75	37.95			8	0.13	52.01			
CLASSROOM 5				27.513					40.14		
26	6	−1.5	26.76			3	−1.33	31.74			
27	8	−2	17.87			8	−1	33.94			
28	6	−1.17	31.93			7	−0.57	40.96			
29	7	−0.14	47.74			3	−2	22.62			
30	8	−1.88	19.88			4	−1.75	24.61			

Table 2. *Cont.*

2010–2011 Number of Goals	Scaled Score	T-Score	Classroom T-Score	School T-Score	2011–2012 Number of Goals	Scaled Score	T-Score	Classroom T-Score	School T-Score	Bell Curve of Adjusted Scores Based on Number of Goals
31	−0.83	37.09			6					

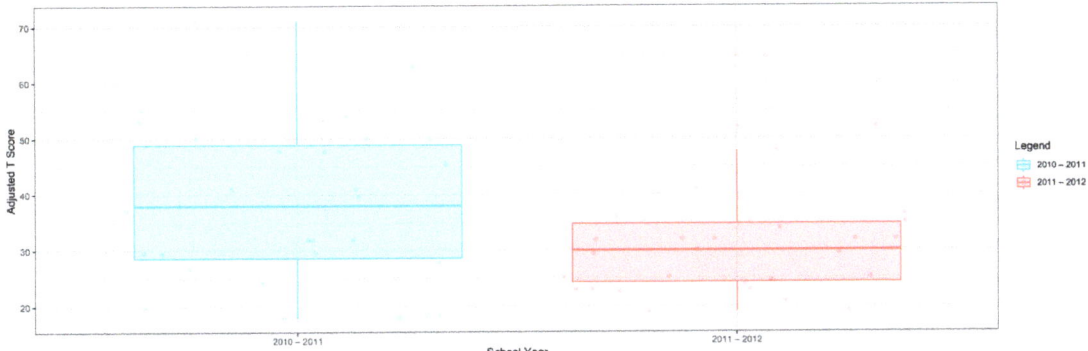

Figure 1. Box plot of adjusted T-scores across school years.

For the 2011–2012 school year, 192 IEP GASs were created for 30 children with disabilities. The average number of goals per student was 6.19, ranging from 5 to 7 goals. Student, classroom, and overall school scores are displayed in Table 2 and Figure 1. Based on summed T-scores, two students demonstrated T-scores of 50 (50 to 71.11), indicating the meeting or exceeding of expectations. Twenty-four children demonstrated improvement beyond baseline below the expected values projected. Five children demonstrated no improvement. Reflective of all student goals, the school effectiveness T-score decreased between school years to 29.45 with only one classroom improving from the 2010–2011 school year to the 2011–2012 school year.

Because the goals of each child may be unique and the number of goals across children can vary, a statistical analysis of GAS scores is challenging and thus there was no statistical test performed to determine whether a significant difference occurred between school years. In this regard, Figure 2 displays the range of scores for GAS and the traditional assessments CPCHILD, FPS-R, DASH, and PEDI for years 2010–2011 and 2011–2012. A noticeable visual difference occurs both in the range and quantiles of scores within the GAS between the school years, as the scores decreased between years. Of the traditional assessments, only the FPS-R assessment depicts a difference in the scores between the two years; however, the scale to which these ranges of scores differ is far less than that of the GAS scores. The CPCHILD, DASH, and PEDI scales display very little difference between the range of scores from one year to the next.

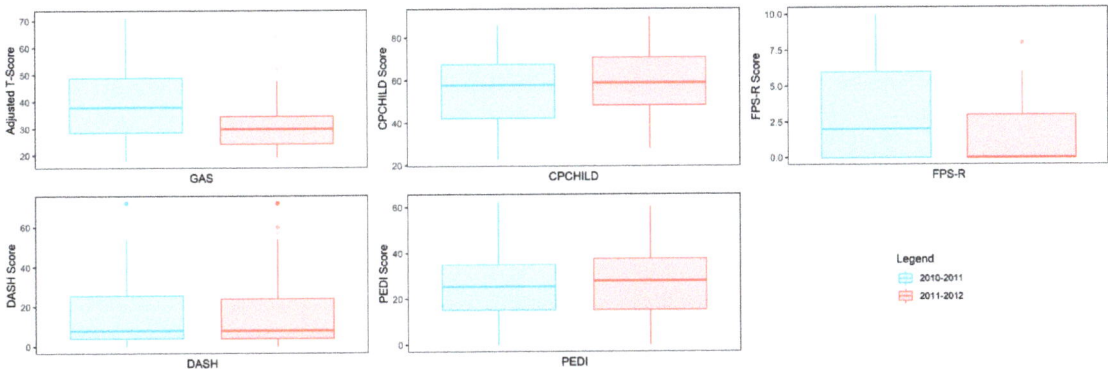

Figure 2. Visualization demonstrating how GAS varies more from year to year relative to traditional assessments (CPCHILD, FPSR, DASH, and PEDI). The vertical axis displays the range of scores for each assessment.

6. Discussion

Goal attainment scaling was able to capture improvement in the majority of CMD. Several or a combination of factors may explain this improvement. First, quality of life discussions with the family provided an opportunity for therapists and teachers to learn what was important from their perspective. Often times in many of these discussions, families highlighted meaningful emerging skills that not only were relevant in the home but also the school and community environments. Second, organizing and prioritizing identified areas of improvement across the ICF allowed family, teachers, and therapists to reach a consensus on goal setting more easily. Third, the use of a battery of assessments, both required and individualized, also helped to recognize and appropriately target emerging skills for goals. Lastly, the weekly formative assessment of goals by scoring the GASs facilitated goal clarification and guided modifications to better target instruction and rehabilitation towards goal success. These explanations for observed GAS improvement are in line with available evidence. In a systematic review of GAS, Haladay and colleagues determined that quantitative, assessment-driven, and patient-initiated goals inclusive of a family-focused approach demonstrated a greater responsiveness than those that were qualitative and provider-initiated [15]. The use of the ICF framework has also documented improved rehabilitation goal setting [40], while goal-directed rehabilitation with regular reassessment has been found to be an effective strategy for achieving goals [41,42].

As stated in the Introduction, measuring change in CMD using traditional educational and rehabilitation measurement tools is challenging, not only because CMD demonstrate varying multi-system impairments and corresponding activity limitations but also because the tools are often unable to capture subtle change that is common in CMD [7–9]. Based on our findings, it appears that GAS may provide an opportunity to overcome measurement challenges in CMD. On the other hand, when these measurement tools are able to capture change, it is important to consider that in the context of the home, community, and school, these changes may not be viewed as meaningful by the family and school team. It has previously been noted that GAS provides a greater responsiveness than other well-recognized measurement tools [15]. In this project's case, although significant improvements were noted for the DASH sensory motor and activities of daily living scales and PEDI Selfcare Caregiver Assistance section, these improvements provide little insight as to each CMD's individual improvement within the actual IEP as well as meaningful change in the home, school, and community settings.

Some of the children demonstrated no improvement in GAS across the IEP. This is especially true for the 2011–2012 school year when students' annual IEP was completed on or near a student's birthday rather than at the beginning of the school year, as was the case in 2010–2011. As such, at the end of the school year when GAS scores were calculated, students with birthdays near the end of the school year had had little time to demonstrate the mastery of goals beyond the current level of performance. Additionally, CMD experience a great number of medical appointments and medical interventions, such as surgeries, hospitalizations, and medication alterations, which often negatively impact school participation and slow the progression of goal achievement. For example, if a CMD were to undergo a posterior spinal fusion in the middle of the school year, then that student may be unable to attend school for 6 weeks. Substantial remediation may also be necessary to regain the preoperative level of function following the return to school. In this case, the progression of skills as defined by goals may be slow because of this absenteeism and/or remediation. Lastly, evidence suggests that in order for teams to create reliable GASs, approximately 3 years of implementation are recommended [19]. Findings from this project spanned across the first and second years of the school's opening, so the GASs developed by teams may have been less effective GASs, which may have interfered with documenting improvement in goals for CMD.

Just as traditional educational and rehabilitation measurement tools can provide an indication of a program's effectiveness, so too can GAS. Classroom and overall school performance T-scores derived from GASs accurately revealed the contextual truth occurring within PACE. One informative finding interpreted from the classroom summative scores was the lower T-score seen in classrooms with earlier career or recently graduated teachers and therapists. In the 2010–2011 year with the opening year of PACE, the intentional decision was made to pair early career or recently graduated teachers and therapists within a classroom to foster team development and growth over time. In reflection, a better strategy may have been to pair senior faculty with junior faculty within a classroom. In spite of this possible misstep, information derived from classrooms with lower scores drove professional development. These lower scores allowed PACE leadership to reflect on all student goals within a lower-performing classroom and to clearly identify areas in which additional instructional or rehabilitation education was needed for classroom teams. For example, by examining students' goals in one of these classrooms, it became quite clear that additional education on cortical visual impairment in CMD was needed. It should be noted that classroom summative scores were never used in a punitive manner as PACE sought to maintain a culture of mutual support with ongoing improvement.

Goal attainment scaling has been effectively implemented in school settings where instruction and rehabilitation co-occur [13,26] and this project adds to this evidence. The previous implementation of GAS in schools has focused on goals specific to the related service areas of physical and occupational therapy within the IEP. The PTCOUNTS [13] study examined physical therapy IEP goals that were related to motor skills and involved children across a variety of diagnostic categories, including CMD. Daly and colleagues [26] also used GAS to successfully measure motor skill improvement following the implementation of an adaptive cycling program for children similar to CMD. This project's findings specific to CMD expand the current level of evidence by demonstrating that GAS can be used to measure goals across all categories of an IEP by an interprofessional team of educators and therapists in the context of a school setting.

One method of capturing meaning is to measure QOL. With a mission of improving QOL for CMD, at the end of each school year, PACE measured QOL using the CPCHILD. Although no significant changes in CPCHILD scores occurred between 2010–2011 and 2011–2012, scores suggested an elevated QOL for CMD attending PACE. In the CPCHILD manual, the mean CPCHILD value for nonambulatory children considered to be mobility-dependent was 44.4. The CPCHILD scores for the end of the 2010–2011 and 2011–2012 school year were 56 and 59, respectively. With a 5- to 9-point MCID for CPCHILD, the greater than 10-point difference between the reported CPCHILD mean and PACE scores indicates that QOL for PACE students may be elevated. No correlation or causation can be reported as related to this elevation, but one possible explanation may be the capacity of GAS to target and measure change in CMD across meaningful life activities and participation. Knowing that pain can negatively impact QOL, it should also be noted that reported pain severity values for CMD that attended PACE were reduced. The values of 2.92 and 2.15 for the 2010–2011 and 2011–2012 years, respectively, are lower than those reported for similar children [43,44].

Several limitations can be noted within this project. Although derived from a conceptual model, the QOL questionnaire used to facilitate discussion between parents and school team members was not validated. Selection bias was also a limitation as parents chose for their CMD to attend PACE and as such other similar populations of CMD may not display the same results. The addition of a control group that was comparable to the CMD attending PACE would have strengthened this project. The administration of the DASH, CPCHILD, FPS-R, and PEDI at the beginning and end of the school year may have captured a greater degree of change than that observed by only administering them once a year. However, this administrative burden would have been quite time consuming for the school team that would have reduced important instruction and rehabilitation for the CMD. A fifth limitation was the different measurement points between the creation and end of the school year scoring of GAS between the 2010–2011 and 2011–2012 years. The lower GAS scores during the second year may be a reflection of this change in which IEPs were created near each child's birthday. As a final limitation, the authors acknowledge that these data are older, but children considered multiply disabled or medically complex are a challenging population to study secondary to their heterogeneity and as such there is limited evidence. In the past 10 years, when completing a quick PubMed search for "special education" or "rehabilitation" in conjunction with children with multiple disabilities or children with medical complexity, there have been eight publications. The majority of publications involving this population of children have explored examining hospitalization, care coordination, nutritional support, and pain. in this population.

7. Conclusions

Findings from this project provide evidence that GAS is an objective and responsive tool for measuring CMD despite their multi-system impairments and activity limitations. The integration of GAS across IEP categories using an interprofessional team of parents, educators, and rehabilitation therapists can also be successfully executed. The use of GAS in CMD has the potential to maximize participation across the school setting where all children in the United States commonly develop and learn skills as well as find meaning. Teams and schools serving CMD should consider incorporating GAS into practice.

Author Contributions: Conceptualization, K.K. and C.D.; methodology, E.K. and C.D.; software, E.K.; validation, no applicable; formal analysis, E.K.; investigation, K.K. and C.D.; resources, C.D.; data curation, K.K., E.K. and C.D.; writing—original draft preparation, K.K. and C.D.; writing—review and editing, K.K., E.K. and C.D.; visualization, E.K.; supervision, C.D.; project administration, K.K. and C.D.; funding acquisition, not applicable. All authors have read and agreed to the published version of the manuscript.

Funding: This research received no external funding.

Institutional Review Board Statement: This statement should be excluded. See Section 2.1.

Informed Consent Statement: This statement should be excluded. See Section 2.1.

Data Availability Statement: The authors may contact the corresponding author for data sharing.

Conflicts of Interest: The authors declare no conflict of interest.

Appendix A.

Appendix A.1. PACE Quality of Life Questionnaire

Questions on the PACE Quality of Life Questionnaire were developed using a QOL model created by Patrick and Chiang [37]. See Figure A1.

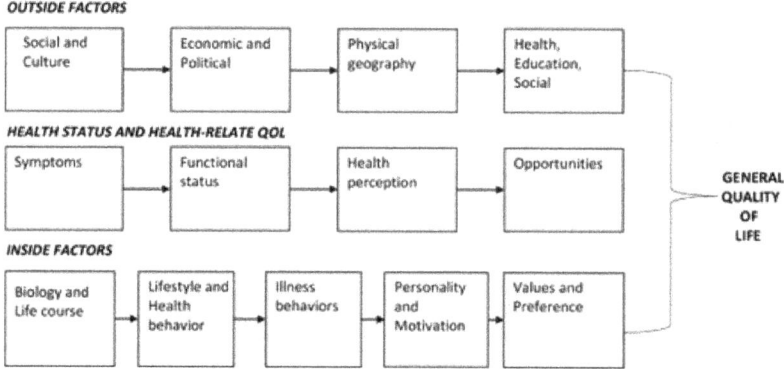

Figure A1. Patrick and Chiang (2000): Relations among quality of life and health concepts.

Appendix A.1.1. Internal Questions
1. What is your child's diagnosis(es) or disease?
2. Do you know how your child's diagnosis or disease affects your child's future?
3. Do you need information on your child's diagnosis(es) or disease and its progression?
4. What can your child do?
5. Do you have any concerns about your child's overall health?
6. Generally, what does your child do each weekday? Weekend?
7. How would you describe your child's personality?
8. What makes your child happy? Sad? Mad? Sick?
9. What does your child enjoy?
10. Does your child have any bad behaviors? If so, what?
11. What good behaviors does your child have?

Appendix A.1.2. Health Status and Health-Related Quality of Life Questions
1. How does your child sleep at night?
2. What position does your child sleep in?
3. Does your child experience pain? If so, how often? Can you explain what causes your child's pain?
4. Are your child's arms and legs tight or loose?
5. Is your child's head and trunk tight or loose?
6. Does your child have seizures? If so, how do you control them? How often do they occur?
7. Is your child's weight good?
8. Does your child move freely and well?
9. Does your child like to move?
10. Does your child see well?
11. Does your child hear well?
12. Does your child like to be touched?
13. Does your child like to touch things?
14. Does your child like to sit?
15. Does your child like to stand?
16. What calms your child?
17. Does your child cough a lot?
18. Does your child vomit a lot?
19. What activities does your child participate in daily? Weekly?
20. Does your child participate in any community activities? (e.g., little league, miracle league, horseback riding, adaptive swimming)
21. How does your child bathe? How often does your child bathe?
22. Who fixes your child's hair?
23. Does your child use diapers? Toilet?
24. How does your child get dressed each day?
25. How does your child eat? Do they enjoy eating? Do you think they get enough calories?
26. Can your child change position in the bed?
27. How does your child get to school?
28. How does your child move about in your home?
29. How does your child move about at the grocery store, doctor's office, or other community locations?
30. How is your child's overall health?
31. How would you rate your child's quality of life?
32. What do you dream of your child doing now?
33. What do you dream of your child doing in the future?
34. What activities would you like to have your child experience or participate in?

Appendix A.1.3. External Questions
1. Do you want us to know anything about you and your child's culture? Religion? Income? Politics?
2. Is there anything in the environment that bothers you or your child? (e.g., Heat? Pools? Horses? Animals?)
3. Is there anything we can do to help with your job? Income? Education?
4. What medications does your child take?
5. What doctors does your child see?
6. What therapies does your child have?
7. Do you like your child's school? What are the pluses of your child's school? What are the minuses of your child's school?
8. What do you and your family like to do? What else would you like to do?
9. How do you transport your child to appointments?
10. Would any changes to your home make it easier to care for them?
11. Do you need any equipment to improve your ability to care for your family and child?
12. How is the health of your family members?
13. How would you rate your family member's quality of life?

Appendix A.1.4. Reference
Source from [38].

Appendix B.
International Classification of Functioning, Disability, and Health
Name: VH
Age: 15 years
Body weight: 118 pounds
Height: 144 inches
Head circumference: 22.44 inches
Primary Nutritional Method: Gastronomy tube
Blood pressure: 118/82
Heart rate: 108
Respiratory rate: 25 breaths per minute
Temperature: 98.6 degrees
Seizure History and Frequency: Yes, and with medication, occurrence of one time annually.
Developmental History: VH was born full-term to married parents, but care was transferred to paternal grandmother by age of 12 months, who was a licensed practical nurse. VH demonstrated hypotonia at birth and was later diagnosed with mitochondrial myopathy. Seizures were also present within the first year of life.
General development level: 3–4 months
Surgeries: Gastronomy tube placement, right femoral head osteotomy, spinal fusion for neuromuscular scoliosis (2009), two femoral fractures without surgical intervention, semi-annual botox to right hamstring and bilateral wrist flexors.
Strengths

- Excellent temperament
- Supportive paternal grandmother support with assistance from father
- Successful access in right hand with button switch
- Improving visual skills, such as seeing more color, greater visual distance
- Loves music and interactions with family and friends
- Receptive greater than expressive language
- Sense of humor
- Healthy body growth
- Tolerates frequent positional changes necessary for skeletal alignment, pain management, nutritional needs, pressure relief, and skin integrity

Body structure and function impairments:

Nervous system

- Cognition
- Cortical visual impairment
- Marked hypotonia (head and trunk)
- Hypertonia (upper extremities' (UEs) and lower extremities' (LEs) flexors)
- Clonus with quick stretch of bilateral plantar flexors
- Selective neuromotor control
- Motor planning and learning
- Pain

Musculoskeletal system

- Marked weakness of oral, head, trunk, UEs', and LEs' musculature
- Initiating and sustaining movement of mouth, head, trunk, UEs, and LEs
- Alignment of UEs, head and trunk, and LEs with postures of flexion of head, shoulder retraction and external rotation, elbow flexion, wrist and finger flexion, hip flexion, abduction, external rotation, knee flexion, and plantar flexion
- Hypermobility of head and trunk
- Hypomobility of UEs and LEs
- Coordination of oral, head, trunk, UEs', and LEs' musculature
- Osteopenia

Circulatory system

- Cardiovascular endurance
- Distal circulatory perfusion with cool distal extremities
- *Pulmonary system*
- Abdominal breathing
- Flared posture of rib cage
- Weakened cough strength
- Sleep apnea

Gastrointestinal system

- Aspiration risk
- Swallowing dysfunction
- Sialorrhea/Drooling

Integumentary

- Potential for skin breakdown
- Spinal and hip scars

Sensory systems

- Vision—cortical visual impairment; latency; see red, yellow, and green primarily; can attend with low levels of background noise; light, reflective qualities, and movements assist with vision; dark background beneficial
- Auditory—intact
- Tactile and proprioception—limited experiences, tolerates input
- Vestibular—limited experiences, tolerates input

Activity Limitations

- Typical learning methods
- Receptive language/communication
- Expressive language/communication
- Swallowing
- Seeing and interpreting complex visual information
- Eating with mouth to meet nutritional needs
- Dependent for bed mobility or positional changes

- Unsupported sitting
- Unsupported standing
- Dependent for mobility
- Dependent for transitions/transfers
- Dependent for dressing
- Dependent for bathing
- Incontinent
- Reaching
- Grasping
- Normal sleeping durations and habits
- Physical activity

Participation Restrictions

- Successful learning of academic and life skills material in a regular education classroom
- Fitness and extracurricular programming in typical school and community environments

Participation desires of parents/caregivers

Active participation in school and community environments where health care and educational needs can be maximized and managed

- Aquatic Therapy
- Attend church
- Go on vacation to Atlanta to visit family
- Family picnic
- *Participation barriers*
- Managing caregiver demands
- Managing health care appointments
- Public transportation for wheelchair
- Wheelchair accessibility in community environments
- Knowledgeable human assistance and assistive technology required to accommodate for impairments, activity limitations, and promotion for active participation
- Life expectations and opportunities set too low by others
- Liability concerns of community organizations
- Funding

Environmental Enhancers

- Grandmother is a licensed practical nurse so the level of care at home is excellent
- BiPAP at night
- Ankle foot orthoses
- Hospital bed in home
- Hoyer lift in home
- Ramp into home
- Roll-in shower
- Certified nursing assistant in home to assist grandmother with activities of daily living
- Stander at school
- Power mobility at school for brief and safe environmental exploration
- Switch assistive technology (simple and brief episodes of communication at school)

Environmental Barriers

- No family-owned wheelchair transportation so dependent on Medicaid transportation
- Lower socioeconomics

Appendix C.

Goal Attainment Scaling Examples for a Child with Multiple Disabilities

	Scale 1—Gross Motor	Scale 2—Feeding	Scale 3—Self-Care	Scale 4—Language with Assistive Technology
Level of Attainment	By September 2012, V will increase her gross motor skills by standing in a vibrating supine stander with bilateral AFOs and immobilizers, 80% of trials over 5 days, as recorded on data sheets by faculty and staff, thus improving health related quality of life which is influenced by health and education.	By September 2012, V will demonstrate oral motor skills by tasting different foods with no facial grimacing, 80% of trials as recorded on data sheets by faculty and staff, thus improving health related quality of life which is influenced by health and education.	By September 2012, V will demonstrate daily living skills by wiping her mouth with a red washcloth, 80% of trials over 5 days, as recorded on data sheets by faculty and staff, thus improving health related quality of life which is influenced by health and education.	By September 2012, V will use a button switch in her right hand (with hands splints on) to socialize with others, 80% of trials over 5 days as recorded on data sheets by faculty and staff, thus improving health related quality of life which is influenced by health and education.
Much Less −2 than expected	V will stand in a vibrating supine stander angled at 70 degrees with bilateral AFOs and immobilizers for 20 min while participating in classroom instruction and interacting with classmates.	During school breakfast and/or lunch time and to enhance oral motor experiences, V will taste 1 different food with no facial grimacing.	When asked and with red washcloth placed in her hand, V will wipe saliva from her mouth within 5 min to promote oral hygiene and social acceptance.	V will use her spec switch in her right hand (with hands splints on) to socialize with others one time throughout the school day.
Somewhat less −1 than expected	V will stand in a vibrating supine stander angled at 70 degrees with bilateral AFOs and immobilizers for 30 min while participating in classroom instruction and interacting with classmates.	During school breakfast and/or lunch time and to enhance oral motor experiences, V will taste 2 different foods with no facial grimacing.	When asked and with red washcloth placed in her hand, V will wipe saliva from her mouth within 4 min to promote oral hygiene and social acceptance.	V will use her spec switch in her right hand (with hands splints on) to socialize with others two times throughout the school day.
Expected level 0 of outcome	V will stand in a vibrating supine stander angled at 70 degrees with bilateral AFOs and immobilizers for 40 min while participating in classroom instruction and interacting with classmates.	During school breakfast and/or lunch time and to enhance oral motor experiences, V will taste 3 different foods with no facial grimacing.	When asked and with red washcloth placed in her hand, V will wipe saliva from her mouth within 3 min to promote oral hygiene and social acceptance.	V will use her spec switch in her right hand (with hands splints on) to socialize with others three times throughout the school day.

	Scale 1—Gross Motor	Scale 2—Feeding	Scale 3—Self-Care	Scale 4—Language with Assistive Technology
Somewhat more +1 than expected	V will stand in a vibrating supine stander angled at 70 degrees with bilateral AFOs and immobilizers for 50 min while participating in classroom instruction and interacting with classmates.	During school breakfast and/or lunch time and to enhance oral motor experiences, V will taste 4 different foods with no facial grimacing.	When asked and with red washcloth placed in her hand, V will wipe saliva from her mouth within 2 min to promote oral hygiene and social acceptance.	V will use her spec switch in her right hand (with hands splints on) to socialize with others four times throughout the school day.
Much more +2 than expected	V will stand in a vibrating supine stander angled at 70 degrees with bilateral AFOs and immobilizers for 60 min while participating in classroom instruction and interacting with classmates.	During school breakfast and/or lunch time and to enhance oral motor experiences, V will taste 5 different foods with no facial grimacing.	When asked and with red washcloth placed in her hand, V will wipe saliva from her mouth within 1 min to promote oral hygiene and social acceptance.	V will use her spec switch in her right hand (with hands splints on) to socialize with others five times throughout the school day.

Appendix D.

Goal Attainment Scaling Data Collection Sheet modified from Murdoch Center Data Sheet

Name: VH Teacher: KLKW				Start date: September 2011		End date: September 2012		
Aim: By September 2012, VH will demonstrate motor skills by using a remote control with her right hand, 80% of trials over 5 days, as recorded on data sheets by team members, thus improving health related quality of life which is influenced by health and education.								
Materials: small red box, streamers, ounce weights				Motivator: red is power color, social interactions, movement				

	I A G P M	I A G P M	I A G P M	I A G P M	I A G P M	I A G P M	I A G P M	I A G P M	I A G P M
When asked, Vanilla will grasp and shake a small 1-pound red box (remote) with red streamers on it with her right hand for 15 seconds within 5 minutes.	I A G P M	I A G P M	I A G P M	I A G P M	I A G P M	I A G P M	I A G P M	I A G P M	I A G P M
	I A G P M	I A G P M	I A G P M	I A G P M	I A G P M	I A G P M	I A G P M	I A G P M	I A G P M
When asked, Vanilla will grasp and shake a small 0.5-pound box (remote) with red streamers attached, using her right hand for 15 seconds.	I A (G) (P) M 09-02-11	I (A) G P M 9/08/11 CD	I A G P M	I A G P M	I A G P M	I A G P M	I A G P M	I A G P M	I A G P M

References

1. United Nations Children's Fund. *Promoting the Rights of Children with Disabilities*; United Nations Children's Fund: Florence, Italy, 2007.
2. National Center for Education Statistics. Students with Disabilities. 2022. Available online: https://nces.ed.gov/programs/coe/indicator/cgg (accessed on 21 February 2023).
3. US Department of Education. *Individuals with Disabilities Education Act*; US Department of Education: Washington, DC, USA, 2018.
4. Cohen, E.; Kuo, D.Z.; Agrawal, R.; Berry, J.G.; Bhagat, S.K.; Simon, T.D.; Srivastava, R. Children with medical complexity: An emerging population for clinical and research initiatives. *Pediatrics* **2011**, *127*, 529–538. [CrossRef] [PubMed]
5. World Health Organization. Classification of Functioning, Disability and Health. 2001. Available online: http://www.who.int/classifications/icf/en/ (accessed on 12 March 2002).
6. Glader, L.; Plews-Ogan, J.; Agrawal, R. Children with medical complexity: Creating a framework for care based on the International Classification of Functioning, Disability and Health. *Dev. Med. Child Neurol.* **2016**, *58*, 1116–1123. [CrossRef] [PubMed]
7. Nelson, C.; van Dijk, J.; McDonnell, A.P.; Thompson, K. The framework for understanding young children with severe disabilities: The van Dijk Approach to Assessment. *Res. Pract. Pers. Sev. Disabil.* **2002**, *27*, 97–111. [CrossRef]
8. Wolf-Schein, E.G. Considerations in Assessment of Children with Severe Disabilities including Deaf-Blindness and Autism. *Int. J. Disabil. Dev. Educ.* **1998**, *45*, 35–55. [CrossRef]
9. Berry, J.G.; Hall, M.; Cohen, E.; O'Neill, M.; Feudtner, C. Ways to Identify Children with Medical Complexity and the Importance of Why. *J. Pediatr.* **2015**, *167*, 229–237. [CrossRef]
10. Sarathy, K.; Doshi, C.; Aroojis, A. Clinical Examination of Children with Cerebral Palsy. *Indian J. Orthop.* **2019**, *53*, 35–44. [CrossRef]
11. Kiresuk, T.J.; Smith, A.; Cardillo, J.E. *Goal Attainment Scaling: Applications, Theory, and Measurement*; Lawrence Erlbaum Associates: New York, NY, USA, 1994.
12. Mailloux, Z.; May-Benson, T.A.; Summers, C.A.; Miller, L.J.; Brett-Green, B.; Burke, J.P.; Cohn, E.S.; Koomar, J.A.; Parham, L.D.; Roley, S.S.; et al. Goal attainment scaling as a measure of meaningful outcomes for children with sensory integration disorders. *Am. J. Occup. Ther.* **2007**, *61*, 254–259. [CrossRef]
13. Chiarello, L.A.; Effgen, S.K.; Jeffries, L.; McCoy, S.W.; Bush, H. Student Outcomes of School-Based Physical Therapy as Measured by Goal Attainment Scaling. *Pediatr. Phys. Ther.* **2016**, *28*, 277–284. [CrossRef]
14. Steenbeek, D.; Gorter, J.W.; Ketelaar, M.; Galama, K.; Lindeman, E. Responsiveness of Goal Attainment Scaling in comparison to two standardized measures in outcome evaluation of children with cerebral palsy. *Clin. Rehabil.* **2011**, *25*, 1128–1139. [CrossRef]
15. Haladay, D.; Swisher, L.; Hardwick, D. Goal attainment scaling for patients with low back pain in rehabilitation: A systematic review. *Health Sci. Rep.* **2021**, *4*, e378. [CrossRef]
16. Hoorntje, A.; Waterval-Witjes, S.; Koenraadt, K.L.; Kuijer, P.P.F.; Blankevoort, L.; Kerkhoffs, G.M.; van Geenen, R.C. Goal Attainment Scaling Rehabilitation Improves Satisfaction with Work Activities for Younger Working Patients After Knee Arthroplasty: Results from the Randomized Controlled ACTION Trial. *J. Bone Jt. Surg. Am. Vol.* **2020**, *102*, 1445–1453. [CrossRef] [PubMed]
17. Harpster, K.; Sheehan, A.; Foster, E.A.; Leffler, E.; Schwab, S.M.; Angeli, J.M. The methodological application of goal attainment scaling in pediatric rehabilitation research: A systematic review. *Disabil. Rehabil.* **2019**, *41*, 2855–2864. [CrossRef] [PubMed]
18. Dodds, C.B.; Bjornson, K.F.; Sweeney, J.K.; Narayanan, U. The effects of supported physical activity on parental-reported health-related quality of life in children with medical complexity. *J. Pediatr. Rehabil. Med.* **2015**, *8*, 83–95. [CrossRef] [PubMed]
19. Doran, G.T. There's a SMART way to write management's goals and objectives. *Manag. Rev.* **1981**, *70*, 35–36.
20. Krasny-Pacini, A.; Pauly, F.; Hiebel, J.; Godon, S.; Isner-Horobeti, M.E.; Chevignard, M. Feasibility of a shorter Goal Attainment Scaling method for a pediatric spasticity clinic—The 3-milestones GAS. *Ann. Phys. Rehabil. Med.* **2017**, *60*, 249–257. [CrossRef] [PubMed]
21. King, G.A.; McDougall, J.; Palisano, R.J.; Gritzan, J.; Tucker, M.A. Goal attainment scaling: Its use in evaluating pediatric therapy programs. *Phys. Occup. Ther. Pediatr.* **1999**, *19*, 31–52. [CrossRef]
22. Gaffney, E.; Gaffney, K.; Bartleson, L.; Dodds, C. Goal Attainment Scaling Made Easy With an App: GOALed. *Pediatr. Phys. Ther.* **2019**, *31*, 225–230. [CrossRef]
23. Portney, L.G.; Watkins, M.P. *Foundations of Clinical Research Applications to Practice*, 2nd ed.; Prentice Hall Heallth, Inc.: Upper Saddle River, NJ, USA, 2000.
24. Dykes, M.K.; Erin, J.N. *Developmental Assessment for Individuals with Severe Disabilities*; Pro-Ed: Austin, TX, USA, 1999.
25. Narayanan, U.G.; Fehlings, D.; Weir, S.; Knights, S.; Kiran, S.; Campbell, K. Initial development and validation of the Caregiver Priorities and Child Health Index of Life with Disabilities (CPCHILD). *Dev. Med. Child Neurol.* **2006**, *48*, 804–812. [CrossRef]
26. Dodds, C.B.; Bjornson, K.F.; Sweeney, J.K.; Narayanan, U.G. The effect of supported physical activity on parental-reported sleep qualities and pain severity in children with medical complexity. *J. Pediatr. Rehabil. Med.* **2016**, *9*, 195–206. [CrossRef]
27. Daly, C.; Moore, C.L.; Johannes, S.; Middleton, J.; Kenyon, L.K. Pilot Evaluation of a School-Based Programme Focused on Activity, Fitness, and Function among Children with Cerebral Palsy at GMFCS Level IV: Single-Subject Research Design. *Physiother. Can.* **2020**, *72*, 195–204. [CrossRef]

28. Bieri, D.; Reeve, R.A.; Champion, G.D.; Addicoat, L.; Ziegler, J.B. The Faces Pain Scale for the self-assessment of the severity of pain experienced by children: Development, initial validation, and preliminary investigation for ratio scale properties. *Pain* **1990**, *41*, 139–150. [CrossRef] [PubMed]
29. Parker, J.; Belew, J.L. Qualitative evaluation of a pain intensity screen for children with severe neurodevelopmental disabilities. *Pain Manag. Nurs.* **2013**, *14*, e115–e123. [CrossRef] [PubMed]
30. Tomlinson, D.; von Baeyer, C.L.; Stinson, J.N.; Sung, L. A systematic review of faces scales for the self-report of pain intensity in children. *Pediatrics* **2010**, *126*, e1168–e1198. [CrossRef] [PubMed]
31. Haley, S.; Coster, W.J.; Ludow, L.; LHaltiwanger, J. *Pediatric Evaluation of Disability Inventory*; Boston University: Boston, MA, USA, 1992.
32. Berg, M.; Jahnsen, R.; Froslie, K.F.; Hussain, A. Reliability of the Pediatric Evaluation of Disability Inventory (PEDI). *Phys. Occup. Ther. Pediatr.* **2004**, *24*, 61–77. [CrossRef]
33. Shore, B.J.; Allar, B.G.; Miller, P.E.; Matheney, T.H.; Snyder, B.D.; Fragala-Pinkham, M. Measuring the Reliability and Construct Validity of the Pediatric Evaluation of Disability Inventory-Computer Adaptive Test (PEDI-CAT) in Children with Cerebral Palsy. *Arch. Phys. Med. Rehabil.* **2019**, *100*, 45–51. [CrossRef]
34. Roman-Lantzy, C. *Cortical Visual Impairment*; American Foundation for the Blind Press: New York, NY, USA, 2007.
35. McConnell, E.L.; Saunders, K.J.; Little, J.A. What assessments are currently used to investigate and diagnose cerebral visual impairment (CVI) in children? A systematic review. *Ophthalmic Physiol. Opt.* **2021**, *41*, 224–244. [CrossRef]
36. Roman-Lantzy, C. *Cortical Visual Impairment: An Approach to Assessment and Intervention*, 2nd ed.; American Foundation for the Blind Press: New York, NY, USA, 2018.
37. Zapf, S.A.; Scherer, M.J.; Baxter, M.F.; D, H.R. Validating a measure to assess factors that affect assistive technology use by students with disabilities in elementary and secondary education. *Disabil. Rehabil. Assist. Technol.* **2016**, *11*, 38–49.
38. Patrick, D.L.; Chiang, Y.P. Measurement of health outcomes in treatment effectiveness evaluations: Conceptual and methodological challenges. *Med. Care* **2000**, *38* (Suppl. S9), II14–II25. [CrossRef]
39. Dodds, C.; Rempel, G. A quality of life model promotes enablement for children with medical complexity. *J. Pediatr. Rehabil. Med.* **2016**, *9*, 253–255. [CrossRef]
40. Autism Classroom Resources. The Murdoch Program Library A Library of Task Analyses Data Sheet. Available online: https://autismclassroomresources.com/murdoch-program-library-a-tool-for-teaching-life-skills/ (accessed on 17 January 2022).
41. Harty, M.; Griesel, M.; van der Merwe, A. The ICF as a common language for rehabilitation goal-setting: Comparing client and professional priorities. *Health Qual Life Outcomes* **2011**, *9*, 87. [CrossRef]
42. Novak, I.; Morgan, C.; Fahey, M.; Finch-Edmondson, M.; Galea, C.; Hines, A.; Langdon, K.; Namara, M.M.; Paton, M.C.B.; Popat, H.; et al. State of the Evidence Traffic Lights 2019: Systematic Review of Interventions for Preventing and Treating Children with Cerebral Palsy. *Curr. Neurol. Neurosci. Rep.* **2020**, *20*, 3. [CrossRef] [PubMed]
43. Pritchard-Wiart, L.; Thompson-Hodgetts, S.; McKillop, A.B.; Rosychuk, R.; Mrklas, K.; Zwaigenbaum, L.; Zwicker, J.; Andersen, J.; King, G.; Firouzeh, P. A multi-center, pragmatic, effectiveness-implementation (hybrid I) cluster randomized controlled trial to evaluate a child-oriented goal-setting approach in paediatric rehabilitation (the ENGAGE approach): A study protocol. *BMC Pediatr.* **2022**, *22*, 375. [CrossRef]
44. Christensen, R.; MacIntosh, A.; Switzer, L.; Fehlings, D. Change in pain status in children with cerebral palsy. *Dev. Med. Child Neurol.* **2017**, *59*, 374–379. [CrossRef] [PubMed]

Disclaimer/Publisher's Note: The statements, opinions and data contained in all publications are solely those of the individual author(s) and contributor(s) and not of MDPI and/or the editor(s). MDPI and/or the editor(s) disclaim responsibility for any injury to people or property resulting from any ideas, methods, instructions or products referred to in the content.

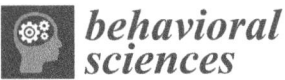

Article

Outcomes Associated with a Single Joystick-Operated Ride-on-Toy Navigation Training Incorporated into a Constraint-Induced Movement Therapy Program: A Pilot Feasibility Study

Sudha Srinivasan [1,2,3,*], Nidhi Amonkar [1,2,3], Patrick Kumavor [4], Kristin Morgan [4] and Deborah Bubela [1,2,3]

1 Physical Therapy Program, Department of Kinesiology, University of Connecticut, Storrs, CT 06268, USA; nidhi.amonkar@uconn.edu (N.A.); deborah.bubela@uconn.edu (D.B.)
2 Institute for Collaboration on Health, Intervention, and Policy (InCHIP), University of Connecticut, Storrs, CT 06268, USA
3 The Institute for the Brain and Cognitive Sciences (IBACS), University of Connecticut, Storrs, CT 06268, USA
4 Biomedical Engineering Department, University of Connecticut, Storrs, CT 06268, USA; patrick.d.kumavor@uconn.edu (P.K.); kristin.2.morgan@uconn.edu (K.M.)
* Correspondence: sudha.srinivasan@uconn.edu; Tel.: +1-860-486-6192

Citation: Srinivasan, S.; Amonkar, N.; Kumavor, P.; Morgan, K.; Bubela, D. Outcomes Associated with a Single Joystick-Operated Ride-on-Toy Navigation Training Incorporated into a Constraint-Induced Movement Therapy Program: A Pilot Feasibility Study. *Behav. Sci.* **2023**, *13*, 413. https://doi.org/10.3390/bs13050413

Academic Editors: Stephanie C. DeLuca and Jill C. Heathcock

Received: 16 March 2023
Revised: 10 May 2023
Accepted: 11 May 2023
Published: 15 May 2023

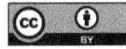

Copyright: © 2023 by the authors. Licensee MDPI, Basel, Switzerland. This article is an open access article distributed under the terms and conditions of the Creative Commons Attribution (CC BY) license (https:// creativecommons.org/licenses/by/ 4.0/).

Abstract: Our research aims to evaluate the utility of joystick-operated ride-on-toys (ROTs) as therapeutic adjuncts to improve upper extremity (UE) function in children with hemiplegic cerebral palsy (HCP). This study assessed changes in affected UE use and function following a three-week ROT navigation training incorporated into an existing constraint-induced movement therapy (CIMT) camp in 11 children (3–14 years old) with HCP. We report changes in scores on the standardized Shriners Hospital Upper Extremity Evaluation (SHUEE) from pretest-to-posttest and changes from early-to-late sessions in percent time spent by the affected arm in: (a) "moderate-to-vigorous activity", "light activity" and "no activity" bouts based on accelerometer data and (b) "independent", "assisted", and "no activity" bouts based on video data. We also explored relationships between standardized measures and training-specific measures of affected UE activity. We found small-to-medium improvements in the SHUEE scores. Between 90 and 100% of children also showed medium-to-large improvements in affected UE activity from early-to-late sessions using accelerometers and small improvements via video-based assessments. Exploratory analyses suggested trends for relationships between pretest-posttest and training-specific objective and subjective measures of arm use and function. Our pilot data suggest that single joystick-operated ROTs may serve as motivating, child-friendly tools that can augment conventional therapies such as CIMT to boost treatment dosing, promote affected UE movement practice during real-world navigation tasks, and ultimately improve functional outcomes in children with HCP.

Keywords: joystick-operated ride-on-toys; children with hemiplegic cerebral palsy; novel technologies for rehabilitation; upper extremity function; wrist-worn accelerometers

1. Introduction

Children with hemiplegic cerebral palsy (HCP) have impaired upper extremity (UE) function on one side of the body with significant hand involvement that leads to considerable limitations in their ability to engage with and learn from their environment [1,2]. Over the last few decades, intensive research on treatment paradigms for improving UE function in children with HCP has led to expanding evidence in favor of task-oriented and intensive approaches [3]. One such evidence-based approach that has evolved out of the adult stroke literature but has also proven to be effective in children with HCP is called constraint-induced movement therapy (CIMT) [4–8]. This paradigm involves constraining the child's unaffected side and encouraging repetitive practice of using the affected UE through structured and intensive UE therapies. Although there is considerable variation within the literature on CIMT in terms of dosing parameters (i.e., duration in weeks of the CIMT program and duration of hours per day of constraint and intensive UE therapy), effective CIMT programs require highly intensive and repetitive active practice using the affected UE during goal-oriented activities [8–11]. While high dosing is critical to producing meaningful improvements in function through CIMT, clinicians frequently struggle to design activities that children find intrinsically motivating and that will promote sustained adherence with therapy [12–15]. In fact, therapists and researchers have long recognized that child motivation is related to gains in function and long-term compliance with therapy [16,17]. Children are more likely to practice activities that they find fun and that are aligned with their interests [18]. Therefore, there is a need to diversify conventional therapeutic activities to include novel training ideas and tools that are child-friendly, promote sensorimotor exploration and affected UE function, and encourage UE practice as part of children's daily play/routines within their naturalistic settings.

Our research team has been exploring the use of modified, commercially available joystick-operated ride-on-toys (ROTs) as therapeutic adjuncts to promote affected UE use and function in children with HCP. Powered ROTs with modified controls (e.g., hand-operated switches instead of leg pedals) have been used previously as early mobility solutions for young children with lower limb impairments, including children with CP and Down syndrome [19,20]. Their use among non-ambulatory children has led to improvements in mobility, social skills, and overall participation [20–24]. However, the use of ROTs to promote UE function has not been explored. We propose that joystick-operated ROTs may serve as engaging adjuncts to conventional care that can be used by clinicians and caregivers to increase treatment dosing and promote children's functional use of their affected UE for goal-directed navigation within a variety of indoor and outdoor naturalistic settings.

This paper is the third in a series of manuscripts that report data from a pilot study exploring the feasibility of implementation and preliminary efficacy of the ROT training integrated into a three-week CIMT-based camp to promote affected UE use/function among children with HCP. Previously, we reported that the ROT training was feasible to implement within the camp setting and was well-received by children, caregivers, and clinicians. Children expressed the desire to repeat the program and both caregivers and clinicians reported observing improvements in children's use of their affected UEs as well as motor function following the training [25]. In the second paper, we report improvements in video-based measures of arm control and navigational accuracy following the ROT training provided within the CIMT camp ([26] under review). In the present manuscript, we report the combined effects of the ROT training and CIMT activities on objective and subjective measures of affected UE function. Specifically, we will report on changes in movement quantity (measured using wrist-worn accelerometers) and quality (assessed using standardized tests and training-specific measures) following the training. We will also explore relationships between affected UE use/control during ROT operation within training sessions and hand-use during everyday functional activities outside the training context.

We hypothesize that children will show improvements in affected UE use and motor function as assessed using qualitative and quantitative measures within the ROT training context as well as outside the training sessions. Moreover, we hypothesize that training-specific measures of motor function will show trends for associations with children's motor performance outside the training context on a standardized test.

2. Materials and Methods

2.1. Participants

Eleven children with HCP (6M, 5F; 8 children with right-sided involvement and 3 children with left-sided involvement) between 3 and 14 years (mean (SD): 6.54 (2.76); 7 Caucasian, 1 Hispanic, 3 of mixed ethnicity), with a moderate level of impairment (mean (SD): 2.64 (0.67), see Table 1 for scores on the manual ability classification system (MACS) [27] participated in the single group pre–post study. The study was conducted within a three-week CIMT-based summer camp. The study was approved by the Institutional Review Board (IRB) at the University of Connecticut, Storrs.

Table 1. Demographic details of study participants.

Child Number	Age at Visit	Gender	Race/Ethnicity	Side of Involvement	MACS Levels
1	3 years 5 months	F	White, Non-Hispanic	L	3
2	13 years 10 months	F	Asian	R	3
3	8 years 11 months	M	White, Non-Hispanic	R	3
4	4 years 6 months	F	White, Non-Hispanic	L	2
5	5 years 28 days	M	Multiracial-Korean, Puerto Rican, Irish, and Polish	R	2
6	8 years 3 months	F	White, Hispanic	R	2
7	6 years 11 months	F	White, Non-Hispanic	R	2
8	8 years 7 months	M	White, Hispanic	R	3
9	4 years 2 months	M	White, Non-Hispanic	L	4
10	6 years 11 months	M	Multiracial-White, Asian	R	2
11	7 years 5 months	M	White, Non-Hispanic	R	3

MACS: Manual ability classification system.

The single joystick-operated ride-on-toy navigation training was incorporated into the Lefty and Righty Camp of Connecticut (LARC), an annually held summer camp for children with HCP, based on principles of the CIMT. The camp activities were designed to provide children with playful movement experiences to improve gross and fine motor function of the affected UE. The ride-on-toy training was offered as one of the daily activities at camp for each child (see details of the camp and the ROT training within the section on procedures). Parental permission and child written/oral assent were obtained prior to any testing or training procedures.

2.2. Outcome Measures and Materials

2.2.1. Pretest–Posttest Measures of Motor Function

The Shriners Hospital Upper Extremity Evaluation (SHUEE) is a standardized, valid, and reliable test to assess movement quality in 3–18-year-old children (inter-rater reliability: 0.89–0.90 (ICC), intra-rater reliability: 0.98–0.99 (ICC)) [28]. The test assesses affected UE use spontaneously and on tester demand during 16 bimanual tasks [29]. The test has 3 parts: spontaneous functional analysis (SFA), dynamic positional analysis (DPA), and grasp-release analysis. At present, there are no data available on standard error of measurement or minimal clinically important difference (MCID) for the SHUEE. However, the SHUEE has been used to assess the efficacy of surgical interventions with children with HCP in multiple studies [30–33]. For this study, we analyzed changes in the total SFA scores (i.e., child's ability to spontaneously use the affected UE during bimanual tasks) and total DPA scores (i.e., segmental alignment of the affected UE at the elbow, forearm, wrist, fingers, and thumb while performing tasks on demand) from pretest (prior to camp) to posttest (following the camp). A single coder coded all the data after establishing intra-rater reliability and inter-rater reliability (with the first and second authors) of over 90% using 20% of the videos.

2.2.2. Training-Specific Measures Assessed during Early and Late Sessions
Objective Accelerometry-Based Assessment of Affected UE Activity during ROT Navigation

Children wore the wGT3X-BT accelerometers (ActiGraph, Pensacola, FL, USA) on the wrist of their affected arm during the entire duration of the ROT training sessions in the first and last weeks of the training program. The wGT3X-BT accelerometer is a small (4.6 × 3.3 × 1.5 cm), lightweight (19 g), 3-axis accelerometer that collects raw acceleration data in all 3 directions with a dynamic range of ±8 g (gravitational units). The accelerometers collected data at a sampling frequency of 30 Hz. Trainers maintained activity diaries of the exact times of the training sessions every day for each child to corroborate the data obtained from the accelerometers. For their data to be included within the analysis, children were required to wear the accelerometer during the ROT training sessions on at least 3 training sessions at each time point (early and late training weeks). Since children were seated in the ROT during the training sessions, data collected through the activity monitor is solely representative of affected UE activity during the training sessions.

At the end of the first and last weeks, data stored in the accelerometers for each child was downloaded using the ActiLife software (ActiGraph, Pensacola, FL, USA). The raw data from the accelerometers were processed using ActiGraph's proprietary algorithms to obtain activity counts (1 count = 0.001664 g, i.e., 0.0163072 m/s^2). Activity counts across 3 axes were summed to calculate vector magnitude (VM) counts as follows:

$$VM = \sqrt{(a\_x^2 + a\_y^2 + a\_z^2)},$$

where a_x, a_y, and a_z are the accelerations in the x-, y-, and z-directions, respectively. We assessed changes in average VM counts (averaged across all training sessions during a week) across early and late training weeks. Moreover, the in-built, Freedson children algorithm was used to classify average activity counts calculated over 60 s epochs during ROT navigation sessions across the entire week into time spent (in minutes) by the affected UE in activities of varying intensity (sedentary: 0–149 counts, light activity: 150–499 counts, and moderate-to-vigorous activity: >500 counts) [30]. The minimal clinically important difference (MCID) for the arm accelerometry is a change of 575–752 counts [31]. Please note that MCID values for arm accelerometry are based on data from adult persons with chronic hemiparesis since no similar data are available from children with HCP. We report changes in the average percent time spent by the affected UE in sedentary, light, and moderate-to-vigorous activity during ROT navigation sessions across early and late training weeks.

Video-Based Assessment of Affected UE Activity during ROT Navigation

Video data of early and late training sessions were coded using Datavyu© behavioral coding software that allows millisecond-to-millisecond coding of behaviors. A single coder coded all data after establishing intra-rater and inter-rater reliability (with a second coder) of over 90% using a subset of videos (20%) from the study. We coded affected UE activity during ROT navigation based on video data from 2 early and 2 late training sessions. Specifically, each ROT session was broken down into time blocks of "independent", "assisted", and "no activity" bouts. "Independent" activity bouts were defined as periods when the child independently maneuvered the joystick of the ROT using their affected UE without any assistance from an adult/external aid. "Assisted" activity bouts included instances where the child required assistance for controlling the joystick with their affected UE. The assistance could be in the form of an external aid (such as a mitt) to help the child grasp the joystick or the adult trainer providing partial or total assistance to help the child push/maneuver the joystick. "No activity" bouts included periods when the child was stationary, and the affected UE was not used to maneuver the joystick of the ROT. We report on the average percent duration of time of independent, assisted, and no activity bouts in the affected UE during early and late training sessions.

2.3. Procedures

2.3.1. Camp Structure and Activities

The three-week intensive, 6 h/day (9 am to 3 pm) summer camp provided group-based CIMT for children with HCP. During the daily six hours at camp, all children wore removable thermoplastic casts on their unaffected UE. Children were encouraged to use their affected side throughout the day during goal-directed gross and fine motor activities/games, as well as functional self-care tasks such as eating and toileting. Each child worked one-on-one with a camp staff who was a trained paraprofessional under the supervision of licensed physical and occupational therapists.

2.3.2. Ride-on-Toy Training Program

The ROT training was incorporated into the camp routine and was offered as one of the daily activities at camp. Each ROT session lasted for around 20–30 min/day. Please note that children received an overall 90 h of CIMT (6 h/day, 5 days/week, 3 weeks) at camp, of which 8 h involved ROT training. Our research team modified a commercially available, dual joystick-operated ROT, the Wild Thing^{TM}, to allow operation in a single joystick mode and provided additional postural support (using PVC pipes for reinforcement of the external frame of the toy; see Figure 1). As part of the ROT training program, children engaged in: (a) incrementally challenging navigation games across different environmental layouts and (b) gross and fine motor UE tasks at intermediate stations along the navigational path. To drive the ROT, children were required to use their affected UE to push/pull and maneuver the joystick in the desired direction of motion. Early sessions focused on teaching the child basic joystick controls for moving forward–backward and making turns. Thereafter, the training was progressed to challenge children to stay on paths of different shapes and sizes (arc, roundabout, slalom, etc.) and avoid obstacles during navigation. Children also completed UE gross and fine tasks at intermediate stations during navigation; the tasks involved multidirectional reaching, catching and throwing objects, different grasps, release, and in-hand manipulation of playful props such as balls and bean bags. The training was based on principles of motor learning and promoted discovery learning, variable practice, active problem-solving, and free play/exploration.

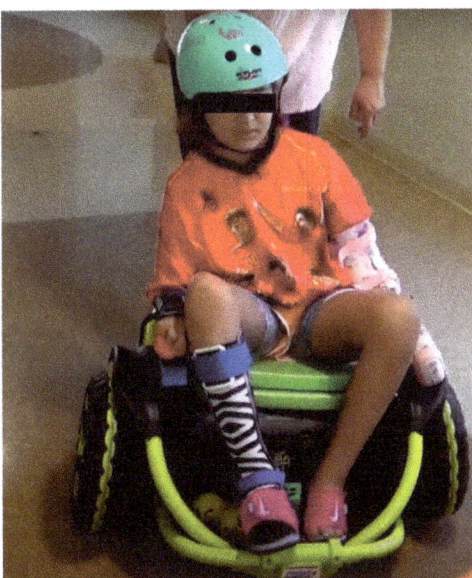

Figure 1. The Wild Thing^{TM} ride-on-toy used for the study.

We focused on promoting functional UE movement patterns during the ROT navigation program. Grasp and operation of the joystick required wrist extensor, finger flexor, and hand intrinsic muscles while the forearm was maintained in pronation. In addition, children used proximal muscles at the elbow and shoulder to control push–pull movements of the joystick in all 4 directions (forward, backward, right turn, and left turn). In our experience, children with poor UE control tend to also use proximal scapular and trunk muscles to move the joysticks. As discussed above, we also incorporated a variety of functional UE tasks within the training program. Children performed these tasks while seated in the ROT at intermediate checkpoints/stations during navigation. These UE tasks involved gross motor activities such as reaching in different directions, overhead throwing, pulling, pushing, lifting, and tossing games as well as fine motor activities such as opening and closing, precision grips, picking, sticking, and releasing objects. While singular joint movements that are typically limited in HCP (forearm supination, wrist extension, and finger extension) were not addressed in isolation, these movements were encouraged as part of multi-joint movement patterns as children engaged in functional UE challenges/games throughout the ROT program.

2.4. Statistical Analyses

Data were checked for assumptions of parametric statistics. Since data satisfied the assumptions of parametric statistics, we used dependent t-tests to assess training-related changes in the standardized SHUEE from the pretest to posttest. We conducted Pillai's trace multivariate analyses of variance (MANOVAs) to evaluate changes in the training-specific measures: (a) wrist-worn accelerometry-based outcomes and (b) video-based estimates of affected UE activity. The MANOVA for accelerometry-based measures included time (early and late sessions) and affected UE activity (percent time spent in sedentary, light, and moderate-to-vigorous activity) as within-subjects factors. The MANOVA for video-based measures included time (early and late sessions) and affected UE activity (percent time engaged in independent, assisted, and no activity bouts) as within-subjects factors. If the analyses found a significant main effect and an interaction effect involving the same factors, post hoc t-tests were conducted to evaluate only the significant interactions. We used dependent t-tests to assess training-related changes in average VM counts/minute. Statistical significance was set at a p-value of <0.05. Effect sizes were calculated using Hedge's standardized mean difference (SMD) [32]. We report on SMD estimates and 95% confidence intervals (CI) surrounding the SMD values. We classified SMD values according to Cohen's conventions of small (0.2–0.49), medium (0.5–0.79), or large (0.8 and above) effects [33].

We also conducted exploratory analyses to evaluate trends for associations between pretest–posttest measures and assessments administered during training sessions (accelerometry and video-based coding of affected UE use). We have used scatter plots to visually represent patterns of associations between measured variables using both pooled data (pooled across early and late sessions or pretest and posttest) and difference data (late–early session or posttest–pretest values). Given the small sample size in this pilot exploratory study, we will not conduct formal tests of significance for these plotted correlations between variables; instead, we interpret the visual data as being suggestive of preliminary trends for relationships between variables that we will confirm in our future studies using larger sample sizes and more robust study designs.

3. Results

3.1. Pretest–Posttest Measures of Affected UE Motor Function

From pretest to posttest, children showed significant medium-sized increases in the SFA scores on the standardized SHUEE (see Figure 2A,B; $t(10) = 4.114$, $p = 0.002$, SMD (95% CI) = 0.5 (−0.21 to 1.21)), with 10 out of 11 children following the group trend. All 11 children also showed small-to-medium increases in DPA scores (see Figure 2A,C; $t(10) = 5.977$, $p \leq 0.001$, SMD (95% CI) = 0.301 (−0.37 to 0.98)), specifically, in the positioning of the elbow ($t(10) = 2.324$, $p = 0.042$, SMD (95% CI) = 0.445 (−0.25 to 1.41)), forearm ($t(10) = 3.184$, $p = 0.010$, SMD (95% CI) = 0.302 (−0.37 to 0.98)) and wrist in the sagittal plane ($t(10) = -2.390$, $p = 0.038$, SMD (95% CI) = 0.152 (−0.51 to 0.81)). Overall, children showed a mean improvement of 9.29% on the SFA and 7.45% in total DPA scores.

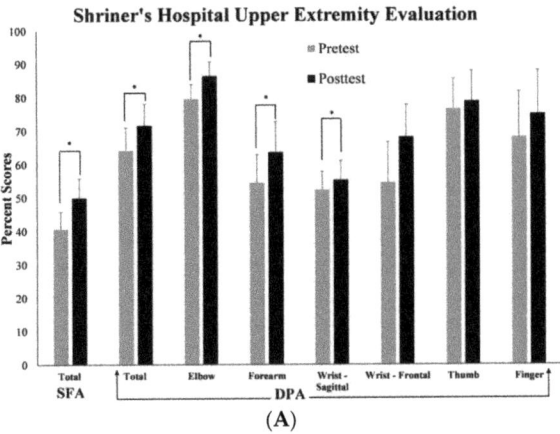

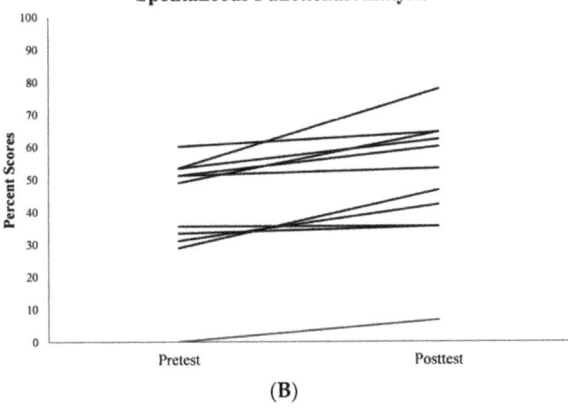

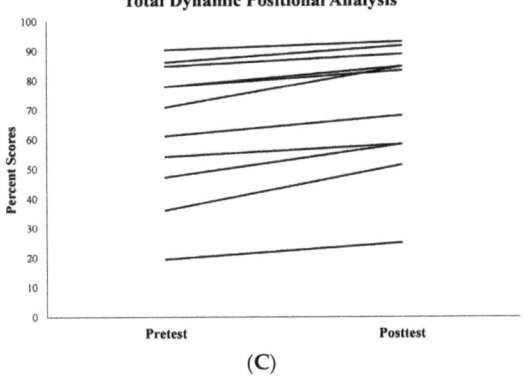

Figure 2. (**A**) Group data on training-related changes on the SHUEE assessed before and after the three-week ROT navigation + CIMT training. (**B**) Individual data on training-related changes in the SFA scores of the SHUEE assessed before and after the three-week ROT navigation + CIMT training. (**C**) Individual data on training-related changes in total DPA scores of the SHUEE assessed before and after the three-week ROT navigation + CIMT training. Please note that * signifies statistically significant differences in measured outcomes at $p \leq 0.05$.

3.2. Objective Accelerometry-Based Measures of Affected UE Activity during Training Sessions

The overall adherence rate with accelerometer wear was 100% and all children wore the monitor on their affected UE for a minimum of three ROT sessions during the week with no complaints. The MANOVA for the intensity of affected arm activity indicated a significant main effect of time ($F (2, 9) = 105.52$, $p < 0.001$, $n_p^2 = 0.95$) and an interaction effect of UE activity × time ($F (2, 9) = 13.48$, $p = 0.002$, $n_p^2 = 0.750$). Post hoc analyses of the significant interaction effect suggested that from early-to-late sessions, the percent time spent by the affected UE in light activity decreased by a large effect size (SMD (95% CI): −0.88 (−1.70 to −0.07)), with a concurrent medium-sized increase in time spent in moderate-to-vigorous activity (see Figure 3A, SMD (95% CI) = 0.72 (−0.04 to 1.49)).

Specifically, 10 out of 11 children decreased the time spent in light activity and all 11 children increased time spent in moderate-to-vigorous arm activity from early-to-late sessions (see Figure 3B,C). Children also showed a statistically significantly large increase in average VM counts/minute from early-to-late sessions (mean (SD): early: 1793.67 (790.7), late: 2490.06 (870.8); SMD (95% CI) = 0.81 (0.018 to 1.6)), with 10 out of 11 children, following these group trends. Overall, children showed a mean increase in VM counts of 696.39 counts/minute following training.

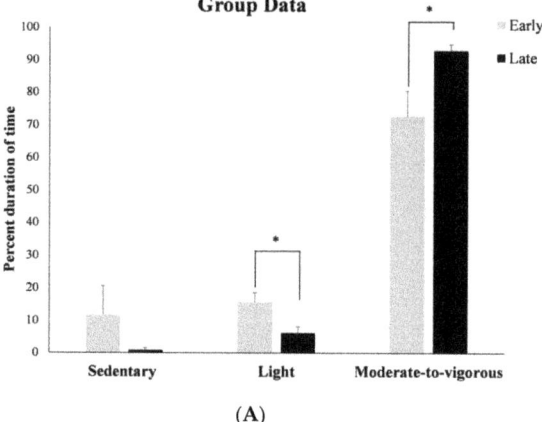

(A)

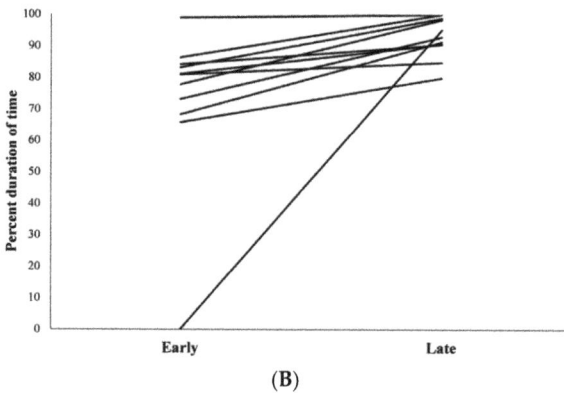

(B)

Figure 3. *Cont.*

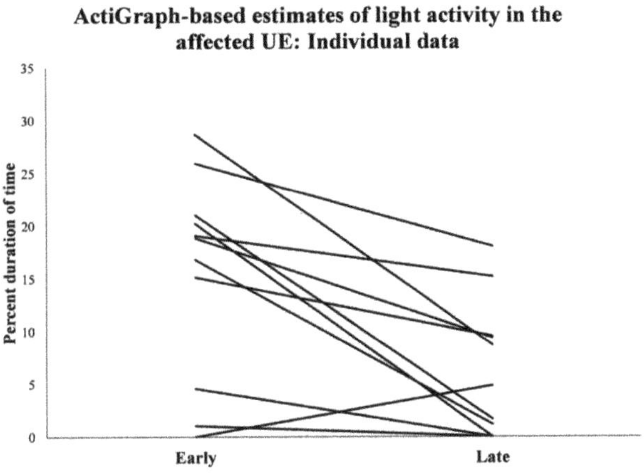

ActiGraph-based estimates of light activity in the affected UE: Individual data

(C)

Figure 3. (A) Group data on training-related changes in affected UE activity during ROT navigation training measured using wrist-worn accelerometers. (B) Individual data on training-related changes in "moderate-to-vigorous" activity in the affected UE during ROT navigation measured using wrist-worn accelerometers (note: the one child who showed a large increase in activity from early-to-late session had to be completely assisted by the trainer in the early session but was able to initiate independent UE activity to push the joystick by the late training weeks). (C) Individual data on training-related changes in "light" activity in the affected UE during ROT navigation measured using wrist-worn accelerometers. Please note that * signifies statistically significant differences in measured outcomes at $p \leq 0.05$.

3.3. Observational Video-Based Assessment of Affected UE Activity during Training Sessions

The MANOVA indicated a significant main effect of affected UE activity ($F(2, 9) = 17.13$, $p < 0.001$, $n_p^2 = 0.981$) and an interaction effect of affected UE activity × time ($F(2, 9) = 2.79$, $p = 0.001$, $n_p^2 = 0.770$). Post hoc testing of the significant interaction suggested that from early to late sessions, there was a significant small increase in the percent duration of "independent" UE activity bouts (SMD (95% CI) = 0.20 (0.19 to 1.95)) and a concurrent decrease in percent time spent by the affected UE in "assisted" activity bouts (SMD (95% CI) = −0.15 (−1.49 to 0.04)) and "no activity" bouts (SMD (95% CI) = −0.16 (−1.61 to −0.02)) (See Figure 4A–C).

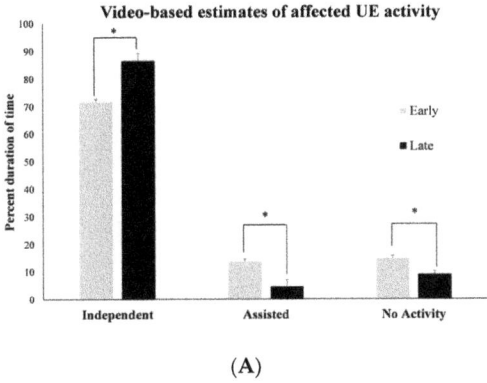

(A)

Figure 4. Cont.

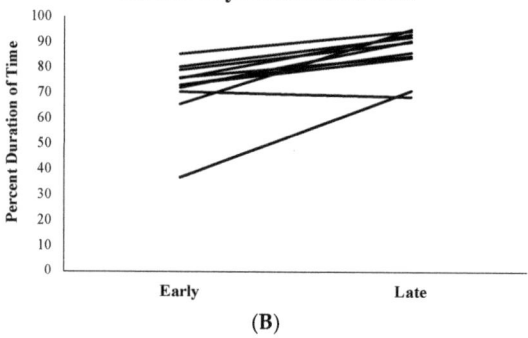

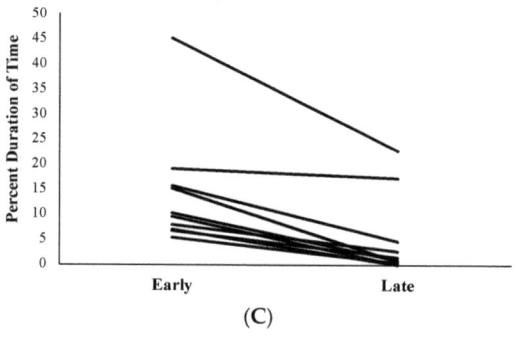

Figure 4. (**A**) Group data on training-related changes in affected UE activity during ROT navigation based on expert ratings of video data. (**B**) Individual data on training-related changes in "independent" use of the affected UE during ROT navigation as measured by video-based observational coding. (**C**) Individual data on training-related changes in "assisted" use of the affected UE activity during ROT navigation as measured by video-based observational coding. Please note that * signifies statistically significant differences in measured outcomes at $p \leq 0.05$.

3.4. Exploratory Analyses of Associations between Pretest–Posttest and Training-Specific Measures of Affected UE Activity

We used scatter plots to explore relationships between standardized and training-specific variables using pooled data (pooled across pretest and posttest or early and late sessions, see Figure 5A) and difference data (i.e., differences between posttest and pretest or late and early session performance; see Figure 5B). For these analyses, please note that we had one child who showed a large improvement with training; this child required complete assistance on their affected side to begin with, but their active use of the affected UE increased over the course of the training. This child's data are visually clearly separated from the rest of the group in some of the graphs (see Figure 5A,B). We therefore conducted exploratory analyses both with and without data from this child. We only report on data trends that showed similar patterns (in terms of direction and magnitude of associations) both with and without this child's data. In other words, we further discuss only preliminary associations between variables that were consistently observed across a majority of the children in the study. For the pooled data, we found a trend for a negative relationship between SHUEE SFA and DPA scores and time spent in assisted navigation, suggesting that children who were less likely to require assistance during ROT navigation had higher SHUEE scores. Moreover, our pilot data suggest preliminary associations between accelerometry-based quantitative measures and video-based subjective measures of affected UE use for navigation (see Figure 5A). Specifically, time spent in moderate-to-vigorous arm activity showed a trend for being positively related with "independent" activity bouts and negatively related with "assisted" navigation (see Figure 5A). On the other hand, time classified as sedentary was related positively with "assisted" mobility bouts. Overall, these exploratory trends suggest that children who were able to drive the ROT independently using their affected UE indicated by video data tended to demonstrate higher levels of moderate-to-vigorous activity with their affected UE and lower levels of sedentary time as measured by wrist-worn accelerometers (see Figure 5A).

Exploratory scatter plots visualizing relationships between variables for difference data (posttest-pretest or late-early sessions) suggested a trend for improvements in SHUEE scores (from pretest to posttest) to be associated with an increase in "independent" activity and a decrease in "no activity" bouts (from early to late sessions) based on video data, as well as a concurrent decrease in percent time spent in light activity as measured by accelerometers from early to late sessions (see Figure 5B).

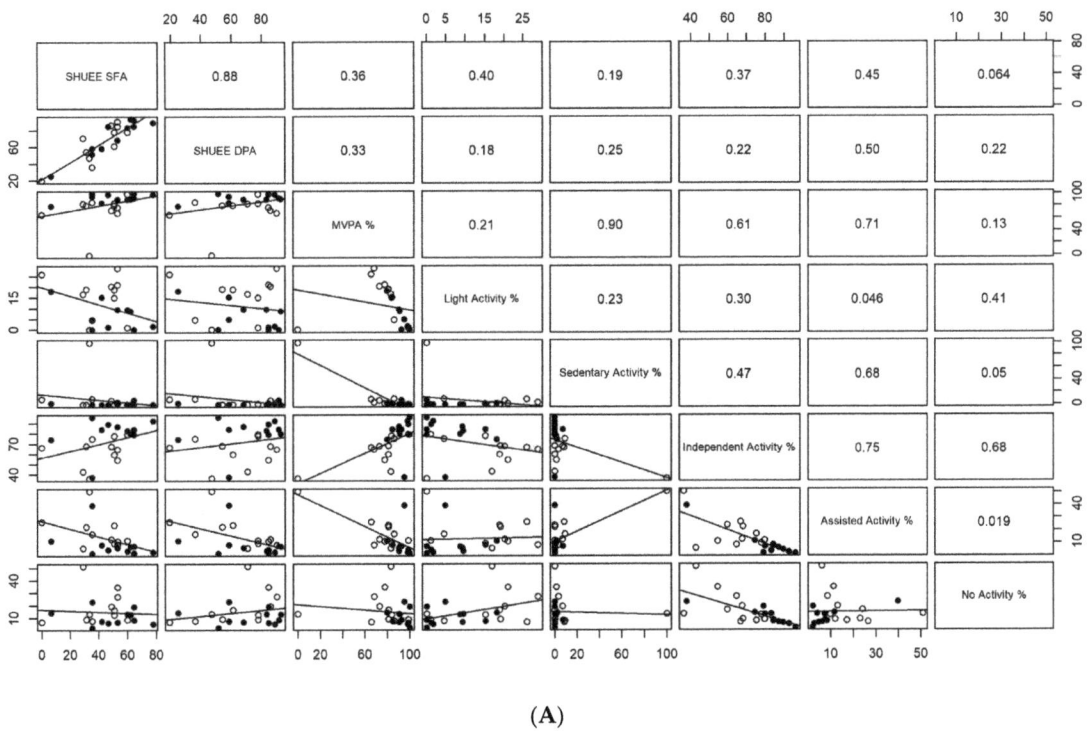

(A)

Figure 5. *Cont.*

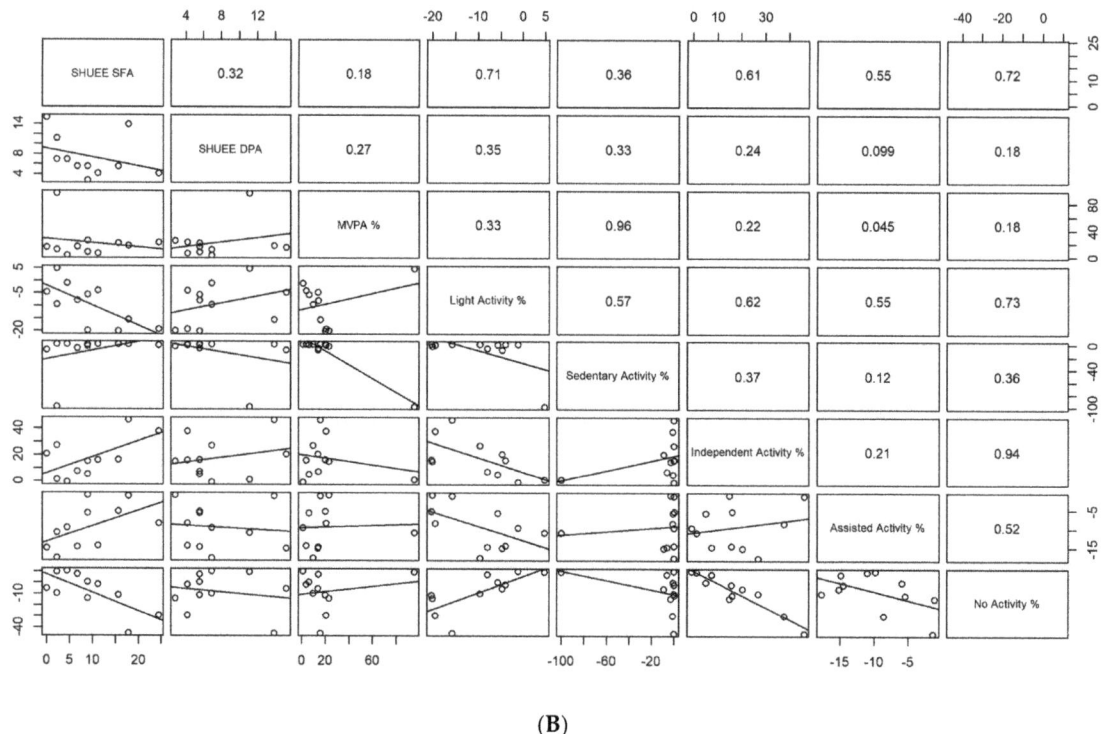

(B)

Figure 5. (**A**) Scatter plots of pooled data from standardized and training-specific measures collected in the study. Closed circles represent data from pretest/early sessions and open circles represent data from posttest/late sessions for each individual participant. The individual plots include regression lines fitted to the data. The numerical values are correlation coefficients exploring relationships between measured variables. Note that formal statistical tests of significance for the correlation coefficients have not been conducted due to the small sample size and pilot nature of the study. (**B**) Scatter plots of training-related improvements in standardized and training-specific measures collected in the study. Each open circle represents data from one participant. The individual plots include regression lines fitted to the data. The numerical values are correlation coefficients exploring relationships between measured variables. Note that formal statistical tests of significance for the correlation coefficients have not been conducted due to the small sample size and pilot nature of the study. Note that in both plots, one of the children in the study showed a significantly larger improvement from pretest to posttest compared to the rest of the children in the study. This child required complete assistance from an adult during testing and training activities and showed high levels of sedentary UE activity; however, with training, the child increased the frequency of affected UE activity and independent navigation. Please note that all preliminary trends discussed further within the manuscript hold true even when these analyses were repeated without this child's data.

4. Discussion

4.1. Summary of Results

Our pilot study suggested that a short three-week ROT navigation training combined with a CIMT program contributed to improvements in affected UE use and motor function during the ROT training sessions with functional carryover outside the training context. Moreover, children showed improvements in both subjective and objective measures that assessed UE movement quality and quantity. Based on our exploratory analyses, we also found trends for associations between measures of UE function assessed during training sessions and a structured standardized test of motor function administered at the pretest and posttest. Moreover, quantitative and qualitative training-specific measures also seemed to be associated with each other, suggesting a corroboration between video-based data and wrist-worn accelerometry to assess affected UE activity in children with HCP. Overall, in conjunction with our previous work in this area [25,26], our findings suggest that joystick-operated ROTs incorporated into a CIMT protocol can serve as effective and child-friendly training tools to promote use of the affected UE among children with HCP. Next, we briefly discuss our findings in the context of the existing literature and the implications of this work.

4.2. Training-Related Changes in Affected UE Activity and Motor Function with ROT Navigation Training

A recent review that assessed the minimum threshold dosing necessary to produce meaningful functional gains in affected UE function among children with HCP indicated that more than 30–40 h of goal-directed functional training is required to produce meaningful improvements [34]. Moreover, the authors also acknowledged that beyond dosing, enjoyment and motivation are key factors that influence outcomes, and that the incorporation of home practice as a supplement to face-to-face therapy is a cost-effective solution to enhance therapeutic success [34–36]. Our goal with this line of research is to explore the utility and efficacy of joystick-operated ride-on-toys as easy-to-use, cost-effective, and intrinsically motivating tools that can be used by clinicians and families to augment dosing/practice of goal-oriented activities and lead to gains in UE function through experience-dependent neuroplastic processes. The novelty of our approach lies in the choice of an unconventional yet age-appropriate and motivating activity to diversify existing activity choices used in CIMT paradigms. It was encouraging to see that ROT combined with conventional therapy led to not only improved navigational skills within the training context, but also the carryover of motor improvements to a standardized functional test outside the training context.

Improvements in movement quantity and quality may be attributed to the nature of the ROT navigation program. Real-world navigation requires a coupling of perceptual, action-based, and cognitive systems, as the child plans their route in space, adapts to changing environmental and task constraints (e.g., different surfaces, obstacles along the path, changes in elevation in the form of slopes), and skillfully maneuvers the joystick in an adaptive manner to move through their physical environment. We observed that children initially required more assistance to control the joystick; however, over the course of the training, children became more independent and engaged in more purposeful and controlled movements of their affected UE to push the joystick. Even children who were more severely involved with limited voluntary control on the affected UE developed new synergies to use proximal shoulder and trunk muscles and body mechanics to achieve success and independence in navigation. Our findings align with a study by Weightman and colleagues that assessed joystick-control abilities in children with HCP and typically developing children; the authors found that children with HCP tend to rely more on their proximal trunk and shoulder muscles compared to their neurotypical peers while operating the joystick [37]. Children in our study persisted with the training activity in order to achieve functional success in self-driven mobility within the environment. The training effects may also be attributed to the incorporation of motor learning principles into our protocol, including variable and repetitive practice, the provision of multimodal feedback and reinforcement, the use of progressively challenging activities that provide a "just-right" challenge, and fostering free play and exploration [38–41]. Other studies have also identified that interventions based on motor learning principles are effective in producing improvements in neuromotor function among children with disabilities [42–44].

Our findings are also in line with studies that used novel activity ideas and technologies to encourage goal-oriented UE practice among children with HCP [45–56]. For instance, Spencer and colleagues used magic-themed activities to incentivize the use of the affected UE in children with HCP to perform magic tricks [50,52,53,57]. They found that a short-term magic-themed camp led to improvements in UE function among children [52]; moreover, children and parents perceived the activities to be fun and motivating while promoting learning and children's willingness to persist with relatively challenging UE activities [52,53]. Other studies have used more high-tech and immersive tools such as virtual reality and robotics to promote the repetitive practice of progressively challenging activities. For instance, Fluet et al. (2010) found small-to-large improvements in the active movements of shoulder abduction, shoulder flexion, and forearm supination, as well as in several measures of reaching kinematics following a short three-week robot-assisted therapy program for children with HCP [49]. Similarly, Acar and colleagues found greater improvements in hand function and movement speed on the standardized Jebsen–Taylor hand function test in a group of children with CP that received six weeks of biweekly Nintendo Wii virtual reality training sessions in addition to conventional therapy compared to a group that only received conventional physical therapy [46]. Overall, our study adds to the body of literature exploring innovative, child-preferred, and diverse types of activities and tools that can be used to incentivize affected UE use and goal-directed practice both as part of conventional therapy as well as outside conventional therapy contexts. By developing activities that align with children's interests and goals, we can maximize their engagement in rehabilitation and overall self-confidence.

Among the types of assessments we used, we found the largest effect sizes for improvements in accelerometer-based estimates of affected UE activity compared to changes in standardized and video-based tests. Improvements in VM counts/minute were greater than the minimal clinically important difference values for arm accelerometry reported in the literature [31], suggesting that the improvements were meaningful and may be reflective of functional changes. Accelerometers have been validated as an outcome measure for assessing the efficacy of behavioral interventions both in adults and children with hemiplegia [58–61]. Accelerometers offer the advantage of being lightweight, non-intrusive, and compact. Moreover, unlike standardized or video-based assessments that provide information on the child's motor performance based on a single snapshot of time often within a structured setting, accelerometers allow the assessment of children's habitual UE activity over long durations across a variety of settings and tasks, therefore reflecting the real-world use of their affected UE. In our study, accelerometer-based measures seemed to be more sensitive to capturing changes in affected UE use and intensity of activity from early to late training sessions. We recommend that clinicians use accelerometers as a sensitive outcome measure to assess the effectiveness of behavioral interventions in promoting affected UE use for activities of daily living as part of the child's daily routines.

4.3. Exploratory Associations between Pretest–Posttest and Training-Specific Measures of Affected UE Activity

Our exploratory analyses suggested some interesting trends for relationships between training-specific variables and a standardized test of motor performance. Although promising, these results must be interpreted with caution given our small sample size and the pilot nature of our study. These associations need to be replicated using larger sample sizes and more rigorous study designs. We found trends for associations between spontaneous use of the affected UE during bimanual tasks on the SHUEE and independent and active use of the affected UE during training sessions. These data provide pilot evidence that improvements within the ROT training context may be related to positive improvements on standardized functional tests conducted outside the training context. Our findings are in line with other studies that evaluated associations between affected UE use as assessed using accelerometry and standardized tests of motor performance [4,59,62]. For instance, Sokal and colleagues reported medium-sized correlations between the intensity of use of the affected arm and a standardized test of motor capacity in children with HCP [62].

Moreover, accelerometer-derived measures of affected UE activity were also related to video-based measures of affected UE activity. Our findings are aligned with other studies that also explored associations between accelerometer-based outcomes and performance on standardized tests and video-based assessments in children and adults with neurological impairments [63–65]. For instance, Poitras and colleagues found good agreement between video-based and accelerometry-based measurements of arm movements during 20 min of free play in a seated position in adults with CP [65]. Similarly, Uswatte et al. found high correlations between threshold-filtered ActiGraph recordings of UE activity and observer ratings of video data in adult patients with unilateral weakness [63]. Our preliminary data add to the previous literature in support of the use of accelerometers as useful outcome measures for assessing UE activity. Video-based measures may be limited to short durations of capture time, limited capture volume, and tedious and time-consuming efforts to code collected video data; in contrast, accelerometer-based estimates offer longer data collection times across a variety of settings without a significant setup, relatively simple postprocessing, and provide accurate and sensitive objective measures of affected UE activity [4,58,66,67]. Overall, we recommend that accelerometers can be used to supplement clinician observations within therapeutic settings and may serve as a sensitive measure to assess the effects of short-term training programs such as a ROT navigation program aimed to improve UE function.

4.4. Limitations & Future Directions

Our study is limited due to the lack of a control group, a small convenience sample, including children with HCP without any history of recent surgeries, a wide age range of ability levels within the participants, lack of sensory testing measures, and the lack of follow-up testing. In this study, we only reported on motor outcomes. However, children with HCP also have sensory impairments that may contribute to their clinical presentation. In our future studies, we will also include measures of sensory function within our test battery. We incorporated our training within a CIMT paradigm; an inherent limitation of CIMT is that it does not allow for mirror movements involving the unaffected UE. The data collected from the accelerometers was analyzed using algorithms that were validated for neurotypical children as there were no validated algorithms available for children with HCP. Moreover, we did not collect accelerometer data outside the training context and at follow-up after completion of the ROT camp. Despite reporting improvements in UE activity during and following ROT navigation when combined with the CIMT program, we were not able to isolate the effects of the ROT training from other camp activities. Our findings also cannot be directly generalized to children with HCP who have undergone surgical procedures such as Botox injections or tendon transfers. Finally, we conducted exploratory analyses that examined trends for relationships between standardized and training-specific variables; these patterns need to be verified using larger sample sizes. In our future studies, we will address some of these limitations by assessing the isolated short-term and long-term effects of a community-based ROT training program using controlled designs and larger homogenous samples.

5. Conclusions

Our pilot study assessed the effects of a three-week joystick-operated ROT navigation training program incorporated as part of a CIMT summer camp on spontaneous use, motor function, and activity of the affected UE in children with HCP using a standardized test, wrist-worn accelerometry, and video-based measures. We found improvements on the standardized test of motor function from pretest to posttest as well as increased activity of the affected UE during ROT navigation from early to late training sessions as indicated by accelerometers and video-based measures of navigation. We also found trends for associations between training-specific and standardized measures of UE activity as well as between quantitative and qualitative measures of affected UE use. Joystick-operated ROTs seem to be effective and child-friendly tools that can be easily incorporated into children's play and conventional therapy by caregivers and clinicians to boost treatment dosing and encourage children with HCP to use their affected UE for purposeful navigation through real-world environments. Our findings have implications for the use of ROTs as therapy adjuncts in UE rehabilitation for children with motor disabilities.

Author Contributions: Conceptualization, S.S. and D.B.; methodology, S.S., P.K. and D.B.; software, P.K.; validation, S.S., D.B. and P.K.; formal analysis, N.A. and S.S.; investigation, N.A., P.K., D.B. and S.S.; resources, S.S.; data curation, S.S.; writing—original draft preparation, N.A. and S.S.; writing—review and editing, P.K., K.M., D.B. and S.S.; visualization, N.A. and S.S.; supervision, P.K., K.M., D.B. and S.S.; project administration, P.K., D.B. and S.S.; funding acquisition, S.S. All authors have read and agreed to the published version of the manuscript.

Funding: This research was funded by a startup grant to the corresponding author through the University of Connecticut.

Institutional Review Board Statement: The study was conducted in accordance with the Declaration of Helsinki and approved by the Institutional Review Board of the University of Connecticut (protocol code H21-0019 and date of approval: 21 April 2021).

Informed Consent Statement: Parental permission and child assent was obtained from all subjects involved in the study.

Data Availability Statement: Data from this project will be made available on request to the corresponding author.

Acknowledgments: The authors thank all the children and families who participated in the study. We would also like to extend our sincere gratitude to Cindy Jackson and her entire team of therapists and staff at the Lefty-Righty Camp of Connecticut (LARC) for supporting this research and accommodating our training within their camp schedule. We thank the UConn biomedical engineering senior design team members Aston Foley, Arshia Puri, Jonathan Rodriguez, and Kyle Vallee for their help in redesigning the ride-on toy with 3D printed parts and modifying the device electronic components. We thank graduate students Julia Lagace, Laura Sweeney, and Taylor Caruso in the Physical Therapy program at the University of Connecticut for their help with data collection. We thank undergraduate students Kathleen Souza, Lauren Granato, and Justina Courgi from the University of Connecticut for their help with data coding and analyses.

Conflicts of Interest: The authors declare no conflict of interest.

References

1. Arner, M.; Eliasson, A.C.; Nichlasson, S.; Sommerstein, K.; Hagglund, G. Hand function in cerebral palsy. Report of 367 children in a population-based longitudinal health care program. *J. Hand Surg.* **2008**, *33*, 1337–1347. [CrossRef]
2. Arnould, C.; Penta, M.; Thonnard, J. Hand impairments and their relationship with manual ability in children with cerebral palsy. *J. Rehabil. Med.* **2008**, *39*, 708–714. [CrossRef]
3. Novak, I.; Morgan, C.; Fahey, M.; Finch-Edmondson, M.; Galea, C.; Hines, A.; Langdon, K.; Mc Namara, M.; Paton, M.C.B.; Popat, H. State of the evidence traffic lights 2019: Systematic review of interventions for preventing and treating children with cerebral palsy. *Curr. Neurol. Neurosci. Rep.* **2020**, *20*, 3. [CrossRef] [PubMed]
4. Taub, D.; Uswatte, G.; Bowman, M.; Mark, V.W.; Delgado, A.; Bryson, C.; Morris, D.; Bishop-McKay, S. Constraint-Induced Therapy Combined with Conventional Neurorehabilitation Techniques in Chronic Stroke Patients with Plegic Hands: A Case Series. *Arch. Phys. Med. Rehabil.* **2012**, *94*, 86–94. [CrossRef] [PubMed]
5. Dong, V.A.; Fong, K.; Chen, Y.F.; Tseng, S.; Wong, L. 'Remind-to-move' treatment versus constraint-induced movement therapy for children with hemiplegic cerebral palsy: A randomized controlled trial. *Dev. Med. Child Neurol.* **2017**, *59*, 160–167. [CrossRef] [PubMed]
6. Gordon, A.M.; Charles, J.; Wolf, S.L. Methods of constraint-induced movement therapy for children with hemiplegic cerebral palsy: Development of a child-friendly intervention for improving upper-extremity function. *Arch. Phys. Med. Rehabil.* **2005**, *86*, 837–844. [CrossRef]
7. Eliasson, A.C.; Bonnier, B.; Krumlinde-Sundholm, L. Clinical experience of constraint induced movement therapy in adolescents with hemiplegic cerebral palsy—A day camp model. *Dev. Med. Child Neurol.* **2003**, *45*, 357–360. [CrossRef]
8. Hoare, B.; Imms, C.; Leeane, C.; Jason, W. Constraint-induced movement therapy in the treatment of the upper limb in children with hemiplegic cerebral palsy: A Cochrane systematic review. *Clin. Rehabil.* **2007**, *21*, 675–685. [CrossRef]
9. Ramey, S.L.; DeLuca, S.C.; Stevenson, R.D.; Conaway, M.; Darragh, A.R.; Lo, W. Constraint-induced movement therapy for cerebral palsy: A randomized trial. *Pediatrics* **2021**, *148*, e2020033878. [CrossRef]
10. Sakzewski, L.; Ziviani, J.; Boyd, R.N. Efficacy of upper limb therapies for unilateral cerebral palsy: A meta-analysis. *Pediatrics* **2014**, *133*, e175–e204. [CrossRef]

11. Sakzewski, L.; Provan, K.; Ziviani, J.; Boyd, R.N. Comparison of dosage of intensive upper limb therapy for children with unilateral cerebral palsy: How big should the therapy pill be? *Res. Dev. Disabil.* **2015**, *37*, 9–16. [CrossRef]
12. Huang, H.; Huang, H.; Chen, Y.; Hsieh, Y.; Shih, M.; Chen, C. Modified ride-on cars and mastery motivation in young children with disabilities: Effects of environmental modifications. *Res. Dev. Disabil.* **2018**, *83*, 37–46. [CrossRef] [PubMed]
13. Tatla, S.K.; Sauve, K.; Jarus, T.; Virji-Babul, N.; Holsti, L. The effects of motivating interventions on rehabilitation outcomes in children and youth with acquired brain injuries: A systematic review. *Brain Inj.* **2014**, *28*, 1022–1035. [CrossRef] [PubMed]
14. El-Shamy, S.M. Efficacy of Armeo® robotic therapy versus conventional therapy on upper limb function in children with hemiplegic cerebral palsy. *Am. J. Phys. Med. Rehabil.* **2018**, *97*, 164–169. [CrossRef] [PubMed]
15. Chen, H.; Lin, S.; Yeh, C.; Chen, R.; Tang, H.; Ruan, S.; Wang, T. Development and Feasibility of a Kinect-Based Constraint-Induced Therapy Program in the Home Setting for Children with Unilateral Cerebral Palsy. *Front. Bioeng. Biotechnol.* **2021**, *9*, 755506. [CrossRef]
16. Majnemer, A.; Shevell, M.; Law, M.; Poulin, C.; Rosenbaum, P. Level of motivation in mastering challenging tasks in children with cerebral palsy. *Dev. Med. Child Neurol.* **2010**, *52*, 1120–1126. [CrossRef] [PubMed]
17. Majnemer, A.; Shikako-Thomas, K.; Lach, L.; Shevell, M.; Law, M.; Schmitz, N. Mastery motivation in adolescents with cerebral palsy. *Res. Dev. Disabil.* **2013**, *34*, 3384–3392. [CrossRef]
18. Bartlett, D.J.; Palisano, R.J. Physical therapists' perceptions of factors influencing the acquisition of motor abilities of children with cerebral palsy: Implications for clinical reasoning. *Phys. Ther.* **2002**, *82*, 237–248. [CrossRef]
19. James, D.; Pfaff, J.; Jeffries, M. Modified ride-on cars as early mobility for children with mobility limitations: A scoping review. *Phys. Occup. Ther. Pediatr.* **2019**, *39*, 525–542. [CrossRef]
20. Logan, S.W.; Hospodar, C.M.; Feldner, H.A.; Huang, H.; Galloway, J.C. Modified Ride-on Car Use by Children with Complex Medical Needs. *Pediatr. Phys. Ther.* **2016**, *28*, 100–107. [CrossRef]
21. Cheung, W.; Meadan, H.; Yang, H. Effects of powered mobility device interventions on social skills for children with disabilities: A systematic review. *J. Dev. Phys. Disabil.* **2020**, *32*, 855–876. [CrossRef]
22. Hospodar, C.; Feldner, H.; Logan, S. Active mobility, active participation: A systematic review of modified ride-on car use by children with disabilities. *Disabil. Rehabil. Assist. Technol.* **2021**, 1–15. [CrossRef] [PubMed]
23. Hospodar, C.M.; Sabet, A.; Logan, S.W.; Catena, M.A.; Galloway, J.C. Exploratory analysis of a developmentally progressive modified ride-on car intervention for young children with Down syndrome. *Disabil. Rehabil. Assist. Technol.* **2021**, *16*, 749–757. [CrossRef] [PubMed]
24. Sabet, A.; Feldner, H.; Tucker, J.; Logan, S.W.; Galloway, J.C. ON Time Mobility: Advocating for Mobility Equity. *Pediatr. Phys. Ther.* **2022**, *34*, 546–550. [CrossRef]
25. Amonkar, N.; Kumavor, P.; Morgan, K.; Bubela, D.; Srinivasan, S. Feasibility of Using Joystick-Operated Ride-on-Toys to Promote Upper Extremity Function in Children with Cerebral Palsy: A Pilot Study. *Pediatr. Phys. Ther.* **2022**, *34*, 508–517. [CrossRef]
26. Amonkar, N.; Sullivan, S.; Kumavor, P.; Morgan, K.; Bubela, D.; Srinivasan, S. Joystick-operated ride-on-toys as playful tools to improve upper extremity activity and function in children with hemiplegic cerebral palsy: Results of a pilot feasibility study. In Proceedings of the 76th Annual Meeting of the American Academy for Cerebral Palsy and Developmental Medicine (AACPDM), Las Vegas, NV, USA, 21–24 September 2022.
27. Eliasson, A.C.; Krumlinde-Sundholm, L.; Rösblad, B.; Beckung, E.; Arner, M.; Öhrvall, A.; Rosenbaum, P. The Manual Ability Classification System (MACS) for children with cerebral palsy: Scale development and evidence of validity and reliability. *Dev. Med. Child Neurol.* **2006**, *48*, 549–554. [CrossRef]
28. Klingels, K.; Jaspers, E.; Van de Winckel, A.; De Cock, P.; Molenaers, G.; Feys, H. A systematic review of arm activity measures for children with hemiplegic cerebral palsy. *Clin. Rehabil.* **2010**, *24*, 887–900. [CrossRef]
29. Davids, J.R.; Peace, L.C.; Wagner, L.V.; Gidewall, M.A.; Blackhurst, D.W.; Roberson, W.M. Validation of the Shriners Hospital for Children Upper Extremity Evaluation (SHUEE) for children with hemiplegic cerebral palsy. *Jbjs* **2006**, *88*, 326–333. [CrossRef]
30. Freedson, P.; Pober, D.; Janz, K.F. Calibration of accelerometer output for children. *Med. Sci. Sports Exerc.* **2005**, *37*, S523. [CrossRef]
31. Chen, H.L.; Lin, K.C.; Hsieh, Y.W.; Wu, C.Y.; Liing, R.J.; Chen, C.L. A study of predictive validity, responsiveness, and minimal clinically important difference of arm accelerometer in real-world activity of patients with chronic stroke. *Clin. Rehabil.* **2018**, *32*, 75–83. [CrossRef]
32. Hedges, L.V. Distribution theory for Glass's estimator of effect size and related estimators. *J. Educ. Stat.* **1981**, *6*, 107–128. [CrossRef]
33. Cohen, J. The effect size. In *Statistical Power Analysis for the Behavioral Sciences*; Lawrence Erlbaum Associates: Hillsdale, NJ, USA, 1988; pp. 77–83.
34. Jackman, M.; Lannin, N.; Galea, C.; Sakzewski, L.; Miller, L.; Novak, I. What is the threshold dose of upper limb training for children with cerebral palsy to improve function? A systematic review. *Aust. Occup. Ther. J.* **2020**, *67*, 269–280. [CrossRef] [PubMed]
35. Polatajko, H.J. Cognitive orientation to daily occupational performance (CO-OP) approach. In *Physical & Occupational Therapy in Pediatrics*; Hinojosa, J., Kramer, P., Royeen, C.B., Eds.; F.A. Davis Company: Philadelphia, PA, USA, 2017; pp. 183–206.
36. Morgan, C.; Novak, I.; Dale, R.C.; Guzzetta, A.; Badawi, N. Single blind randomised controlled trial of GAME (Goals Activity Motor Enrichment) in infants at high risk of cerebral palsy. *Res. Dev. Disabil.* **2016**, *55*, 256–267. [CrossRef]

37. Weightman, A.; Preston, N.; Levesley, M.; Bhakta, B.; Holt, R.; Mon-Williams, M. The nature of arm movement in children with cerebral palsy when using computer-generated exercise games. *Disabil. Rehabil. Assist. Technol.* **2014**, *9*, 219–225. [CrossRef]
38. Shumway-Cook, A.; Woollacott, M.H. *Motor Control: Translating Research into Clinical Practice*; Wolters Kluwer Health: Lippincott Williams & Wilkins: Philadelphia, PA, USA, 2007.
39. Diamond, A. Close interrelation of motor development and cognitive development and of the cerebellum and prefrontal cortex. *Child Dev.* **2000**, *71*, 44–56. [CrossRef]
40. Gibson, J.J. *The Theory of Affordances*; Lawrence Erlbaum Associates: Hillsdale, NJ, USA, 1977; Volume 1, pp. 67–82.
41. Thelen, E.; Schöner, G.; Scheier, C.; Smith, L.B. The dynamics of embodiment: A field theory of infant perseverative reaching. *Behav. Brain Sci.* **2001**, *24*, 1–34. [CrossRef]
42. Demers, M.; Fung, K.; Subramanian, S.K.; Lemay, M.; Robert, M.T. Integration of motor learning principles into virtual reality interventions for individuals with cerebral palsy: Systematic review. *JMIR Serious Games* **2021**, *9*, e23822. [CrossRef] [PubMed]
43. Levin, M.F.; Weiss, P.; Keshner, E.A. Emergence of virtual reality as a tool for upper limb rehabilitation: Incorporation of motor control and motor learning principles. *Phys. Ther.* **2015**, *95*, 415–425. [CrossRef] [PubMed]
44. Taghizadeh, A.; Webster, K.E.; Bhopti, A.; Carey, L.; Hoare, B. Are they really motor learning therapies? A scoping review of evidence-based, task-focused models of upper limb therapy for children with unilateral cerebral palsy. *Disabil. Rehabil.* **2022**, *9*, 1–13. [CrossRef]
45. Goyal, C.; Vardhan, V.; Naqvi, W.; Arora, S. Effect of virtual reality and haptic feedback on upper extremity function and functional independence in children with hemiplegic cerebral palsy: A research protocol. *Pan Afr. Med. J.* **2022**, *41*, 155. [CrossRef]
46. Acar, G.; Altun, G.P.; Yurdalan, S.; Polat, M.G. Efficacy of neurodevelopmental treatment combined with the Nintendo® Wii in patients with cerebral palsy. *J. Phys. Ther. Sci.* **2016**, *28*, 774–780. [CrossRef] [PubMed]
47. Arps, K.; Darr, N.; Katz, J. Effect of adapted motorized ride-on toy use on developmental skills, quality of life, and driving competency in nonambulatory children age 9–60 months. *Assist. Technol.* **2021**, *35*, 83–93. [CrossRef] [PubMed]
48. Fasoli, S.E.; Fragala-Pinkham, M.; Hughes, R.; Hogan, N.; Stein, J.; Krebs, H.I. Upper limb robot-assisted therapy: A new option for children with hemiplegia. *Technol. Disabil.* **2010**, *22*, 193–198. [CrossRef]
49. Fluet, G.G.; Qiu, Q.; Kelly, D.; Parikh, H.D.; Ramirez, D.; Saleh, S.; Adamovich, S.V. Interfacing a haptic robotic system with complex virtual environments to treat impaired upper extremity motor function in children with cerebral palsy. *Dev. Neurorehabilit.* **2010**, *13*, 335–345. [CrossRef]
50. Spencer, K.; Yuen, H.K.; Jenkins, G.R.; Kirklin, K.; Vogtle, L.K.; Davis, D. The 'magic' of magic camp from the perspective of children with hemiparesis. *J. Exerc. Rehabil.* **2021**, *17*, 15–20. [CrossRef]
51. Green, D.; Schertz, M.; Gordon, A.M.; Moore, A.; Schejter Margalit, T.; Farquharson, Y.; Ben Bashat, D.; Weinstein, M.; Lin, J.; Fattal-Valevski, A. A multi-site study of functional outcomes following a themed approach to hand–arm bimanual intensive therapy for children with hemiplegia. *Dev. Med. Child Neurol.* **2013**, *55*, 527–533. [CrossRef]
52. Spencer, K.; Yuen, H.K.; Jenkins, G.R.; Kirklin, K.; Griffin, A.R.; Vogtle, L.K.; Davis, D. Evaluation of a magic camp for children with hemiparesis: A pilot study. *Occup. Ther. Health Care* **2020**, *34*, 155–170. [CrossRef]
53. Hines, A.; Bundy, A.C.; Black, D.; Haertsch, M.; Wallen, M. Upper limb function of children with unilateral cerebral palsy after a magic-themed HABIT: A pre-post-study with 3-and 6-month follow-up. *Phys. Occup. Ther. Pediatr.* **2019**, *39*, 404–419. [CrossRef]
54. Chang, H.J.; Ku, K.H.; Park, Y.S.; Park, J.G.; Cho, E.S.; Seo, J.S.; Kim, C.W. Effects of virtual reality-based rehabilitation on upper extremity function among children with cerebral palsy. *Healthcare* **2020**, *8*, 391. [CrossRef]
55. Menekseoglu, A.K.; Capan, N.; Arman, A.; Aydin, A.R. Effect of a Virtual Reality-Mediated Gamified Rehabilitation Program on Upper Limb Functions in Children with Hemiplegic Cerebral Palsy: A Prospective, Randomized Controlled Study. *Am. J. Phys. Med. Rehabil.* **2023**, *102*, 198–205. [CrossRef]
56. Roberts, H.; Shierk, A.; Clegg, N.J.; Baldwin, D.; Smith, L.; Yeatts, P.; Delgado, M.R. Constraint induced movement therapy camp for children with hemiplegic cerebral palsy augmented by use of an exoskeleton to play games in virtual reality. *Phys. Occup. Ther. Pediatr.* **2020**, *41*, 150–165. [CrossRef] [PubMed]
57. Hines, A.; Bundy, A.C.; Haertsch, M.; Wallen, M. A magic-themed upper limb intervention for children with unilateral cerebral palsy: The perspectives of parents. *Dev. Neurorehabilit.* **2019**, *22*, 104–110. [CrossRef] [PubMed]
58. Lang, C.E.; Waddell, K.J.; Klaesner, J.W.; Bland, M.D. A method for quantifying upper limb performance in daily life using accelerometers. *JoVE (J. Vis. Exp.)* **2017**, *122*, e55673.
59. Coker-Bolt, P.; Downey, R.J.; Connolly, J.; Hoover, R.; Shelton, D.; Seo, N.J. Exploring the feasibility and use of accelerometers before, during, and after a camp-based CIMT program for children with cerebral palsy. *J. Pediatr. Rehabil. Med.* **2017**, *10*, 27–36. [CrossRef] [PubMed]
60. Beani, E.; Maselli, M.; Sicola, E.; Perazza, S.; Cecchi, F.; Dario, P.; Braito, I.; Boyd, R.; Cioni, G.; Sgandurra, G. Actigraph assessment for measuring upper limb activity in unilateral cerebral palsy. *J. Neuroeng. Rehabil.* **2019**, *16*, 30. [CrossRef]
61. Goodwin, B.M.; Sabelhaus, E.K.; Pan, Y.; Bjornson, K.F.; Pham, K.; Walker, W.O.; Steele, K.M. Accelerometer measurements indicate that arm movements of children with cerebral palsy do not increase after constraint-induced movement therapy (CIMT). *Am. J. Occup. Ther.* **2020**, *74*, 7405205100p1–7405205100p9. [CrossRef]
62. Sokal, B.; Uswatte, G.; Vogtle, L.; Byrom, E.; Barman, J. Everyday movement and use of the arms: Relationship in children with hemiparesis differs from adults. *J. Pediatr. Rehabil. Med.* **2015**, *8*, 197–206. [CrossRef] [PubMed]

63. Uswatte, G.; Miltner, W.; Foo, B.; Varma, M.; Moran, S.; Taub, E. Objective measurement of functional upper-extremity movement using accelerometer recordings transformed with a threshold filter. *Stroke* **2000**, *31*, 662–667. [CrossRef]
64. Gordon, A.M.; Schneider, J.A.; Chinnan, A.; Charles, J.R. Efficacy of a hand–arm bimanual intensive therapy (HABIT) in children with hemiplegic cerebral palsy: A randomized control trial. *Dev. Med. Child Neurol.* **2007**, *49*, 830–838. [CrossRef]
65. Poitras, I.; Clouâtre, J.; Campeau-Lecours, A.; Mercier, C. Accelerometry-Based Metrics to Evaluate the Relative Use of the More Affected Arm during Daily Activities in Adults Living with Cerebral Palsy. *Sensors* **2022**, *22*, 1022. [CrossRef]
66. Hayward, K.S.; Eng, J.J.; Boyd, L.A.; Lakhani, B.; Bernhardt, J.; Lang, C.E. Exploring the role of accelerometers in the measurement of real world upper-limb use after stroke. *Brain Impair.* **2016**, *17*, 16–33. [CrossRef]
67. Wang, T.; Lin, K.; Wu, C.; Chung, C.; Pei, Y.; Teng, Y. Validity, responsiveness, and clinically important difference of the ABILHAND questionnaire in patients with stroke. *Arch. Phys. Med. Rehabil.* **2011**, *92*, 1086–1091. [CrossRef] [PubMed]

Disclaimer/Publisher's Note: The statements, opinions and data contained in all publications are solely those of the individual author(s) and contributor(s) and not of MDPI and/or the editor(s). MDPI and/or the editor(s) disclaim responsibility for any injury to people or property resulting from any ideas, methods, instructions or products referred to in the content.

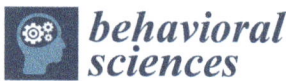

Article

Combining Unimanual and Bimanual Therapies for Children with Hemiparesis: Is There an Optimal Delivery Schedule?

Ka Lai K. Au [1], Julie L. Knitter [1], Susan Morrow-McGinty [1], Talita C. Campos [2], Jason B. Carmel [3] and Kathleen M. Friel [4,5,*]

[1] Blythedale Children's Hospital, Valhalla, NY 10595, USA
[2] School of Nursing, Columbia University Irving Medical Center, New York, NY 10032, USA
[3] Weinberg Family Cerebral Palsy Center, Department of Neurology, Columbia University Irving Medical Center, New York, NY 10032, USA
[4] Burke Neurological Institute, White Plains, NY 10605, USA
[5] Brain Mind Research Institute, Weill Cornell Medical College, New York, NY 10021, USA
* Correspondence: kaf3001@med.cornell.edu; Tel.: +1-914-368-3116

Citation: Au, K.L.K.; Knitter, J.L.; Morrow-McGinty, S.; Campos, T.C.; Carmel, J.B.; Friel, K.M. Combining Unimanual and Bimanual Therapies for Children with Hemiparesis: Is There an Optimal Delivery Schedule? *Behav. Sci.* 2023, *13*, 490. https://doi.org/10.3390/bs13060490

Academic Editors: Stephanie C. DeLuca and Jill C. Heathcock

Received: 13 April 2023
Revised: 1 June 2023
Accepted: 6 June 2023
Published: 9 June 2023

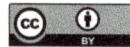

Copyright: © 2023 by the authors. Licensee MDPI, Basel, Switzerland. This article is an open access article distributed under the terms and conditions of the Creative Commons Attribution (CC BY) license (https:// creativecommons.org/licenses/by/ 4.0/).

Abstract: Constraint-induced movement therapy (CIMT) and bimanual therapy (BT) are among the most effective hand therapies for children with unilateral cerebral palsy (uCP). Since they train different aspects of hand use, they likely have synergistic effects. The aim of this study was to examine the efficacy of different combinations of mCIMT and BT in an intensive occupational therapy program for children with uCP. Children (n = 35) participated in intensive modified CIMT (mCIMT) and BT, 6 weeks, 5 days/week, 6 h/day. During the first 2 weeks, children wore a mitt over the less-affected hand and engaged in functional and play activities with the affected hand. Starting in week 3, bimanual play and functional activities were added progressively, 1 hour/week. This intervention was compared to two different schedules of block interventions: (1) 3 weeks of mCIMT followed by 3 weeks of BT, and (2) 3 weeks of BT followed by 3 weeks of mCIMT. Hand function was tested before, after, and two months after therapy with the Assisting Hand Assessment (AHA), Pediatric Evaluation of Disability Inventory (PEDI), and Canadian Occupational Performance Measure (COPM). All three groups of children improved in functional independence (PEDI; $p < 0.031$), goal performance (COPM Performance; $p < 0.0001$) and satisfaction (COPM Satisfaction; $p < 0.0001$), which persisted two months post-intervention. All groups showed similar amounts of improvement, indicating that the delivery schedule for mCIMT and BT does not significantly impact the outcomes.

Keywords: hemiplegia; occupational therapy; cerebral palsy; constraint

1. Introduction

Intensive hand therapy is among the most effective, evidence-based therapies for children with hemiplegia [1]. A key question in hemiplegia therapy is whether the affected hand should be trained alone or in tandem with the other hand. In constraint-induced movement therapy (CIMT), a participant's less-affected upper extremity is restricted with a sling, cast, or mitt, while the participant actively uses the affected arm and hand in skill-based therapeutic activities [2]. Bimanual training (BT), in contrast, engages both hands in therapeutic movement [3]. These two interventions have shown equivalence in most studies and Cochrane reviews [4–10], though some studies show that BT is more effective in improving functional use of the affected hand [9,11]. Since most functional activities of daily living require bimanual coordination, BT is thought to be most effective at improving performance of these activities [12]. Alternatively, there is evidence that CIMT may be more effective in home- and school-based environments [13], isolated hand movements [14], and may produce stronger improvements in head and reach control [15] than BT.

Since CIMT and BT target different aspects of hand use, they likely have synergistic effects on hand function [16]. By requiring children to use the more-affected arm, CIMT is especially useful for overcoming "developmental disuse" [2]. The sensorimotor experience of CIMT improves function and may "prime" the affected hand by increasing a child's awareness and engagement of the affected hand. This may then make subsequent bimanual therapy more effective. A combined approach of CIMT followed by bimanual therapy has been found to improve outcomes [17] beyond CIMT alone [18].

While most therapies have directly compared CIMT and BT, either by comparing one therapy against the other or administering both therapies in a block design, other combinations have not been well-studied. We developed a six-week occupational therapy program that combines CIMT and BT over the course of treatment. The goal was to engage the affected arm and hand using modified constraint-induced movement therapy (mCIMT), then to focus on functional activities that require both hands. We rationalized that an optimal therapy would first increase awareness and engagement of the impaired arm and hand, then train that hand in functional bimanual tasks. We compared this approach to two groups who received blocks of interventions. One of these groups completed three weeks of mCIMT, followed by three weeks of BT, following the same rationale of first focusing on improving the skill of the impaired upper limb and then introducing bimanual training. For a comparison, one other group completed three weeks of BT, followed by three weeks of mCIMT. This group was included to control for the order of the types of training. The goal of this study was to determine if efficacy is impacted by the schedule of delivery of mCIMT versus BT. We hypothesized that children who received mCIMT before BT would show a greater improvement in hand function at the end of the intervention, as focusing on strengthening the more-affected hand first would optimize the efficacy of the subsequent BT.

2. Materials and Methods

2.1. Participants

Thirty-five children participated in the study during the summers of 2011–2018. Five to eleven children participated each summer. Demographics and clinical characteristics of participants are shown in Table 1. Children were recruited from the outpatient service at Blythedale Children's Hospital and through community outreach.

Table 1. Baseline Participant Characteristics.

Child/Group	Sex	Age (Y, M)	Paretic Side	AHA Baseline	COPM Baseline	PEDI Baseline
Step01	M	3, 11	R	21	3.2 (P), 2.8 (S)	58
Step02	F	7, 9	R	47	3.8 (P), 4.5 (S)	74.7
Step03	M	9, 1	R	53	3.5 (P), 2.5 (S)	72.6
Step04	F	6, 6	R	38	4.2 (P), 3.6 (S)	57.4
Step05	M	8, 1	R	35	3.4 (P), 2.6 (S)	66
Step06	F	12, 5	L	30	4.0 (P), 3.4 (S)	79
Step07	M	8, 1	R	17	4.8 (P), 4.0 (S)	66
Step08	F	10, 4	R	58	3.4 (P), 3.8 (S)	77.3
Step09	F	10, 7	R	44	1.6 (P), 1.8 (S)	74.7
Step10	M	5, 2	L	44	1.8 (P), 2.6 (S)	55.6
Step11	M	6, 7	L	24	2.0 (P), 1.6 (S)	71.7
Step12	M	5, 8	R	27	3.0 (P), 3.4 (S)	61.2
Step13	M	6, 3	R	58	3.0 (P), 2.4 (S)	58.6
Step14	M	9, 5	L	58	1.6 (P), 1.0 (S)	75.9
BC01	M	12, 0	L	50	4 (P), 7.2 (S)	65.3
BC02	F	5, 8	R	59	2 (P), 5 (S)	53.7

Table 1. Cont.

Child/Group	Sex	Age (Y, M)	Paretic Side	AHA Baseline	COPM Baseline	PEDI Baseline
BC03	M	5, 3	R	30	2 (P), 4.8 (S)	55.6
BC04	M	4, 9	R	61	1.8 (P), 5 (S)	59.9
BC05	M	5, 2	L	7	1.4 (P), 2.8 (S)	51.7
BC06	F	9, 0	L	52	2.2 (P), 5.8 (S)	61.2
BC07	F	8, 8	R	59	3.2 (P), 3 (S)	75.9
BC08	M	4, 11	L	55	2.4 (P), 1.4 (S)	55.6
BC09	M	5, 9	L	52	1.8 (P), 2.2 (S)	70
BC10	M	5, 5	R	43	2.4 (P), 2.6 (S)	54.9
CB01	M	4, 8	R	87	4.2 (P), 6.8 (S)	63.9
CB02	M	5, 9	R	33	3.4 (P), 6.6 (S)	59.9
CB03	M	10, 2	R	50	1.8 (P), 5.2 (S)	75.9
CB04	F	4, 9	L	65	2 (P), 5.2 (S)	60.5
CB05	F	11, 2	R	50	3.8 (P), 3.4 (S)	60.5
CB06	F	5, 8	R	52	4.6 (P), 4.2 (S)	62.5
CB07	M	11, 0	L	47	2.2 (P), 1.6 (S)	77.3
CB08	M	9, 8	L	52	3 (P), 1.8 (S)	65.3
CB09	F	5, 1	L	66	2 (P), 2 (S)	63.2
CB10	M	7, 6	R	84	4 (P), 2 (S)	56.2
CB11	M	5, 9	R	42	3 (P), 2.2 (S)	53
Summaries	Counts	Avg ± SD	Counts	Avg ± SD	Avg ± SD	Avg ± SD
Step (n = 14)	9M/5F	7.4 ± 2.3	10R/4L	39.6 ± 14.3	3.1 ±1.0 (P), 2.8 ± 1.0 (S)	67.8 ± 8.3
BC (n = 10)	7M/3F	6.8 ± 2.5	5R/5L	46.8 ± 16.7	2.3 ± 0.8 (P), 4.0 ± 1.8 (S)	60.4 ± 7.8
CB (n = 11)	7M/4F	7.5 ± 2.7	7R/4L	57.1 ± 16.8	3.1 ± 1.0 (P), 3.7 ±2.0 (S)	63.5 ± 7.4

Abbreviations: Step, stepwise progression group; BC, bimanual training followed by modified constraint-induced movement therapy; CB, modified constraint-induced movement therapy followed by bimanual training; M, male; F, female; R, right; L, left; AHA, Assisting Hand Assessment; COPM, Canadian Occupational Performance Measure; P, performance; S, satisfaction; PEDI, The Pediatric Evaluation of Disability Inventory; Avg, average; SD, standard deviation.

Inclusion criteria: (1) unilateral brain injury resulting in impairment of one side of the body, (2) ability to move all joints of affected upper extremity, (3) age 4–12 years, and (4) ability to comply with study protocol. Exclusion criteria: health problems or uncorrected vision that would interfere with study participation. The study was approved by the Institutional Review Board of Blythedale Children's Hospital.

The interventions were offered as part of a clinical program in the Department of Occupational Therapy. IRB approval was obtained to analyze data from the intervention for the group that received the blended intervention. Children in the crossover groups were prospectively enrolled and provided written assent. Their caregiver provided written informed consent. The study was registered on clinicaltrials.gov (NCT02840643) before the first child was randomized to one of the crossover groups.

2.2. Interventions

All intervention groups used combinations of modified constraint-induced movement therapy (mCIMT) and bimanual therapy (BT). Therapy was conducted in a large room, such that all children and occupational therapists had the opportunity to interact throughout the program. The program was coordinated by an experienced occupational therapist, who was in the therapy room during the duration of the program. Each intervention took place for 6 h per day, 5 days per week, for 6 weeks (180 h).

Three different interventions were tested:

1. 3 weeks of mCIMT followed by 3 weeks of BT (group CB);
2. 3 weeks of BT followed by 3 weeks of mCIMT (group BC);
3. 2 weeks of mCIMT followed by stepwise incorporation of BT, increasing the amount of BT by 1 h per day for each of the next 4 weeks (group Step).

Materials: Both mCIMT and BT used toys, board games, art supplies, craft supplies, and sports equipment selected and structured by occupational therapists. Children brought items to the intervention for practicing caregiver/child-identified self-care and functional goals, such as a shirt with buttons or shoes with laces.

Participants engaged in age-appropriate training 6 h/day for 30 days (180 h).

Providers and Location: Therapy was provided in one room at a pediatric rehabilitation center. Therapy was provided by occupational therapists. The ratio of therapists to children was approximately 1:4. For 60 min daily, each child received 1:1 training with an OT. In addition to the OTs, there were 1–2 volunteers and/or OT interns always present in the therapy room.

Duration of therapy and therapy regimen: Therapy was provided 6 h/day for six weeks (30 days, 180 h total). The CB group received three weeks of mCIMT, followed by three weeks of BT. The BC group received three weeks of BT, followed by three weeks of mCIMT.

The Step group had a stepwise integration of BT after starting the intervention with mCIMT. During the first two weeks of the intervention, children received mCIMT. During the third week of the intervention, children received mCIMT for the first five hours of each day, then received one hour of BT. In each subsequent week of intervention, the duration of mCIMT was reduced by one hour per day, while the duration of BT was increased by one hour per day. Thus, in week four of the intervention, children began each day with four hours of mCIMT, followed by two hours of BT. In week five of the intervention, children began each day with three hours of mCIMT, followed by three hours of BT. In the sixth and final week of the intervention, children began each day with two hours of mCIMT, followed by four hours of BT (Figure 1).

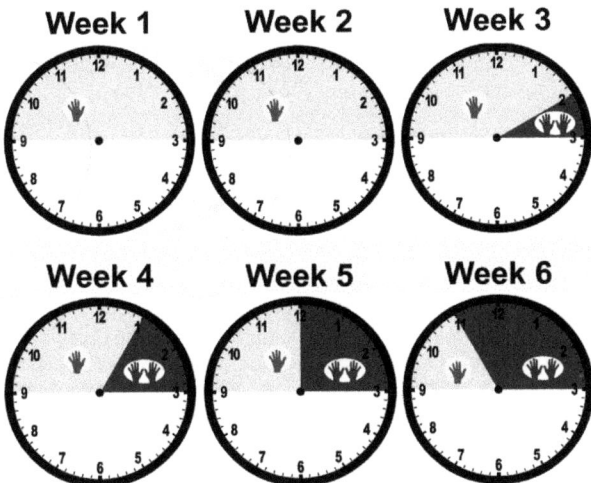

Figure 1. Delivery schedule for the Step group. Each clock represents a day's schedule, with the same schedule used each day that week. The intervention ran from 9 am to 3 pm, five days per week. During the first two weeks, children received mCIMT for the entire six hours, represented by a single hand icon and a shaded region on the clock, corresponding to the time of day. In week 3, children received mCIMT

for 5 h, 9 am to 2 pm, followed by one hour of bimanual training, represented by two hand icons. In each subsequent week of intervention, the duration of mCIMT was reduced by one hour per day, while the duration of BT was increased by one hour per day. Throughout the intervention, mCIMT was always given first in the day, followed by BT. By week 6, children received two hours per day of mCIMT (9 am to 11 am) followed by BT (11 am to 3 pm).

During mCIMT, children wore a mitt over their less-affected hand, which restricted use of that hand. Children engaged in intensive therapy to improve the active range of motion, strength, motor control, and sensory awareness of the affected hand. Activities were functional and play-based. Daily structure included: morning gym, fine motor, gross motor, sensory motor, therapeutic feeding, sports, and self-care activities. During training, children performed play-based and functional activities with the affected hand. Example activities included playing card and board games, arts and crafts, and activities that provided sensory stimulation to the affected hand, such as finger painting. Activities also included stretching and strengthening, and reciprocal coordination exercises.

During BT, children did not wear a mitt over the less-affected hand. Children were provided individualized activities that facilitated active use of both hands. Therapists adapted and graded activities and guided children to problem-solve for success. Bimanual activities included self-care (tying shoes, zippering, cutting food), sports activities, and manipulation of classroom tools (cutting with scissors).

Tailoring of therapy: Activities were selected for each participant based on the child's preferences, interest, and functional goals. Examples of the children's preferred interests include sports, arts and crafts, model construction, music, dancing, and computer games. Some examples of functional goals include donning and doffing clothing, using eating utensils, pouring liquid into a cup, carrying a lunch tray, and opening zippered food storage bags.

2.3. Group Allocation

This study began as a clinical program at Blythedale Children's Hospital, held once annually during the summer. From 2011 to 2015, the Step protocol was used exclusively. In 2016, we decided to add the CB and BC groups. In 2016–2018, only the CB and BC protocols were used. During this time, children were randomized to either of the two groups. Thus, the Step group was not randomized, while the CB and BC groups were randomized. Each cohort was split into two equally sized, age-matched groups. Then, each group was randomized to either the CB or BC interventions. Randomization was done off site by a scientist not otherwise associated with the study.

2.4. Outcome Measures

All study participants were evaluated at three time points: before the first day of treatment, within two days of the end of treatment, and two months after treatment. Bimanual performance was tested for in the CB and BC groups after week three of the intervention, when they switched between mCIMT and BT. Three outcome measures were chosen to quantify bimanual performance, motor function of the impaired upper extremity, and functional goal performance.

The Assisting Hand Assessment (AHA) was used to measure how children use the two hands together. The AHA quantifies how well children with unimanual upper limb impairments use their impaired hand when performing bimanual activities. The AHA shows excellent validity, reliability (0.97–0.99) and responsiveness to change [19]. The test was videotaped and scored by a trained evaluator. Scores were computed as logit-based AHA units. The functionally meaningful difference in score for the AHA is 4 points [20].

The Canadian Occupational Performance Measure (COPM) was used to measure performance and satisfaction levels in functional goals in self-care, productivity, and leisure domains [21]. The COPM is a standardized test in which a child's caregiver identifies a child's functional goals during a structured interview [22]. The caregiver rates satisfaction and performance on a scale of 1 (poor) to 10 (excellent), on a maximum of five goals.

The minimal clinically important difference is 2 points. Mean performance and caregiver satisfaction scores were analyzed.

The Pediatric Evaluation of Disability Inventory (PEDI) was used to assess each child's functional independence with activities of daily living. For this study, only the PEDI self-care domain was used, as evaluated by a caregiver. Scaled performance scores ranging from 0 (poor) to 100 (excellent) were used to assess change over time. The MCID is 11 points [23]. It has very good inter-rater reliability, with an intra-class coefficient of 0.7–0.98 [24].

The AHA was conducted by staff who were not therapists in the intervention. The AHA was scored by a blinded, trained, certified evaluator who was not involved in any other aspect of this study. The COPM and PEDI were given by one of the therapists, who may or may not have worked with a particular child.

2.5. Statistical Analyses

A group × time repeated-measured analysis of variance (ANOVA) was used to evaluate differences in outcome measures after the intervention and a two-month follow-up, for each intervention group, using SPSS Software (IBM, version 21). Missing data were interpolated based on average changes in measures from pre- and immediate post-intervention to 2 months follow-up. Two-month AHA follow-up data were missing for two children in the Step group, one child in the BT group, and two children in the CB group. Two-month COPM follow-up data were missing for one child in the Step group, one child in the BC group, and two children in the CB group. Two-month PEDI follow-up data were missing for seven children in the Step group, one child in the BC group, and two children in the CB group. Analyses were done with and without the inclusion of the missing data estimates, and the statistical outcomes were not different between these methods. The findings presented below include the missing data estimates. When main ANOVA effects were found, post-hoc analyses were performed, using Bonferroni corrections to correct for multiple comparisons. The Fisher's exact test was used to compare baseline categorical variables, sex, and side of lesion, among the groups. A p-value of less than 0.05 was considered statistically significant.

3. Results

Thirty-five children with unilateral CP participated in a six-week intensive occupational therapy program that combined unimanual and bimanual training. Participant demographics and baseline clinical measures are presented in Table 1. We examined differences among baseline characteristics of the groups. There were no significant differences in sex (Fisher's Exact, $p = 1.0$), lesion side (Fisher's Exact, $p = 0.61$), age ($F(2,32) = 0.48$, $p = 0.63$), COPM-Performance ($F(2,32) = 2.4$, $p = 0.11$), COPM-Satisfaction ($F(2,32) = 1.75$, $p = 0.19$), or the PEDI ($F(2,32) = 2.6$, $p = 0.087$). There was a difference in baseline AHA among groups ($F(2,31) = 3.7$, $p = 0.037$)), which was a limitation of this study. The AHA for the CB group was significantly higher than the AHA for the Step group ($p = 0.033$). The BC group AHA scores were not significantly different from the other groups ($p > 0.45$).

3.1. Improvements in Bimanual Hand Function after Intervention

Bimanual hand function was measured before, after, and two months after intervention with the Assisting Hand Assessment (AHA; Figure 2A). There was no main effect of the intervention on AHA scores ($F(2,39) = 1.03$, $p = 0.37$). We assessed how many children per group met the functionally meaningful difference for the AHA, which is 4 points. In the Step group, 71.4% children improved by 4 or more points, while 70% of children in the BC group and 36% of children in the CB group reached the functionally meaningful difference.

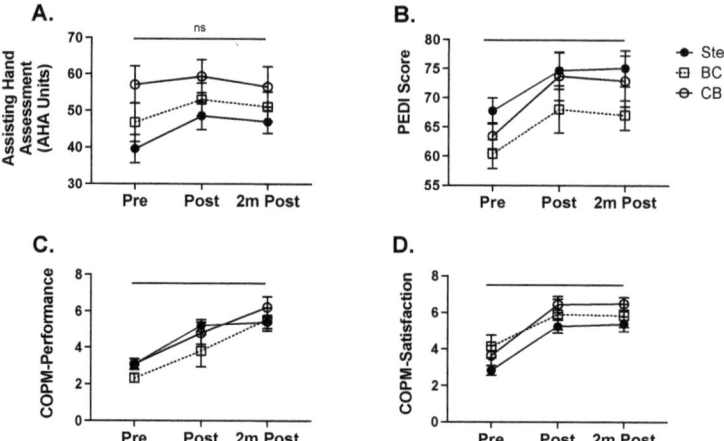

Figure 2. Outcome measures assessed before, immediately after, and two months after the intervention. (**A**). There were no statistically significant differences in the AHA between the time points or groups. (**B**). There was an overall improvement in the PEDI ($p < 0.031$), with the Step group improving more than the BC group ($p = 0.0022$). There was an overall improvement in the COPM Performance ($p < 0.0001$, (**C**)) and in the COPM Satisfaction ($p < 0.0001$, (**D**)). For COPM Performance, the CB group improved more than the BC group ($p = 0.034$).

3.2. Improvements in Self-Care Skills Independence after Intervention

Changes in self-care skills performance were measured before, after, and two months after intervention with the Pediatric Evaluation of Disability Inventory (PEDI). Caregiver reports of self-care skills performance were obtained. There was a significant improvement in skill performance (Figure 2B) outcomes after intervention ($F(2,39) = 4.2$, $p < 0.031$). For COPM Performance, the CB group improved slightly more than the BC group ($p = 0.034$), while the Step group did not differ from the CB ($p = 0.89$) or BC ($p = 0.24$) groups. For COPM Satisfaction, there were no significant differences in improvement among the groups ($p > 0.1$).

3.3. Improvements in Functional Goal Performance and Satisfaction after Intervention

Changes in functional goal performance and satisfaction were measured before, after, and two months after intervention with the Canadian Occupational Performance Measure (COPM). Caregiver reports of goal performance and satisfaction with performance were obtained. There was a significant improvement in both performance (Figure 2C) and caregiver satisfaction (Figure 2D) outcomes after intervention (Performance: $F(2,39) = 19.1$, $p < 0.0001$; Satisfaction: $F(2,39) = 35.2$, $p < 0.0001$) that was retained two months after intervention. These represent clinically meaningful improvements in both functional goal performance and satisfaction.

3.4. Midpoint Analysis of Bimanual Function in BC and CB Groups

In the BC and CB groups, we measured bimanual function using the AHA after three weeks of the intervention. We examined whether bimanual function changed differently if children received mCIMT or BT in the first block of the intervention (Figure 3). The AHA significantly improved for both groups after three weeks ($F(3,57) = 3.49$, $p = 0.034$). There were no significant differences between groups ($F(3,57) = 1.31$, $p = 0.28$), meaning that the order of mCIMT or BT delivery did not impact efficacy.

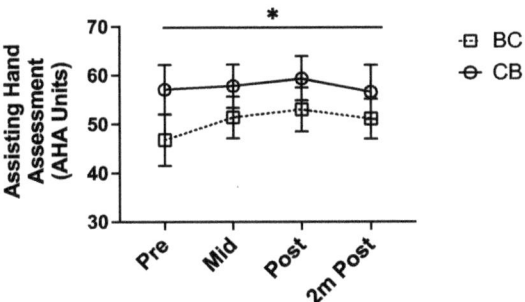

Figure 3. Comparison of bimanual function for the BC and CB groups, including a midpoint measure done at the end of week 3 of the intervention. There was an overall improvement in AHA scores across all time points ($p = 0.034$), with no difference in AHA scores between the groups ($p = 0.28$). * $p < 0.05$.

4. Discussion

This study compared the efficacy of different combinations of mCIMT and BT for improving hand function in children with uCP. The intervention improved self-care skills independence and performance and satisfaction in caregiver-rated functional goals. Improvements were maintained two months after therapy.

While many clinical trials have shown that CIMT and bimanual therapy have equivalent efficacy in children with hemiplegia [6–10], a recent focus has been to select the hypothesized key ingredients from each therapy and combine these two approaches. CIMT provides focused training of the impaired hand, which may be optimal for improving strength of that hand [13,14]. Bimanual therapy has been shown to be slightly better than CIMT at improving functional, bimanual hand use [25].

In our study, we did not find clinically meaningful differences in outcomes among the three groups. We had hypothesized that children receiving mCIMT before BT would have the greatest improvements. In our comparison of pre-, post-, and two-month follow-up time points for all three groups, we found some group differences, but these did not differ by a clinically meaningful amount. Children in the CB group improved in COPM Performance more than the BC group, by a difference on 0.8 points, whereas the clinically meaningful difference is 2 points. Children in the Step group improved in the PEDI more than the BC group, by a difference of 7.3 points, while the clinically meaningful difference is 11 points. Thus, we conclude that the three interventions are not meaningfully different in their efficacy. This could indicate that at the intensity delivered, either type of training was sufficient to drive change.

Despite the abundance of research into the optimal therapies for children with uCP, all available therapies remain unable to ameliorate impairments. Children, and their families, invest a massive amount of time, effort, and hope in the best available therapies. Nevertheless, these children spend a lifetime with movement impairments. Much more work is needed to develop effective therapies that enable children to sustain long-term improvements in function.

Further study is needed to better understand the optimal combination, schedule, and intensity of therapeutic strategies. There are a wide variety of factors that contribute to movement, and even the best available therapies do not address all factors. For example, many children with uCP have impairments in motor planning and motor imagery [26–29]. Adding action-observation training to CIMT can improve the efficacy of CIMT [30]. The role of sensory impairments in improvement of movement needs to be further studied, as the sensory system plays an essential role in accurate voluntary movement [31].

Moreover, a better understanding of individual differences in responsiveness to therapy is needed. There is a high variability in responses among children in the studies cited in this manuscript. Efficacy can depend on how engaged a child is in the intervention [32], the intensity of training [33], and a myriad of other factors. One study suggests, for example, that a child may be more responsive to CIMT or bimanual therapy based on whether their impaired hand is controlled via contralateral connections from the injured motor cortex, or via ipsilateral connections from the uninjured motor cortex [34], while others did not find a difference in efficacy based on motor system connectivity [35]. Gender may also affect efficacy, though the key ingredient may be the active engagement of each child in the training. When conducting group interventions, it is important to have a variety of fun activities that will be appealing to children of varied genders, ages, ability levels, and interests.

There were several limitations to this study that pertain to how the study was done, and how the findings can be interpreted. First, we will discuss limitations regarding how the study was done. The study is underpowered to be an efficacy study or a non-inferiority study. However, our results are consistent with prior studies comparing unimanual and bimanual training [6,9,10,36,37]. A limitation is that the Step group was completed before the CB and BC groups were developed. Ideally, all three interventions would have been tested at the same time, and children would have been randomized to each of the groups. The length of time between the delivery of the three intervention types may have affected the outcomes. Another limitation is the large number of children in the Step group who did not complete the two-month follow-up PEDI evaluation. The PEDI and COPM findings also have a limitation, since therapists associated with the intervention conducted these surveys. Finally, a limitation is that the CB group had a higher baseline AHA score than the Step group.

There are also limitations regarding how our findings can be interpreted. The children in this study were school aged between 4 and 12 years old. We chose this age group because they are capable of remaining engaged in training tasks for 6 h/day, but it is possible that younger children may show greater improvements in a similar intervention, since neuroplasticity is greater in young children [38]. Our findings cannot be generalized to younger children, teens, or adults with uCP.

Moreover, our conclusions are limited by the length of follow-up of this study. We included a two-month follow-up evaluation, but ideally the effects would be sustained long-term. In the future, longer follow-ups, such as six months later, would provide important information about the longevity of improvements. It is possible that our three schedules of the intervention led to different rates of long-term retention of improved function.

In this study, we hypothesized that children who received unimanual training before bimanual training would improve more than children who did not receive unimanual training first. Our findings indicate, however, that the order of training strategies does not significantly affect outcomes. The optimal schedule of training approaches is likely to be specific to an individual's impairments and other unknown factors. More work is needed to better understand how to optimize a child's improvements.

5. Conclusions

This study compared the efficacy of blocks of mCIMT and BT or progressive shift from mCIMT to BT for improving hand function in children ages 4–12 with uCP. All groups improved equally in self-care skills independence and performance and satisfaction in caregiver-rated functional goals. This interpretation is limited by a small sample size, lack of long-term follow up, and differences in baseline bimanual function among the three groups.

Author Contributions: Conceptualization, K.L.K.A., J.L.K., S.M.-M., J.B.C. and K.M.F.; methodology, K.L.K.A., J.L.K., S.M.-M., T.C.C., J.B.C. and K.M.F.; formal analysis, T.C.C. and K.M.F.; investigation, K.L.K.A., J.L.K. and S.M.-M.; writing—original draft preparation, K.M.F.; writing—review and editing, K.L.K.A., J.L.K., S.M.-M., T.C.C., J.B.C. and K.M.F.; visualization, K.M.F.; supervision, K.L.K.A., J.L.K. and S.M.-M.; project administration, K.L.K.A., J.L.K. and S.M.-M.; funding acquisition, K.L.K.A., J.L.K., S.M.-M., J.B.C. and K.M.F. All authors have read and agreed to the published version of the manuscript.

Funding: This research was funded by Blythedale Children's Hospital, NIH R01 HD076436 (K.M.F.), NIH K08 NS073796 (J.B.C.), Thomas and Agnes Carvel Foundation (K.M.F. and J.B.C.). The National Institutes of Health and the Thomas and Agnes Carvel Foundation provided funding to J.B.C. and K.M.F. that paid for a portion of the time these authors spent working on this manuscript. These grantors were not involved in study design, data collection, analysis, manuscript preparation, and publication decisions.

Institutional Review Board Statement: The study was conducted in accordance with the Declaration of Helsinki, and approved by the Institutional Review Board of Blythedale Children's Hospital (IRB #15-0309KF).

Informed Consent Statement: Written informed consent was obtained from a parent/caregiver for each participant involved in the BC and CB groups. Written assent was obtained from each participant involved in the BC and CB groups. The Step group was done as a clinical program, therefore informed consent was not obtained. We received IRB approval to analyze and include data from the Step group for this study.

Data Availability Statement: Requests for data can be made to Kathleen Friel, kaf3001@med.cornell.edu.

Acknowledgments: We thank the OTs at Blythedale, especially Tara Sullivan, Fran Sotirhos, Diana Ryan who provided interventions, and the OT volunteers who supported the program. We thank Linda Monterroso for assistance with data tabulation. We thank the participants and their families.

Conflicts of Interest: The authors declare no conflict of interest.

References

1. Novak, I.; Morgan, C.; Fahey, M.; Finch-Edmondson, M.; Galea, C.; Hines, A.; Langdon, K.; Mc Namara, M.; Paton, M.C.; Popat, H.; et al. State of the Evidence Traffic Lights 2019: Systematic Review of Interventions for Preventing and Treating Children with Cerebral Palsy. *Curr. Neurol. Neurosci. Rep.* **2020**, *20*, 3. [CrossRef] [PubMed]
2. Charles, J.R.; Wolf, S.L.; Schneider, J.A.; Gordon, A. Efficacy of a child-friendly form of constraint-induced movement therapy in hemiplegic cerebral palsy: A randomized control trial. *Dev. Med. Child Neurol.* **2006**, *48*, 635–642. [CrossRef] [PubMed]
3. Charles, J.; Gordon, A.M. Development of hand–arm bimanual intensive training (HABIT) for improving bimanual coordination in children with hemiplegic cerebral palsy. *Dev. Med. Child Neurol.* **2006**, *48*, 931–936. [CrossRef] [PubMed]
4. Hoare, B.; Imms, C.; Carey, L.; Wasiak, J. Constraint-induced movement therapy in the treatment of the upper limb in children with hemiplegic cerebral palsy: A Cochrane systematic review. *Clin. Rehabil.* **2007**, *21*, 675–685. [CrossRef]
5. Hoare, B.J.; Wasiak, J.; Imms, C.; Carey, L. Constraint-induced movement therapy in the treatment of the upper limb in children with hemiplegic cerebral palsy. *Cochrane Database Syst. Rev.* **2007**, CD004149. [CrossRef]
6. Sakzewski, L.; Ziviani, J.; Abbott, D.F.; MacDonell, R.A.L.; Jackson, G.; Boyd, R.N. Equivalent Retention of Gains at 1 Year After Training with Constraint-Induced or Bimanual Therapy in Children with Unilateral Cerebral Palsy. *Neurorehabilit. Neural Repair* **2011**, *25*, 664–671. [CrossRef]
7. Sakzewski, L.; Ziviani, J.; Abbott, D.; MacDonell, R.A.L.; Jackson, G.D.; Boyd, R.N. Randomized trial of constraint-induced movement therapy and bimanual training on activity outcomes for children with congenital hemiplegia. *Dev. Med. Child Neurol.* **2011**, *53*, 313–320. [CrossRef]
8. Dong, V.A.-Q.; Tung, I.H.-H.; Siu, H.W.-Y.; Fong, K.N.-K. Studies comparing the efficacy of constraint-induced movement therapy and bimanual training in children with unilateral cerebral palsy: A systematic review. *Dev. Neurorehabilit.* **2012**, *16*, 133–143. [CrossRef]
9. Gordon, A.M.; Hung, Y.-C.; Brandao, M.; Ferre, C.L.; Kuo, H.-C.; Friel, K.; Petra, E.; Chinnan, A.; Charles, J.R. Bimanual Training and Constraint-Induced Movement Therapy in Children with Hemiplegic Cerebral Palsy. *Neurorehabilit. Neural Repair* **2011**, *25*, 692–702. [CrossRef]
10. Friel, K.M.; Ferre, C.L.; Brandao, M.; Kuo, H.-C.; Chin, K.; Hung, Y.-C.; Robert, M.T.; Flamand, V.H.; Smorenburg, A.; Bleyenheuft, Y.; et al. Improvements in Upper Extremity Function Following Intensive Training Are Independent of Corticospinal Tract Organization in Children with Unilateral Spastic Cerebral Palsy: A Clinical Randomized Trial. *Front. Neurol.* **2021**, *12*, 660780. [CrossRef]
11. Brandão, M.D.B.; Gordon, A.M.; Mancini, M.C. Functional Impact of Constraint Therapy and Bimanual Training in Children with Cerebral Palsy: A Randomized Controlled Trial. *Am. J. Occup. Ther.* **2012**, *66*, 672–681. [CrossRef]
12. Gordon, A. Two hands are better than one: Bimanual skill development in children with hemiplegic cerebral palsy. *Dev. Med. Child Neurol.* **2010**, *52*, 315–316. [CrossRef]
13. Bingöl, H.; Günel, M.K. Comparing the effects of modified constraint-induced movement therapy and bimanual training in children with hemiplegic cerebral palsy mainstreamed in regular school: A randomized controlled study. *Arch. Pediatr.* **2022**, *29*, 105–115. [CrossRef]
14. Deppe, W.; Thuemmler, K.; Fleischer, J.; Berger, C.; Meyer, S.; Wiedemann, B. Modified constraint-induced movement therapy versus intensive bimanual training for children with hemiplegia—A randomized controlled trial. *Clin. Rehabil.* **2013**, *27*, 909–920. [CrossRef]
15. Hung, Y.-C.; Spingarn, A.; Friel, K.M.; Gordon, A.M. Intensive Unimanual Training Leads to Better Reaching and Head Control than Bimanual Training in Children with Unilateral Cerebral Palsy. *Phys. Occup. Ther. Pediatr.* **2020**, *40*, 491–505. [CrossRef]
16. Hoare, B.; Greaves, S. Unimanual versus bimanual therapy in children with unilateral cerebral palsy: Same, same, but different. *J. Pediatr. Rehabil. Med.* **2017**, *10*, 47–59. [CrossRef]
17. de Brito Brandao, M.; Mancini, M.C.; Vaz, D.V.; de Melo, A.P.P.; Fonseca, S.T. Adapted version of constraint-induced movement therapy promotes functioning in children with cerebral palsy: A randomized controlled trial. *Clin. Rehabil.* **2010**, *24*, 639–647. [CrossRef]

18. Klingels, K.; Feys, H.; Molenaers, G.; Verbeke, G.; Van Daele, S.; Hoskens, J.; Desloovere, K.; De Cock, P. Randomized Trial of Modified Constraint-Induced Movement Therapy with and Without an Intensive Therapy Program in Children with Unilateral Cerebral Palsy. *Neurorehabil. Neural Repair* **2013**, *27*, 799–807. [CrossRef]
19. Krumlinde-Sundholm, L.; Holmefur, M.; Kottorp, A.; Eliasson, A.-C. The Assisting Hand Assessment: Current evidence of validity, reliability, and responsiveness to change. *Dev. Med. Child Neurol.* **2007**, *49*, 259–264. [CrossRef]
20. Holmefur, M.; Krumlinde-Sundholm, L.; Eliasson, A.-C. Interrater and Intrarater Reliability of the Assisting Hand Assessment. *Am. J. Occup. Ther.* **2007**, *61*, 79–84. [CrossRef]
21. Verkerk, G.J.Q.; Wolf, M.J.M.A.G.; Louwers, A.M.; Meester-Delver, A.; Nollet, F. The reproducibility and validity of the Canadian Occupational Performance Measure in parents of children with disabilities. *Clin. Rehabil.* **2006**, *20*, 980–988. [CrossRef] [PubMed]
22. Law, M.; Baptiste, S.; McColl, M.; Opzoomer, A.; Polatajko, H.; Pollock, N. The Canadian Occupational Performance Measure: An Outcome Measure for Occupational Therapy. *Can. J. Occup. Ther.* **1990**, *57*, 82–87. [CrossRef] [PubMed]
23. Iyer, L.V.; Haley, S.M.; Watkins, M.P.; Dumas, H.M. Establishing minimal clinically important differences for scores on the pediatric evaluation of disability inventory for inpatient rehabilitation. *Phys. Ther.* **2003**, *83*, 888–898. [CrossRef] [PubMed]
24. Berg, M.; Jahnsen, R.; Frøslie, K.F.; Hussain, A. Reliability of the Pediatric Evaluation of Disability Inventory (PEDI). *Phys. Occup. Ther. Pediatr.* **2004**, *24*, 61–67. [CrossRef]
25. Gordon, A.M.; Schneider, J.A.; Chinnan, A.; Charles, J.R. Efficacy of a hand–arm bimanual intensive therapy (HABIT) in children with hemiplegic cerebral palsy: A randomized control trial. *Dev. Med. Child Neurol.* **2007**, *49*, 830–838. [CrossRef]
26. Mutsaarts, M.; Steenbergen, B.; Bekkering, H. Anticipatory planning deficits and task context effects in hemiparetic cerebral palsy. *Exp. Brain Res.* **2006**, *172*, 151–162. [CrossRef]
27. Steenbergen, B.; Jongbloed-Pereboom, M.; Spruijt, S.; Gordon, A. Impaired motor planning and motor imagery in children with unilateral spastic cerebral palsy: Challenges for the future of pediatric rehabilitation. *Dev. Med. Child Neurol.* **2013**, *55* (Suppl. S4), 43–46. [CrossRef]
28. Martinie, O.; Mercier, C.; Gordon, A.M.; Robert, M.T. Upper Limb Motor Planning in Individuals with Cerebral Palsy Aged between 3 and 21 Years Old: A Systematic Review. *Brain Sci.* **2021**, *11*, 920. [CrossRef]
29. Gutterman, J.; Lee-Miller, T.; Friel, K.M.; Dimitropoulou, K.; Gordon, A.M. Anticipatory Motor Planning and Control of Grasp in Children with Unilateral Spastic Cerebral Palsy. *Brain Sci.* **2021**, *11*, 1161. [CrossRef]
30. Simon-Martinez, C.; Mailleux, L.; Hoskens, J.; Ortibus, E.; Jaspers, E.; Wenderoth, N.; Sgandurra, G.; Cioni, G.; Molenaers, G.; Klingels, K.; et al. Randomized controlled trial combining constraint-induced movement therapy and action-observation training in unilateral cerebral palsy: Clinical effects and influencing factors of treatment response. *Ther. Adv. Neurol. Disord.* **2020**, *13*, 1756286419898065. [CrossRef]
31. Gupta, D.; Barachant, A.; Gordon, A.; Ferre, C.; Kuo, H.-C.; Carmel, J.B.; Friel, K.M. Effect of sensory and motor connectivity on hand function in pediatric hemiplegia. *Ann. Neurol.* **2017**, *82*, 766–780. [CrossRef]
32. Delfing, D.; Chin, K.; Hentrich, L.; Rachwani, J.; Friel, K.M.; Santamaria, V.; Imms, C.; Gordon, A.M. Assessing engagement in rehabilitation: Development, validity, reliability, and responsiveness to change of the Rehabilitation Observation Measure of Engagement (ROME). *Disabil. Rehabil.* **2023**, *10*, 1–10. [CrossRef]
33. Friel, K.M.; Kuo, H.-C.; Fuller, J.; Ferre, C.L.; Brandão, M.; Carmel, J.B.; Bleyenheuft, Y.; Gowatsky, J.L.; Stanford, A.D.; Rowny, S.B.; et al. Skilled Bimanual Training Drives Motor Cortex Plasticity in Children with Unilateral Cerebral Palsy. *Neurorehabil. Neural Repair* **2016**, *30*, 834–844. [CrossRef]
34. Kuhnke, N.; Juenger, H.; Walther, M.; Berweck, S.; Mall, V.; Staudt, M. Do patients with congenital hemiparesis and ipsilateral corticospinal projections respond differently to constraint-induced movement therapy? *Dev. Med. Child Neurol.* **2008**, *50*, 898–903. [CrossRef]
35. Smorenburg, A.R.P.; Gordon, A.M.; Kuo, H.-C.; Ferre, C.L.; Brandao, M.; Bleyenheuft, Y.; Carmel, J.B.; Friel, K.M. Does Corticospinal Tract Connectivity Influence the Response to Intensive Bimanual Therapy in Children with Unilateral Cerebral Palsy? *Neurorehabil. Neural Repair* **2016**, *31*, 250–260. [CrossRef]
36. Gelkop, N.; Burshtein, D.G.; Lahav, A.; Brezner, A.; Al-Oraibi, S.; Ferre, C.L.; Gordon, A. Efficacy of Constraint-Induced Movement Therapy and Bimanual Training in Children with Hemiplegic Cerebral Palsy in an Educational Setting. *Phys. Occup. Ther. Pediatr.* **2014**, *35*, 24–39. [CrossRef]
37. Klepper, S.E.; Krasinski, D.C.; Gilb, M.C.; Khalil, N. Comparing Unimanual and Bimanual Training in Upper Extremity Function in Children with Unilateral Cerebral Palsy. *Pediatr. Phys. Ther.* **2017**, *29*, 288–306. [CrossRef]
38. Rice, D.; Barone, S., Jr. Critical periods of vulnerability for the developing nervous system: Evidence from humans and animal models. *Environ. Health Perspect.* **2000**, *108* (Suppl. S3), 511–533. [CrossRef]

Disclaimer/Publisher's Note: The statements, opinions and data contained in all publications are solely those of the individual author(s) and contributor(s) and not of MDPI and/or the editor(s). MDPI and/or the editor(s) disclaim responsibility for any injury to people or property resulting from any ideas, methods, instructions or products referred to in the content.

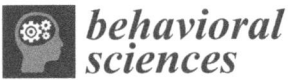

Article

Bimanual Movement Characteristics and Real-World Performance Following Hand–Arm Bimanual Intensive Therapy in Children with Unilateral Cerebral Palsy

Shailesh S. Gardas [1], Christine Lysaght [1], Amy Gross McMillan [1], Shailesh Kantak [2,3], John D. Willson [1], Charity G. Patterson [4] and Swati M. Surkar [1,*]

1. Department of Physical Therapy, East Carolina University, Greenville, NC 27834, USA; gardass21@students.ecu.edu (S.S.G.); lysaghtc@ecu.edu (C.L.); grossmcmillana@ecu.edu (A.G.M.); willsonj@ecu.edu (J.D.W.)
2. Moss Rehabilitation Research Institute, Elkins Park, PA 19027, USA
3. Department of Physical Therapy, Arcadia University, Glenside, PA 19038, USA
4. Department of Physical Therapy and School of Health and Rehabilitation Sciences Data Center, University of Pittsburgh, Pittsburgh, PA 15260, USA; cgp22@pitt.edu
* Correspondence: surkars19@ecu.edu

Abstract: The purpose of this study was to quantify characteristics of bimanual movement intensity during 30 h of hand–arm bimanual intensive therapy (HABIT) and bimanual performance (activities and participation) in real-world settings using accelerometers in children with unilateral cerebral palsy (UCP). Twenty-five children with UCP participated in a 30 h HABIT program. Data were collected from bilateral wrist-worn accelerometers during 30 h of HABIT to quantify the movement intensity and three days pre- and post-HABIT to assess real-world performance gains. Movement intensity and performance gains were measured using six standard accelerometer-derived variables. Bimanual capacity (body function and activities) was assessed using standardized hand function tests. We found that accelerometer variables increased significantly during HABIT, indicating increased bimanual symmetry and intensity. Post-HABIT, children demonstrated significant improvements in all accelerometer metrics, reflecting real-world performance gains. Children also achieved significant and clinically relevant changes in hand capacity following HABIT. Therefore, our findings suggest that accelerometers can objectively quantify bimanual movement intensity during HABIT. Moreover, HABIT enhances hand function as well as activities and participation in real-world situations in children with UCP.

Keywords: training intensity; bimanual coordination; real-world activity; actigraphs; upper extremity

1. Introduction

Unilateral cerebral palsy (UCP) is a leading cause of childhood disability [1]. Children with UCP have difficulty with bimanual coordination, which further restricts the child's independence in daily activities and impairs quality of life [2]. Hand–arm bimanual intensive therapy (HABIT) is a well-established intervention to improve hand function and bimanual coordination in children with UCP [3]. Traditionally, the intensity of HABIT has been quantified as the number of hours of therapy [4,5]. Despite the reported improvements in upper extremity (UE) function, discrepancies exist in the intensity of training protocols [6,7]. Evidence indicates that greater intensities in terms of hours result in larger gains in UE motor outcomes [4,8]. However, time is recognized as a proxy measure of training intensity since it does not reveal specific information about the goal-directed UE or bimanual movements occurring during training [9]. Hence, it is crucial to develop objective methods to quantify the intensity of HABIT in terms of bimanual movement characteristics that would provide insights into bimanual training intensity.

Citation: Gardas, S.S.; Lysaght, C.; McMillan, A.G.; Kantak, S.; Willson, J.D.; Patterson, C.G.; Surkar, S.M. Bimanual Movement Characteristics and Real-World Performance Following Hand–Arm Bimanual Intensive Therapy in Children with Unilateral Cerebral Palsy. *Behav. Sci.* **2023**, *13*, 681. https://doi.org/10.3390/bs13080681

Academic Editors: Stephanie C. DeLuca and Jill C. Heathcock

Received: 16 June 2023
Revised: 8 August 2023
Accepted: 10 August 2023
Published: 13 August 2023

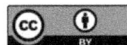

Copyright: © 2023 by the authors. Licensee MDPI, Basel, Switzerland. This article is an open access article distributed under the terms and conditions of the Creative Commons Attribution (CC BY) license (https://creativecommons.org/licenses/by/4.0/).

Accelerometers have been accepted as a valid tool to objectively capture UE movement characteristics in the real-world environment [10–12]. They measure accelerations of UE movements along the predefined axes in gravitational units called activity counts. The gold standard methods to monitor quality and quantity of UE use, such as 3D kinematic [13] and human-observed coding [14] of video recordings, can be time-consuming and expensive to quantify the intensity of HABIT. Accelerometer metrics overcome these problems and provide a convenient option to measure movement characteristics during intensive therapy as well as in the real-world environment, thus capturing the activities and participation domains per the International Classification of Functioning, Disability, and Health—Children and Youth Version (ICF-CY) [15]. Acceleration metrics that reflect UE movement characteristics are broadly classified into three categories [16]. The first category indicates the relative contributions of the affected and less affected UE movements using use ratio, magnitude ratio, and bilateral magnitude [16]. The second category comprises characteristics specific to the accelerations of the affected extremity through median acceleration and acceleration variability. The third category provides the number of accelerations using activity counts for both extremities [16]. Our novel approach capitalized on these three categories to quantify the characteristics of a 30 h (intensity) HABIT. An understanding of bimanual movement characteristics can provide clinically meaningful information regarding the contribution of the affected vs. less affected extremity to bimanual activities during HABIT and thereby guide clinical dosing criteria and capture gains in bimanual performance in real-world activities.

Performance refers to what a person actually does in a real-world environment, whereas capacity refers to what a person can do in a controlled environment such as a clinic [17]. The International Classification of Functioning, Disability, and Health—Children and Youth Version (ICF-CY) by the World Health Organization, provides a clear differentiation between performance and capacity within the domains of activities and participation [15]. Activity refers to the execution of a task or action by an individual, whereas participation is involvement in a life situation. Performance qualifier, according to ICF-CY, refers to what a person does in a current (real-world or lived experience) environment, signifying participation, whereas capacity refers to what a person can do in a controlled (standard) environment such as in a clinic, signifying activity [17]. Traditionally, studies examining the efficacy of HABIT have assessed changes in UE capacity using standardized clinical tests such as the Assisting Hand Assessment (AHA), Box and Block Test (BBT), Nine-Hole Peg Test (NHPT), Jebsen Hand Function Test (JHFT), etc., that primarily capture body function and activity per ICF-CY [18]. UE performance (activity and participation) has been assessed using self-reported measures such as the Canadian Occupational Performance Measure, the Pediatric Evaluation and Disability Inventory, and ABILHAND [18]. Collectively, these studies indicate that HABIT improves UE capacity as well as the performance of children with UCP. However, self-reported measures are prone to subjective and social desirability biases, which raise questions about whether in-clinic improvements are indicative of changes in real-world bimanual activities and participation [19]. Recent evidence supports this conjecture since discrepancies between parents' perceptions of their child's performance using self-reported measures and therapists' assessments of capacity have been reported [20]. Furthermore, changes in standardized assessments may not translate to improvements in the affected UE use in daily life when assessed with accelerometers in children with UCP [21,22] as well as the adult stroke population [23]. Therefore, capturing the performance of the affected UE during daily bimanual activities using accelerometers is crucial to elucidate whether improvements in capacity with HABIT translate to gains in performance in real-world bimanual activities and participation in children with UCP.

In the last decade, accelerometers have been primarily used to assess UE performance after intervention in adult stroke survivors [24,25] and to detect motor asymmetries in children with UCP [26]. Only a few studies have used accelerometers to monitor UE gains in children with UCP following intensive therapy such as constraint-induced movement therapy (CIMT) [21,27]. Collectively, the results of the studies in adults with stroke [16] as well as in children with UCP [21,27] indicate that despite improvements in UE capacity, UE performance in daily life showed little to no improvement. Despite the excellent capacity of accelerometers to capture activity counts and movement characteristics in a real-world environment, none of the studies have utilized accelerometers to measure real-world bimanual performance post-HABIT.

Therefore, the primary purpose of this novel study was to objectively quantify the characteristics of bimanual movements during 30 h (intensity) of HABIT using bilateral wrist-worn accelerometers. The second purpose was to examine the gains in real-world bimanual performance following HABIT using accelerometer-derived variables reflecting activities and participation. We hypothesize that accelerometers will accurately capture the UE movement characteristics reflecting bimanual use during HABIT. Furthermore, 30 h of HABIT will enhance children's affected UE contributions to the performance of real-world bimanual activities.

2. Materials and Methods

2.1. Study Design and Setting

This study is an ancillary analysis [28] of a double-blind, randomized controlled trial (NCT05355883). It was a prospective pre- and post-training study conducted at the Pediatric Assessment and Rehabilitation Laboratory (PeARL) at East Carolina University (ECU), NC. The University and Medical Center Institutional Review Board, ECU, approved the study. We obtained parental consent and child assent. The assessors were blinded to the pre- and post-testing assessments. The study was conducted between November 2021 and January 2023.

2.2. Participants

Twenty-five children with UCP, ages 6–16 years (mean age = 11.20 ± 3.59 years), and Manual Ability Classification System levels I–III participated in this study. Figure 1 shows the CONSORT diagram, describing the flow of participants through the study, withdrawals, and inclusion in analyses.

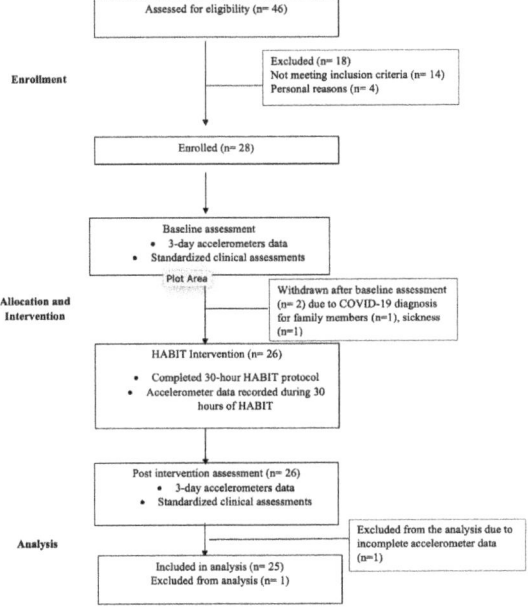

Figure 1. CONSORT flow chart.

Children with other neuromotor disabilities, cognitive and communication deficits, cardiorespiratory dysfunctions, metabolic disorders, neoplasms, and a history of botulinum neurotoxin injections on the affected UE in the past 6 months were excluded. Table 1 describes further details about participant characteristics.

Table 1. Demographic details of the participants.

Characteristics	Participants
	Children with Unilateral Cerebral Palsy ($n = 25$)
Sex, n (%)	
Male	18 (72)
Females	7 (28)
Age, mean (SD)	11.20 (3.59)
Side of hemiplegia, n (%)	
Left	10 (40)
Right	15 (60)
Race, n (%)	
White	21 (84)
African American	1 (4)
Asian	3 (12)
Multiracial	-
MACS Level, n (%)	
I	1 (4)
II	9 (36)
III	15 (60)

MACS indicates Manual ability classification system.

2.3. Procedures

2.3.1. Hand–Arm Bimanual Intensive Therapy (HABIT) Protocol

HABIT is a well-established intervention shown to improve bimanual coordination in children with UCP [3]. We administered HABIT in a camp-based setting with a pre-determined duration of a total of 30 h of structured, task-specific, bimanual activities, six hours per day for five consecutive days. The therapy included age-appropriate bimanual gross and fine motor tasks in a playful context (please see Supplementary Material S1). The child-to-interventionist ratio (trained physical and occupational therapy students) was 1:4. Individualized therapy goals were formulated based on the pre-training behavioral hand function tests as well as parent–child identified bimanual goals. Interventionists progressively increased the complexity of bimanual activities. The task demands were graded based on the task performance to allow the child to complete the task successfully. Children were encouraged to use the affected and the less affected UE in a coordinated manner. Positive reinforcement and knowledge of performance were provided to motivate and reinforce desired goal-directed activities. Emphasis was placed on different roles of the affected UE, such as stabilizer, manipulator, and assistor, depending on the child's ability and task goal. Sessions comprised whole-task and part-task practice. Throughout the HABIT, three licensed physical therapists supervised the interventionists to ensure the fidelity of therapy. Activities performed by the children were documented by the interventionists [7].

2.3.2. Accelerometry Methodology

Bilateral wrist-worn accelerometers (Actigraphy GT9X Link, Pensacola, FL, USA) were used to quantify the movement characteristics during the five days of HABIT and the performance (real-world UE activity) gains post-HABIT. Actigraph GT9X Link measures accelerations in activity counts along three axes, with one count equaling 0.001664 g [29]. Accelerometer data were sampled at 30 Hz, and activity counts were binned into 1 s epochs for each axis using ActiLifeTM 6 software. Data was then processed in MATLAB (Mathworks Inc, Natick, MA, USA) using custom-written software developed by Lang et al. [29]. To determine movement characteristics during HABIT days, children wore accelerometers for 5 days of HABIT (30 h total wear time). To measure UE performance gains, children wore accelerometers for three consecutive days pre- and post-HABIT during their daily activities, which included home, school, and play. This approach was designed to capture bimanual activities throughout the day in a natural, real-world environment. Moreover, the three-day accelerometer wearing time pre- and post-HABIT was chosen since it produces a reliable estimate of performance in children with CP [30]. Detailed instructions were provided to both parents and children on the proper wearing and usage of accelerometers. Specifically, they were instructed to keep the Actigraphs on during waking hours, but to remove them while bathing or engaging in water-related activities.

2.4. Outcome Measures

2.4.1. Bimanual Movement Intensity Characteristics and Performance Measures

Accelerometer-derived metrics [16,29]: Activity and Participation Domains of ICF-CY

We quantified the bimanual movement characteristics using six standard accelerometry derived variables: (1) use ratio (UR), (2) magnitude ratio (MR), (3) bilateral magnitude (BM), (4) median acceleration (MA), (5) acceleration variability (AV), and (6) affected UE activity counts (AAC). Changes in UE performance pre- and post-HABIT reflecting real-world performance (activity and participation) were assessed using (1) UR, (2) MR, (3) BM, (4) MA, and (5) AV [15]. Figure 2 explains the accelerometry-derived variables.

(1) The use ratio reflects the contribution of the affected UE relative to the less affected UE and is calculated as the ratio of the active duration of the affected arm to that of the less affected arm. The UR value ranges between 0 and 1. A value close to or equal to 1 indicates symmetrical use of the extremities, whereas a value closer to zero indicates less affected UE use.

(2) The magnitude ratio is the ratio of acceleration magnitude (range of movement) of both UEs and is calculated by dividing the acceleration magnitude of the affected and the less affected UE. The value of MR ranges from -7 to $+7$. A value closer to 0 indicates equal contributions from both UEs; positive values indicate greater movement magnitude of the affected UE, and negative values indicate greater movement magnitude of the less affected UE.

(3) Bilateral magnitude reflects the magnitude of accelerations across both UEs and is calculated by summing the smoothed vector magnitudes of both UEs for each second of activity. Zero indicates no activity, and an increasing value indicates greater magnitudes of bilateral UE activity.

(4) Median acceleration and acceleration variability are variables that reflect movement characteristics considering only the affected UE. The median acceleration represents the acceleration of the affected UE magnitude over the entire wear time.

(5) Acceleration variability is the variance of the mean acceleration and represents the average distance of the affected UE accelerations from the mean acceleration. A higher score for both of these variables indicates better overall UE movement and variability, respectively [16,21].

(6) Affected extremity activity counts quantify the number of affected extremity accelerations (activity counts) during therapy.

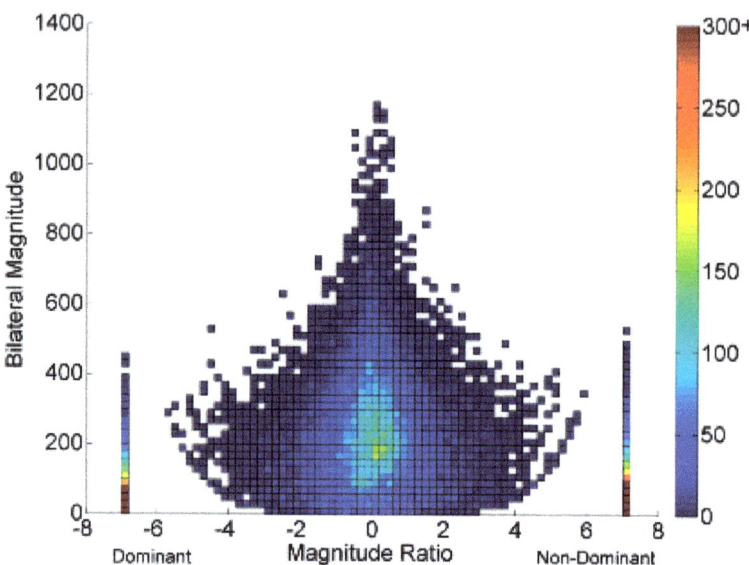

Figure 2. A representative example of a density plot, which is a graphical representation of accelerometer data obtained from both upper extremities (UE) of a typically developing child. The plot shows accelerations on a second-by-second basis recorded over a total wear time of three days, both pre- and post-HABIT in our study. The x-axis represents the magnitude ratio, indicating the contribution of each UE to the task, while the y-axis represents the overall intensity or magnitude of movement. The right and left halves of the plot represent the use of the right and left UEs, respectively. The dots visible in the graph indicate the counts or number of movements (accelerations) performed by each UE. The large color bar scale on the right of the plot displays the frequency of movements, with brighter colors indicating greater frequencies and vice versa. The plot is noticeably symmetrical, indicating that the typically developing child used both UEs equally in terms of hours, which is called the use ratio. The magnitude ratio indicates the contribution of the affected UE relative to the less affected UE in terms of the intensity of movements. The dots seen in both halves of the plot appear at similar heights, suggesting a symmetrical magnitude of movements with both UEs in a typically developing child. Bilateral magnitude is the overall intensity of both UEs, which is determined by the height of the density plot. A taller density plot indicates better bilateral magnitude. Median acceleration and acceleration variability are measures reflecting the mean accelerations and variance in the accelerations of the affected UE, which are shown in only one half of the density plot, depending on the affected side.

2.4.2. Capacity Measures

Standardized Clinical Assessments—Body Function and Activity Domains of ICF-CY

Standardized clinical assessments were used to measure changes in UE capacity pre- and post-HABIT in a controlled laboratory setting [15]. The AHA assesses the affected hand function and bimanual coordination in children with UCP [31]. An improvement of 5 units is considered clinically meaningful [32]. JHFT (reliability; interrater = 0.94, test–retest = 0.91 [33]) and NHPT (reliability; interrater = 0.99, test–retest = 0.81 [34]) measure unimanual dexterity and speed. BBT (reliability; interrater = 0.99, test–retest = 0.85 [35]) assesses the unimanual speed.

2.5. Statistical Analysis

Data were analyzed using IBM Statistical Package for Social Sciences Version 28.0.0. Data are presented as mean ± SD for continuous variables and n (%) for categorical variables. The intensity of UE movement characteristics during 5 days of HABIT were quantified using descriptive statistics for UR, MR, BM, MA, AV, and AAC. Repeated measures analysis of variance (ANOVA) was used with time (five days) as a within-group variable to determine variability in training using UR, MR, BM, MA, AV, and AAC. Considering the repetitive measurements, the significance level for the ANOVA was set at p value ≤ 0.01 using the Bonferroni method. Capacity and performance outcomes were assessed for normality using the Shapiro–Wilk test. Pre- and post-HABIT changes in the capacity and performance measures were assessed using a paired t-test for all the variables, except for MR and BBT scores. The Wilcoxon signed rank test was used to analyze changes in MR and BBT scores pre- and post-HABIT as the data violated the assumption of normality. The significance level was set at a p value = 0.05 for the paired t-test.

3. Results

Twenty-eight participants were enrolled, and twenty-six completed the study intervention. However, data were analyzed for only 25 participants due to incomplete accelerometer data from one participant. There were no adverse events reported during HABIT. Power was derived based on Goodwin et al.'s [21] study and computed using G*Power [36]. To detect the mean difference of 0.25 ($\mu_1 = 1.36$, $\mu_2 = 1.61$; SD1 = 0.12, SD2 = 0.21) in the primary outcome use ratio (UR), a total of 26 participants provides 94% power to detect an effect size of 1.46 at a significance level of 0.05. The sample size was calculated based on a two-sided t-test.

3.1. Characteristics of Bimanual Movement Intensity during HABIT

Accelerometer metrics, UR, MR, BM, MA, AV, and AAC, representing the bimanual movement characteristics during HABIT days, are summarized as descriptive statistics in Table 2. All the children participated in 30 h of HABIT training across five days. Overall, during HABIT, the affected UE use was 47.26% as compared to 53.73% of the less affected UE use.

(1) Magnitude ratio (MR): The average MR across five days of HABIT was -0.56 ± 0.26 (range: -0.97 to 0.05, Figure 3b). There was no significant main effect of time ($F(4,96) = 1.688$, $p = 0.159$) for MR.

(2) Bilateral Magnitude (BM): The average BM across five days of HABIT was 167.25 ± 39.83 (range: 101.98–267.51, Figure 3c). There was no significant main effect of time ($F(4,96) = 1.923$, $p = 0.113$) for BM.

(3) Median acceleration (MA): The average MA across five days of HABIT was 56.99 ± 21.21 (range: 28.49–115.07, Figure 3d). There was no significant main effect of time ($F(4,96) = 2.004$, $p = 0.1$) for MA.

(4) Acceleration variability (AV): The average AV across five days of HABIT was 110.27 ± 18.63 (range: 69.07–143.05, Figure 3e). There was a significant main effect of time ($F(4,96) = 3.666$, $p = 0.008$). Table 3 shows significant post hoc analysis results using Bonferroni multiple comparisons for acceleration variability across five days of HABIT.

(5) Affected extremity activity counts (AAC): The average daily number of affected UE accelerations during 6 h across five days of HABIT were (mean ± SD) $15,399 \pm 2477$ (range: 9863–20,057 counts) (Figure 3f). The total affected UE accelerations reflecting UE use (sum of the means of daily affected UE accelerations) during 30 h of HABIT was 76,997 movements. There was a significant main effect of time ($F(4,96) = 2.633$, $p = 0.03$) for the AAC. Table 3 shows significant post hoc analysis results using Bonferroni multiple comparisons for AAC across five days of HABIT.

Table 2. Descriptive statistics of accelerometer-derived variables across five days of HABIT.

Accelerometer Variables	Minimum	Maximum	Mean	Std Deviation
Use Ratio				
Day 1	0.81	1.13	0.91	0.07
Day 2	0.80	0.99	0.89	0.05
Day 3	0.78	1.00	0.89	0.06
Day 4	0.81	1.08	0.92	0.06
Day 5	0.77	1.05	0.89	0.07
Average	0.79	1.05	0.90	0.06
Magnitude Ratio				
Day 1	−0.96	0.69	−0.52	0.33
Day 2	−1.09	−0.13	−0.58	0.24
Day 3	−1.03	−0.27	−0.61	0.22
Day 4	−0.91	−0.01	−0.50	0.25
Day 5	−0.87	−0.04	−0.57	0.25
Average	−0.97	0.05	−0.56	0.26
Bilateral Magnitude				
Day 1	93.78	268.94	161.99	43.80
Day 2	102.43	296.16	164.69	41.04
Day 3	98.53	240.82	163.87	35.36
Day 4	114.13	257.18	172.56	32.44
Day 5	101.02	274.46	173.16	46.50
Average	101.98	267.51	167.25	39.83
Median Acceleration				
Day 1	25.00	117.14	55.85	24.82
Day 2	28.44	134.99	55.04	22.69
Day 3	25.30	101.24	53.56	18.64
Day 4	37.16	104.35	60.61	16.50
Day 5	26.57	117.63	59.89	23.40
Average	28.49	115.07	56.99	21.21
Acceleration Variability				
Day 1	73.44	142.26	107.28	18.65
Day 2	79.14	140.00	112.29	17.26
Day 3	63.44	132.51	105.49	17.63
Day 4	73.08	158.11	117.40	19.09
Day 5	56.25	142.36	108.89	20.53
Average	69.07	143.05	110.27	18.63
Affected Use count				
Day 1	10,198	20,283	15,325	2745
Day 2	11,100	20,823	15,531	2280
Day 3	3790	19,760	14,714	3275
Day 4	12,903	19,996	16,160	1767
Day 5	11,322	19,425	15,267	2317
Average	9863	20,057	15,399	2477

Use ratio (UR): The average use ratio across five days of HABIT was 0.90 ± 0.06 (range: 0.79–1.00, Figure 3a). There was no significant main effect of time ($F_{(4,96)} = 1.873$, $p = 0.121$) for UR.

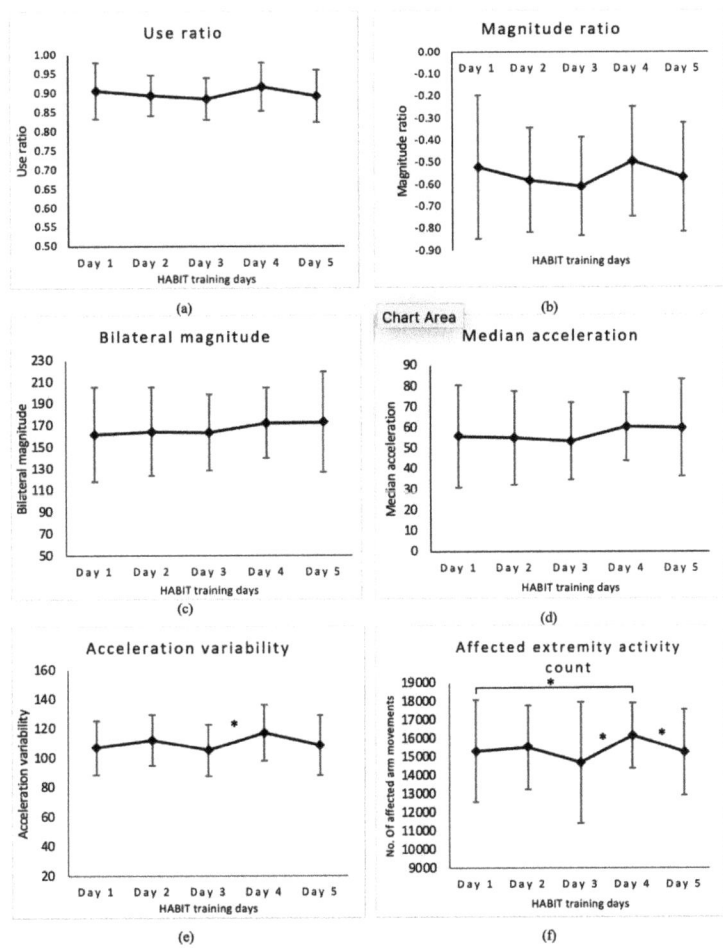

Figure 3. HABIT intensity across 5 days of training using accelerometer-derived variables. Values are means ± SD for each day of HABIT: (**a**) use ratio, (**b**) magnitude ratio, (**c**) bilateral magnitude, (**d**) median acceleration, (**e**) acceleration variability, and (**f**) affected extremity use count. Variability is observed in all the accelerometer variables during the five training days. * denotes a significant p value at $\alpha = 0.05$.

Table 3. Pairwise comparison of the accelerometer metrics between different HABIT training days.

	Bonferroni Pairwise Comparison							
Variables	Mean	vs.	Mean	Significance	Mean Difference	Standard Error of Difference	Lower Bound	Upper Bound
Acceleration variability	Day3	vs.	Day4	0.001 *	−11.9	3.6	−19.3	−4.6
Affected extremity activity counts	Day1	vs.	Day5	0.04 *	−835.3	385.0	−1629.9	−40.7
	Day3	vs.	Day5	0.024 *	−1445.6	601.9	−2687.9	−203.2
	Day4	vs.	Day5	0.036 *	893.5	402.7	62.5	1724.6

Post hoc analysis results with Bonferroni multiple comparisons between training days; * indicates a significant p value at $\alpha = 0.05$.

3.2. Pre- and Post-HABIT Change in Upper Extremity Performance Measures: Activity and Participation

There was a significant improvement in UR ($p = 0.002$, Figure 4a), MR ($p = 0.018$, Figure 4b), bilateral magnitude ($p = 0.006$, Figure 4c), median acceleration ($p = 0.002$, Figure 4d), and acceleration variability ($p = 0.024$, Figure 4e) post-HABIT. These findings indicate that 30 h of HABIT enhanced children's use of the affected arm in terms of movement symmetry, magnitude, and variability. Supplementary Material S2 shows exemplary data from a study participant with pre- and post-HABIT changes in these performance measures. Supplementary Material S3 shows the inter- and intra-individual differences in accelerometer-derived variables for all the participants across time points.

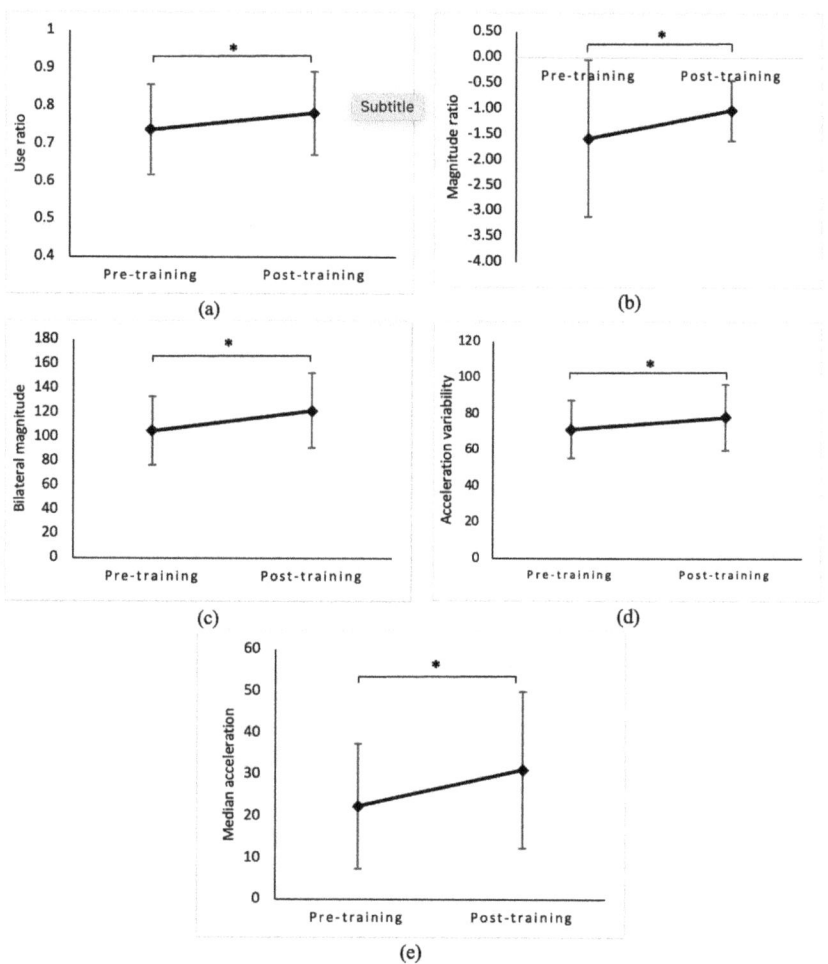

Figure 4. Comparison of differences in the mean scores of accelerometer-derived variables to assess performance gains (activity and participation) pre- and post-HABIT training. Values reported are means ± SD or median (range) as determined by the distribution of data during each assessment time point. Pre-training refers to baseline assessment, and post-training refers to assessment within one week following HABIT. There was a significant change in the average (**a**) use ratio, (**b**) magnitude ratio, (**c**) bilateral magnitude, (**d**) acceleration variability, and (**e**) median acceleration from pre- to post-HABIT. * indicates a significant p value at $\alpha = 0.05$.

3.3. Pre- and Post-HABIT Change in Capacity Measures of the Affected Upper Extremity: Body Function and Activity

There was significant improvement in the mean scores of the AHA ($p = 0.001$, Figure 5a), the JHFT ($p = 0.001$, Figure 5b), the BBT ($p = 0.002$, Figure 5c), and the NHPT ($p = 0.011$, Figure 5d) from pre- to post-HABIT. The mean scores of AHA and BBT exceeded the minimal clinically important difference (MCID) of five logit scores [32] and two blocks [37]. The mean score of the JHFT was very close (53.4 s) to the MCID of 55 s [37]. These findings indicate that post-HABIT, children showed an increase in bimanual coordination, dexterity, and speed of the affected hand use.

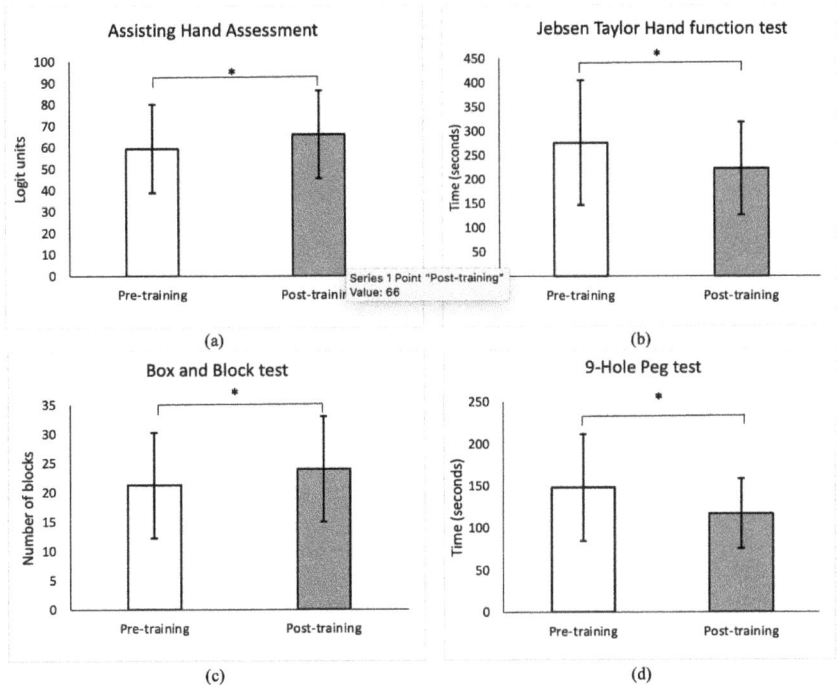

Figure 5. Comparison of differences in the mean scores of capacity (body function and activity) measures pre- and post-HABIT. Values reported are means ± SD as determined by the distribution of data during each assessment time point. Pre-training refers to baseline assessment, and post-training refers to assessment within one week following HABIT. There were significant changes seen in the mean scores of (**a**) Assisting Hand Assessment (>MCID of 5 logit scores), (**b**) Jebsen Taylor Hand Function Test [very close (53.4 s) to MCID of 55 s], (**c**) Box and Block Test (>MCID of 2 blocks), and (**d**) Nine Hole Peg Test pre- vs. post-training. Children demonstrated significant improvement in bimanual coordination, speed, and dexterity as reflected by a greater AHA score, faster speeds in JHFT and NHPT, and a greater number of blocks transferred in BBT, respectively, during post-training assessment compared to baseline. * indicates a significant p value at $\alpha = 0.05$.

4. Discussion

Our primary aim was to quantify the characteristics of bimanual movement intensity during 30 h of HABIT utilizing bilateral wrist-worn accelerometers. Our findings illustrate that the standard accelerometer-derived variables can quantify the contribution of the affected UE to bimanual activities and hence can provide an objective metric for the intensity of bimanual movements practiced during HABIT. Moreover, our results indicate that children performed a total of 76,997 accelerations with their affected UE during HABIT. Our secondary aim was to examine gains in bimanual performance (activity and participation in a real-world environment) and capacity (body function and activity in a clinical setting) post-HABIT using accelerometer-derived metrics and standardized outcomes, respectively. We found significant gains in real-world performance of bimanual activities post-HABIT, suggesting improved activities and participation in the child's natural, real-world environment. Furthermore, consistent with prior studies, our results indicate improvements in UE capacity following HABIT. Overall, this is the first study that utilized wearable technology to quantify the intensity of HABIT and demonstrated that accelerometers can objectively quantify bimanual movement characteristics reflecting the intensity of UE use during HABIT. Moreover, 30 h of HABIT has the potential to improve the UE capacity as well as real-world bimanual performance in children with UCP.

Time is a dominant measure used to define the intensity of arm use during intensive therapies [4,5]. However, time does not indicate the actual number of movements or movement characteristics performed during a particular session [9,38]. In this study, we overcame this limitation using accelerometers and demonstrated a more accurate method to objectively quantify UE movement characteristics during HABIT. UR and MR signify the contributions of the affected relative to the less affected UE considering the duration and magnitude (range of movement) during bimanual activities. Children in our study attained an average UR of 0.90 during HABIT, which was 22% higher than pre-training. The UR being close to 1 suggests that there was nearly equal use of both UEs during HABIT. The average MR during HABIT was −0.56, which was 64.6% higher than pre-training. The value of MR moved substantially closer to 0, indicating a greater magnitude of the affected UE during training. Likewise, the average BM reflecting the combined magnitudes of accelerations from both UEs during HABIT was 167.25, which was 58.8% higher than pre-training. The average MA and AV reflecting mean accelerations of the affected UE and variability of accelerations also increased (MA = 56.9, AV = 110.3) noticeably during HABIT by 154.36% and 54.4% compared to pre-training. Collectively, these results indicate greater symmetry in UE use and higher affected arm use during HABIT. These improvements can be attributed to the intensive nature of bimanual, task-specific activities incorporated in HABIT. Notably, the UR and MR attained during training were comparable to those reported in accelerometer studies in typically developing children of 0.96 and −0.28, respectively, which suggests that the bimanual activities incorporated in HABIT were comparable with the amount of typical bimanual activities [21,26]. Overall, our findings provide preliminary evidence for using accelerometers to quantify movement characteristics during HABIT. These findings could serve as the foundation for future studies to understand the relationship between accelerometer metrics and motor outcomes in children with UCP.

Affected UE activity counts (AAC) during 6 h of HABIT ranged from 14,714 to 16,160, and a total of nearly 76,997 accelerations occurred during 30 h of HABIT. The use of repetitions to quantify intensity is limited in rehabilitation research and clinical practice. Some studies on stroke survivors have investigated repetitions of UE training by observing video recordings of therapy sessions [14,39]. Lang and colleagues used repetitions to quantify the intensity of upper limb exercise during stroke rehabilitation and inpatient hospital stays [40]. These observational studies, however, focused on routine therapy sessions, which are invariably of shorter duration. Although this is the gold standard method for monitoring repetitions, manual coding by human observers could be exceedingly strenuous, especially for extended hours of therapy such as HABIT. Despite the differences regarding the inability of accelerometers to isolate purposeful movements, UE movement characteristics derived from accelerometer metrics could still provide clinically relevant data about UE use during prolonged hours of training. Moreover, previous studies have found an agreement between the affected UE activity counts and human-observed purposeful repetitions during group [41] and individual therapy [39] sessions, suggesting that accelerometer measures have concurrent validity. As a result, this study is unique in two ways: (1) for the first time, we provide objective data on bimanual movement characteristics reflecting the intensity of arm use during HABIT; and (2) we were able to quantify the number of affected UE activity counts during 30 h of HABIT, which, while an overestimation, could still be considered a key component to influence motor learning.

Our results demonstrated significant improvements on all standardized clinical tests, reflecting enhanced UE capacity and suggesting improvements in body function and activity measured in a constrained clinical environment post-HABIT. Notably, the AHA scores exceeded the minimal clinically important (MCID) difference of five units [32]. Children were able to transfer a greater number of blocks (>2 blocks compared to pre-training, MCID = 2 [37]) with their affected UE (12% increase in BBT) and complete the NHPT (21.04% faster) and JHFT (19.35% faster, pre-to-post-HABIT difference = 53.4 s, very close to MCID of 55 s) [37] in less time, indicating greater speed and dexterity post-HABIT. These findings are consistent with previous studies that demonstrated an increase in hand capacity following intensive therapies [18].

Our study results also indicate gains in UE performance following HABIT, which indicates enhanced activities and participation in a natural, real-world environment in these participants [15]. Children demonstrated increases in UR, MR, and BM of 6.85%, 34.81%, and 15.84%, respectively, indicating greater symmetry and contribution of the affected UE in terms of hours of use and magnitude of real-world bimanual activities. Additionally, post-HABIT, MA and AV increased by 39.56% and 9.48%, respectively, which indicates an increase in the affected UE speed and variations in movement speed following HABIT. However, our accelerometer measures also revealed a significant degree of variability at pre- and post-HABIT time points, aligning with previous studies that employed similar methods [21,27]. This variability can be attributed to the heterogeneity of our study population, including differences in age, gender, and functional level as measured by MACS. Further analysis of the individual profile plots depicting inter-individual differences (Supplementary Material Figure S2a) revealed that a few participants with MACS level III exhibited higher UR (>0.8) at baseline. This could be due to involuntary and mirror movements in their more affected UE, resulting in higher accelerometer readings indicating increased affected UE use. Additionally, the profile plot of MR (Supplementary Material Figure S2b) indicated that the changes in the magnitude of movement of the more affected UE following HABIT were significantly driven by three participants. These three participants were relatively older (≥15 years) compared to younger children and likely had higher motivation for high-amplitude activities, such as overhead catch and throw with a soccer ball or hitting a baseball, etc., which plausibly led to greater improvements in MR post-HABIT. The profile plots for BM, MA, and AV (Supplementary Material Figure S2c–e) revealed similar trends: participants with MACS level III, who initially had lower baseline scores, exhibited more pronounced improvements after undergoing HABIT compared to those with MACS levels I and II. Similar to MR, the profile plots for BM and MA indicated that a small subset of participants with MACS level III, who were comparatively older demonstrated pronounced changes post-HABIT. Despite the observed variability, which is typical in clinical populations, collectively, our study findings demonstrated improvements in real-world bimanual performance, which contradict the findings of previous studies that utilized accelerometers to assess UE performance gains post-CIMT [21,27]. The limited gains reported in those studies could be due to the lack of a bimanual training component in the CIMT approach. We believe the intensity of HABIT administered in our study, as seen by improved UE movement characteristics, was potentially adequate to drive changes in UE capacity beyond a specific threshold required to produce a change in UE performance.

Study Limitations: We recognize a few study limitations and propose future study directions. First, wrist-worn accelerometers capture only arm and forearm accelerations (gross motor function), but they are limited in capturing finger accelerations (fine motor function). Thus, future studies could use finger-worn inertial sensors to quantify fine movements in this population. Second, although we attempted to perform bimanual activities during HABIT training to achieve purposeful movements, a part of our data may contain non-purposeful movements occurring during non-therapy time, such as normal walking, washroom breaks, etc. Therefore, caution should be used when interpreting the results of this study. Third, we did not measure long-term retention of the UE performance gains in this study. We suggest that future studies address this limitation by conducting follow-up assessments to determine the persistence of immediate gains in performance, which could provide insight into the retention and transfer components of motor skill learning. Finally, the generalizability of our study findings could be limited due to heterogeneous study participants and a lack of a control group.

5. Conclusions

Accelerometers can be used to quantify the movement characteristics of UE during HABIT, which could provide an objective measure regarding the intensity of UE use. Thirty hours of HABIT has the potential to improve UE function in real-world bimanual activities, indicating improvements in activities and participation in the natural environment, and to enhance the speed and dexterity of the affected UE, indicating improvements in body function and activity in a clinical environment. Overall, the accelerometer is a valuable tool for clinicians to conveniently quantify the different aspects of UE movements and monitor in-clinic as well as real-world improvements in UE use in children with UCP.

Supplementary Materials: The following supporting information can be downloaded at: https://www.mdpi.com/article/10.3390/bs13080681/s1, Supplementary Material S1. Activities included in the HABIT protocol; Supplementary Material S2. Figure S1A,B: Representative example of pre- and post-HABIT density plots of a child with unilateral cerebral palsy, Table S1 shows the pre- and post-HABIT changes in the accelerometer derived variables following 30-hours HABIT in this representative participant data; Supplementary Material S3. Figure S2a–e: Profile plots illustrating individual differences in accelerometer-derived variables.

Author Contributions: Conceptualization, S.M.S.; methodology, S.S.G., S.M.S. and S.K.; software, S.S.G. and S.M.S.; validation, S.M.S.; formal analysis, S.S.G., C.G.P. and S.M.S.; investigation, S.S.G., C.L., A.G.M., J.D.W. and S.M.S.; resources, C.L., A.G.M., J.D.W. and S.M.S.; data curation, S.S.G. and S.M.S.; writing—original draft preparation, S.S.G.; writing—review and editing, S.S.G., C.L., A.G.M., S.K., J.D.W., C.G.P. and S.M.S.; visualization, S.S.G. and S.M.S.; supervision, S.M.S.; project administration, S.M.S.; funding acquisition, S.M.S. All authors have read and agreed to the published version of the manuscript.

Funding: The research reported in this publication was supported in part by the Eunice Kennedy Shriner National Institute of Child Health & Human Development of the National Institutes of Health under Award Number R03HD107644 and APTA's Pediatric Physical Therapy (grant no. 21-0810).

Institutional Review Board Statement: The study was conducted in accordance with the Declaration of Helsinki, and approved by the University and Medical Center Institutional Review Board of East Carolina University, NC (protocol code 21-001913, and approval date 29 September 2021).

Informed Consent Statement: Informed consent was obtained from all subjects involved in the study. Written informed consent has been obtained from the patient(s) to publish this paper.

Data Availability Statement: The data presented in this study are available on request from the corresponding author.

Acknowledgments: We thank the children and their families who participated in the study and all the volunteer (physical and occupational therapy students) interventionists for their contributions to the HABIT camp. We sincerely thank the graduate research assistants Casey Burroughs, David Turnure, Mary Scott Faircloth, Caroline Pusey-Brown, Katie Woosley, Natalie McBryde, Grant Kirkman, Jovanna Zapata, and Brody Morton for their contributions to this project.

Conflicts of Interest: The authors have no conflict of interest to declare. All co-authors have seen and agree with the contents of the manuscript, and there is no financial interest to report. We certify that the submission is original work and is not under review at any other publication. The funders had no role in the design of the study; in the collection, analyses, or interpretation of data; in the writing of the manuscript; or in the decision to publish the results.

References

1. Stavsky, M.; Mor, O.; Mastrolia, S.A.; Greenbaum, S.; Than, N.G.; Erez, O. Cerebral Palsy-Trends in Epidemiology and Recent Development in Prenatal Mechanisms of Disease, Treatment, and Prevention. *Front. Pediatr.* **2017**, *5*, 21. [CrossRef]
2. Hung, Y.-C.; Charles, J.; Gordon, A.M. Bimanual Coordination during a Goal-Directed Task in Children with Hemiplegic Cerebral Palsy. *Dev. Med. Child Neurol.* **2004**, *46*, 46–53. [CrossRef] [PubMed]
3. Novak, I.; Mcintyre, S.; Morgan, C.; Campbell, L.; Dark, L.; Morton, N.; Stumbles, E.; Wilson, S.-A.; Goldsmith, S. A Systematic Review of Interventions for Children with Cerebral Palsy: State of the Evidence. *Dev. Med. Child Neurol.* **2013**, *55*, 885–910. [CrossRef] [PubMed]
4. Sakzewski, L.; Provan, K.; Ziviani, J.; Boyd, R.N. Comparison of Dosage of Intensive Upper Limb Therapy for Children with Unilateral Cerebral Palsy: How Big Should the Therapy Pill Be? *Res. Dev. Disabil.* **2015**, *37*, 9–16. [CrossRef]
5. Brandão, M.B.; Mancini, M.C.; Ferre, C.L.; Figueiredo, P.R.P.; Oliveira, R.H.S.; Gonçalves, S.C.; Dias, M.C.S.; Gordon, A.M. Does Dosage Matter? A Pilot Study of Hand-Arm Bimanual Intensive Training (HABIT) Dose and Dosing Schedule in Children with Unilateral Cerebral Palsy. *Phys. Occup. Ther. Pediatr.* **2018**, *38*, 227–242. [CrossRef]
6. Gordon, A.M.; Hung, Y.C.; Brandao, M.; Ferre, C.L.; Kuo, H.C.; Friel, K.; Petra, E.; Chinnan, A.; Charles, J.R. Bimanual Training and Constraint-Induced Movement Therapy in Children with Hemiplegic Cerebral Palsy: A Randomized Trial. *Neurorehabil. Neural. Repair.* **2011**, *25*, 692–702. [CrossRef]
7. Surkar, S.M.; Hoffman, R.M.; Willett, S.; Flegle, J.; Harbourne, R.; Kurz, M.J. Hand-Arm Bimanual Intensive Therapy Improves Prefrontal Cortex Activation in Children with Hemiplegic Cerebral Palsy. *Pediatr. Phys. Ther.* **2018**, *30*, 93–100. [CrossRef]
8. Gordon, A.M. To Constrain or Not to Constrain, and Other Stories of Intensive Upper Extremity Training for Children with Unilateral Cerebral Palsy. *Dev. Med. Child Neurol.* **2011**, *53*, 56–61. [CrossRef]
9. Lang, C.E.; Macdonald, J.R.; Reisman, D.S.; Boyd, L.; Jacobson Kimberley, T.; Schindler-Ivens, S.M.; Hornby, T.G.; Ross, S.A.; Scheets, P.L. Observation of Amounts of Movement Practice Provided during Stroke Rehabilitation. *Arch. Phys. Med. Rehabil.* **2009**, *90*, 1692–1698. [CrossRef]
10. Urbin, M.A.; Bailey, R.R.; Lang, C.E. Validity of Body-Worn Sensor Acceleration Metrics to Index Upper Extremity Function in Hemiparetic Stroke. *J. Neurol. Phys. Ther.* **2015**, *39*, 111–118. [CrossRef]
11. Uswatte, G.; Giuliani, C.; Winstein, C.; Zeringue, A.; Hobbs, L.; Wolf, S.L. Validity of Accelerometry for Monitoring Real-World Arm Activity in Patients With Subacute Stroke: Evidence From the Extremity Constraint-Induced Therapy Evaluation Trial. *Arch. Phys. Med. Rehabil.* **2006**, *87*, 1340–1345. [CrossRef]
12. Uswatte, G.; Foo, W.L.; Olmstead, H.; Lopez, K.; Holand, A.; Simms, L.B. Ambulatory Monitoring of Arm Movement Using Accelerometry: An Objective Measure of Upper-Extremity Rehabilitation in Persons With Chronic Stroke. *Arch. Phys. Med. Rehabil.* **2005**, *86*, 1498–1501. [CrossRef]
13. Kwakkel, G.; Van Wegen, E.; Burridge, J.H.; Winstein, C.J.; van Dokkum, L.; Alt Murphy, M.; Levin, M.F.; Krakauer, J.W. Standardized Measurement of Quality of Upper Limb Movement after Stroke: Consensus-Based Core Recommendations from the Second Stroke Recovery and Rehabilitation Roundtable. *Int. J. Stroke* **2019**, *14*, 783–791. [CrossRef] [PubMed]
14. Lang, C.E.; MacDonald, J.R.; Gnip, C. Counting Repetitions: An Observational Study of Outpatient Therapy for People with Hemiparesis Post-Stroke. *J. Neurol. Phys. Ther.* **2007**, *31*, 3–10. [CrossRef] [PubMed]
15. *International Classification of Functioning, Disability and Health: Children and Youth Version: ICF-CY*; World Health Organization: Geneva, Switzerland, 2007; Available online: https://apps.who.int/iris/handle/10665/43737 (accessed on 10 May 2023).
16. Waddell, K.J.; Strube, M.J.; Bailey, R.R.; Klaesner, J.W.; Birkenmeier, R.L.; Dromerick, A.W.; Lang, C.E. Does Task-Specific Training Improve Upper Limb Performance in Daily Life Poststroke? *Neurorehabil. Neural. Repair* **2017**, *31*, 290–300. [CrossRef] [PubMed]
17. Holsbeeke, L.; Ketelaar, M.; Schoemaker, M.M.; Gorter, J.W. Capacity, Capability, and Performance: Different Constructs or Three of a Kind? *Arch. Phys. Med. Rehabil.* **2009**, *90*, 849–855. [CrossRef] [PubMed]
18. Ouyang, R.G.; Yang, C.N.; Qu, Y.L.; Koduri, M.P.; Chien, C.W. Effectiveness of Hand-Arm Bimanual Intensive Training on Upper Extremity Function in Children with Cerebral Palsy: A Systematic Review. *Eur. J. Paediatr.* **2020**, *25*, 17–28. [CrossRef]
19. Adams, S.A. The Effect of Social Desirability and Social Approval on Self-Reports of Physical Activity. *Am. J. Epidemiol.* **2005**, *161*, 389–398. [CrossRef]
20. Elad, D.; Barak, S.; Eisenstein, E.; Bar, O.; Givon, U.; Brezner, A. Discrepancies between Mothers and Clinicians in Assessing Functional Capabilities and Performance of Children with Cerebral Palsy. *Res. Dev. Disabil.* **2013**, *34*, 3746–3753. [CrossRef]
21. Goodwin, B.M.; Sabelhaus, E.K.; Pan, Y.C.; Bjornson, K.F.; Pham, K.L.D.; Walker, W.O.; Steele, K.M. Accelerometer Measurements Indicate That Arm Movements of Children with Cerebral Palsy Do Not Increase after Constraint-Induced Movement Therapy (CIMT). *Am. J. Occup. Ther.* **2020**, *74*, p1–p7405205100. [CrossRef]
22. Mitchell, L.E.; Ziviani, J.; Boyd, R.N. A Randomized Controlled Trial of Web-Based Training to Increase Activity in Children with Cerebral Palsy. *Dev. Med. Child Neurol.* **2016**, *58*, 767–773. [CrossRef]
23. Doman, C.A.; Waddell, K.J.; Bailey, R.R.; Moore, J.L.; Lang, C.E. Changes in Upper-Extremity Functional Capacity and Daily Performance During Outpatient Occupational Therapy for People with Stroke. *Am. J. Occup. Ther.* **2016**, *70*, p1–p7003290040. [CrossRef] [PubMed]
24. Waddell, K. Exploring the Complexities of Real-World Upper Limb Performance after Stroke. 2019. Available online: https://openscholarship.wustl.edu/art_sci_etds/1800 (accessed on 11 January 2023).

25. Bailey, R.R.; Klaesner, J.W.; Lang, C.E. Quantifying Real-World Upper-Limb Activity in Nondisabled Adults and Adults with Chronic Stroke. *Neurorehabil. Neural. Repair* **2015**, *29*, 969–978. [CrossRef] [PubMed]
26. Hoyt, C.R.; Brown, S.K.; Sherman, S.K.; Wood-Smith, M.; Van, A.N.; Ortega, M.; Nguyen, A.L.; Lang, C.E.; Schlaggar, B.L.; Dosenbach, N.U.F. Using Accelerometry for Measurement of Motor Behavior in Children: Relationship of Real-World Movement to Standardized Evaluation. *Res. Dev. Disabil.* **2020**, *96*, 103546. [CrossRef] [PubMed]
27. Coker-Bolt, P.; Downey, R.J.; Connolly, J.; Hoover, R.; Shelton, D.; Seo, N.J. Exploring the Feasibility and Use of Accelerometers before, during, and after a Camp-Based CIMT Program for Children with Cerebral Palsy. *J. Pediatr. Rehabil. Med.* **2017**, *10*, 27–36. [CrossRef]
28. National Institute of Allergy and Infectious Diseases (NIAID). For Ancillary Studies, Consider NIH Definitions Carefully. Available online: https://www.niaid.nih.gov/grants-contracts/ancillary-studies-definitions (accessed on 23 May 2023).
29. Lang, C.E.; Waddell, K.J.; Klaesner, J.W.; Bland, M.D. A Method for Quantifying Upper Limb Performance in Daily Life Using Accelerometers. *J. Vis. Exp.* **2017**, *122*, 55673.
30. Mitchell, L.E.; Ziviani, J.; Boyd, R.N. Variability in Measuring Physical Activity in Children with Cerebral Palsy. *Med. Sci. Sport. Exerc.* **2015**, *47*, 194–200. [CrossRef] [PubMed]
31. Krumlinde-Sundholm, L.; Holmefur, M.; Kottorp, A.; Eliasson, A.-C. The Assisting Hand Assessment: Current Evidence of Validity, Reliability, and Responsiveness to Change. *Dev. Med. Child Neurol.* **2007**, *49*, 259–264. [CrossRef]
32. Krumlinde-Sundholm, L. Reporting Outcomes of the Assisting Hand Assessment: What Scale Should Be Used? *Dev. Med. Child Neurol.* **2012**, *54*, 807–808. [CrossRef]
33. Tofani, M.; Castelli, E.; Sabbadini, M.; Berardi, A.; Murgia, M.; Servadio, A.; Galeoto, G. Examining Reliability and Validity of the Jebsen-Taylor Hand Function Test Among Children with Cerebral Palsy. *Percept Mot. Ski.* **2020**, *127*, 684–697. [CrossRef]
34. Poole, J.L.; Burtner, P.A.; Torres, T.A.; McMullen, C.K.; Markham, A.; Marcum, M.L.; Anderson, J.B.; Qualls, C. Measuring Dexterity in Children Using the Nine-Hole Peg Test. *J. Hand Ther.* **2005**, *18*, 348–351. [CrossRef] [PubMed]
35. Jongbloed-Pereboom, M.; Nijhuis-van der Sanden, M.W.G.; Steenbergen, B. Norm Scores of the Box and Block Test for Children Ages 3–10 Years. *Am. J. Occup. Ther.* **2013**, *67*, 312–318. [CrossRef] [PubMed]
36. Faul, F.; Erdfelder, E.; Lang, A.-G.; Buchner, A. G*Power 3: A Flexible Statistical Power Analysis Program for the Social, Behavioral, and Biomedical Sciences. *Behav. Res. Methods* **2007**, *39*, 175–191. [CrossRef] [PubMed]
37. Araneda, R.; Ebner-Karestinos, D.; Paradis, J.; Saussez, G.; Friel, K.M.; Gordon, A.M.; Bleyenheuft, Y. Reliability and Responsiveness of the Jebsen-Taylor Test of Hand Function and the Box and Block Test for Children with Cerebral Palsy. *Dev. Med. Child Neurol.* **2019**, *61*, 1182–1188. [CrossRef] [PubMed]
38. Lang, C.E.; Lohse, K.R.; Birkenmeier, R.L. Dose and Timing in Neurorehabilitation: Prescribing Motor Therapy after Stroke. *Curr. Opin. Neurol.* **2015**, *28*, 549–555. [CrossRef]
39. Connell, L.A.; McMahon, N.E.; Simpson, L.A.; Watkins, C.L.; Eng, J.J. Investigating Measures of Intensity During a Structured Upper Limb Exercise Program in Stroke Rehabilitation: An Exploratory Study. *Arch. Phys. Med. Rehabil.* **2014**, *95*, 2410–2419. [CrossRef]
40. Lang, C.E.; Wagner, J.M.; Edwards, D.F.; Dromerick, A.W. Upper Extremity Use in People with Hemiparesis in the First Few Weeks after Stroke. *J. Neurol. Phys. Ther.* **2007**, *31*, 56–63. [CrossRef]
41. Rand, D.; Givon, N.; Weingarden, H.; Nota, A.; Zeilig, G. Eliciting Upper Extremity Purposeful Movements Using Video Games. *Neurorehabil. Neural. Repair* **2014**, *28*, 733–739. [CrossRef]

Disclaimer/Publisher's Note: The statements, opinions and data contained in all publications are solely those of the individual author(s) and contributor(s) and not of MDPI and/or the editor(s). MDPI and/or the editor(s) disclaim responsibility for any injury to people or property resulting from any ideas, methods, instructions or products referred to in the content.

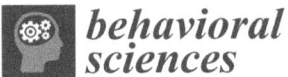

Article

Preoperative Biopsychosocial Assessment and Length of Stay in Orthopaedic Surgery Admissions of Youth with Cerebral Palsy

Nancy Lennon, Carrie Sewell-Roberts, Tolulope Banjo , Denver B. Kraft , Jose J. Salazar-Torres, Chris Church * and M. Wade Shrader

Nemours Children's Health, Wilmington, NC 19803, USA; nancy.lennon@nemours.org (N.L.);
carrie.sewellroberts@nemours.org (C.S.-R.); tolulope.banjo1@gmail.com (T.B.); denverkraft@gmail.com (D.B.K.);
jose.salazar@nemours.org (J.J.S.-T.); wade.shrader@nemours.org (M.W.S.)
* Correspondence: chris.church@nemours.org; Tel.: +1-302-651-4614

Abstract: Caregivers of children with cerebral palsy (CP) experience stress surrounding orthopaedic surgery related to their child's pain and recovery needs. Social determinants of health can affect the severity of this stress and hinder health care delivery. A preoperative biopsychosocial assessment (BPSA) can identify risk factors and assist in alleviating psychosocial risk. This study examined the relationship between the completion of a BPSA, hospital length of stay (LOS), and 30-day readmission rates for children with CP who underwent hip reconstruction (HR) or posterior spinal fusion (PSF). Outcomes were compared with a matched group who did not have a preoperative BPSA. The BPSA involved meeting with a social worker to discuss support systems, financial needs, transportation, equipment, housing, and other services. A total of 92 children (28 HR pairs, 18 PSF pairs) were identified. Wilcoxon analysis was statistically significant ($p = 0.000228$) for shorter LOS in children who underwent PSF with preoperative BPSA (median = 7.0 days) vs. without (median = 12.5 days). Multivariate analysis showed that a BPSA, a lower Gross Motor Function Classification System level, and fewer comorbidities were associated with a shorter LOS after both PSF and HR ($p < 0.05$). Identifying and addressing the psychosocial needs of patients and caregivers prior to surgery can lead to more timely discharge postoperatively.

Keywords: cerebral palsy; biopsychosocial assessment; orthopaedics

1. Introduction

Background

Cerebral palsy (CP) is the most common pediatric motor disability, affecting an estimated 1 in 345 children in the United States [1]. The neurological pathology of CP involves a brain injury or disruption occurring before birth, during delivery, or in early childhood [2]. Motor disability in children with CP is described using a five-level classification system, the Gross Motor Function Classification System (GMFCS) [3]. Symptoms of CP differ among children, ranging from minor motor difficulties to major physical disabilities that negatively impact independent movement. Often, individuals with CP have co-occurring medical conditions and developmental disabilities alongside the musculoskeletal impairments [4].

The experience of parenting a child with CP can be stressful due to the child's need for support in activities of daily living, need for ongoing therapies, educational advocacy, higher financial strain, and barriers to caregivers maintaining employment [5–9]. While every parent/caregiver of a person with CP experiences some level of stress that is higher (on average) than a parent of a typically developing child [6,10], this level of stress is greater for parents with other risks associated with social determinants of health (SDOH) [11,12]. These determinants may include financial hardship, housing and food insecurity, lack of access to quality education, environmental and neighborhood safety concerns, racism, ableism, discrimination based on sexual identity, and lack of employment opportunity [13].

Children and adolescents with CP often require orthopaedic surgery to maintain or improve their function, reduce pain, and improve quality of life [14–18]. Common orthopaedic surgeries for children functioning at GMFCS levels IV and V include posterior spinal fusion (PSF) and hip reconstruction (HR) [17,18]. The experience of surgery, a hospital stay, rehabilitative therapies, and recovery is stressful for both patients and their parents/caregivers [19,20]. The stress caused by these surgical events is multi-faceted: concern about the risks and long-term outcomes of surgery, the experience of pain and recovery from the surgical procedure itself, the financial strain of a hospitalization, disruption to daily routine and parent employment, and childcare concerns for siblings [21].

If medical teams can evaluate the family system's SDOH and baseline stress load, the team may be able to support the family in minimizing these factors and making the stress of a surgical event more manageable. One avenue for capturing the SDOH of families is through the administration of a biopsychosocial assessment (BPSA), a tool utilized by medical social workers to develop treatment and intervention plans [22]. A BPSA reveals a family's basic composition; strengths such as resilience, family/community support, and health literacy; as well as areas of risk, including SDOH barriers and access to needed therapies, benefits, and services.

The aim of this study was to examine the relationship between the completion of a preoperative BPSA and hospital discharge metrics including length of stay (LOS) and 30-day readmission rate (RR) for children with CP undergoing PSF or HR surgeries.

2. Materials and Methods

This Institutional-Review-Board-approved retrospective cohort study included children with CP who underwent hip or spine surgery. Potential cases were identified from a historical database from the authors' institution. Inclusion criteria were (a) diagnosis of CP classified at GMFCS levels IV and V, (b) underwent PSF or HR at the authors' institution between 2017 and 2021, and (c) aged 2 to 21 years. Children whose families completed a BPSA were selected from this group and were then matched according to surgery type (hip or spine), age (within 2 years), number of comorbid conditions, and GMFCS level to a group that did not have a preoperative BPSA. Comorbidities were categorized as seizures, gastrostomy tube, tracheostomy, or non-verbal [23]. Based on chart review, the number of comorbidities for each patient was identified and, for statistical analysis, was ranked as none = 0, small = 1 or 2, and large = 3 or 4.

2.1. Biopsychosocial Assessment

The BPSA utilized by the social work team was developed based on the guidelines set by the National Association of Social Workers Standards for Social Work Practice in Health Care Settings [24]. It includes the assessment of patient and caregiver strengths, such as self-efficacy, access to family, faith and community supports and resources, and resilience. The BPSA also identifies SDOH risks such as transportation, food, housing, employment, income, access to government benefits, homecare services, home accessibility, access to needed durable medical equipment, access to therapies, and mental health care (see the Supplementary Material). The BPSA was utilized as a guide for the medical social worker to provide interventions for the family to mitigate the stress burden of specific areas of risk. For example, if the BPSA identified that a family had housing insecurity, the social worker would assist the family in contacting the state housing authority to check housing vouchers. If the BPSA identified that the family had transportation barriers ahead of the surgery, the social worker would assist the family in scheduling Medicaid transportation for preoperative appointments and on the day of the surgery. If the family identified a need for mental health therapy to cope with stress, anxiety, or depressive symptoms, the social worker would assist the family in accessing mental health care. The roll out of the BPSA in late 2018 was controlled by the CP division chief, beginning with his own patients, and limited in scope by social work resources. The referral process for BPSA was formalized and social work resources were increased in 2019. By 2020, all children (GMFCS IV and V preoperative for HR PSF) were referred for preoperative BPSA.

Primary outcome variables included postoperative LOS (number of days), rate of extended LOS (ELOS), and 30-day RR. Length of stays over the median (6 days for HR and 10 days for PSF) were considered ELOS. For any child with a readmission within 30 days, a chart review was performed to determine reasons for readmission.

2.2. Statistical Analysis

Chi-squared analysis was completed to examine differences in matching criteria between BPSA and no-BPSA groups. The median LOS, rate of ELOS, and 30-day RR for each type of surgery (hip or spine) were compared between BPSA and no-BPSA groups. Statistical analyses were carried out with a Wilcoxon test for LOS and a chi-squared analysis for ELOS and 30-day RR.

A general linear regression model (GLM) with a Poisson distribution and a stepwise function to select relevant variables was used to predict LOS in days for each type of surgery. Variables in the model included BPSA (yes, no), number of comorbidities (none = 0, small = 1 or 2, large = 3 or 4), age, sex, and GMFCS level. Similarly, a GLM with a binomial distribution and a stepwise function to select relevant variables was used to determine the effect of these same factors on whether LOS was within the median range (≤ 6 days for HR, 10 days for PSF) or extended (>6 days for HR, >10 days for PSF). An additional GLM with a binomial distribution and a stepwise function to select relevant variables was used to determine whether these factors influenced 30-day RR. All statistical analyses were performed using R [25]. Significance level for all tests was set at $p < 0.05$.

3. Results

Forty-six children with CP who had a BPSA were matched with forty-six children who did not have a BPSA with similar age, GMFCS level, and number of comorbidities (Table 1). Fifty-six children had HR and thirty-six had PSF. Table 2 shows the LOS median, interquartile range, confidence interval, and 30-day readmission ($n = 10$) for the 92 children included in this analysis and the distribution according to preoperative BPSA, type of surgery, and number of comorbidities.

Table 1. Distribution of matching variables for children who underwent spinal surgery and had preoperative biopsychosocial assessment (BPSA) or no BPSA.

Variable		BPSA No	BPSA Yes	p Value	Test
Age	Median (CI)	10.6 (0.94)	10.9 (0.97)	0.72	Wilcoxon
Race	Asian	1	0	0.68	Chi-squared
	Asian Indian	1	0		
	Black or African American	13	13		
	Guamanian or Chamorro	0	1		
	Some other race	3	4		
	White or Caucasian	28	28		
GMFCS	IV	16	17	0.83	Chi-squared
	V	30	29		
Surgery type	Hip	28	28	1	Chi-squared
	Spine	18	18		

Table 1. Cont.

Variable		BPSA No	BPSA Yes	p Value	Test
Range of medical issues	None = 0	6	8		
	Small = 1,2	24	23	0.84	Chi-squared
	Large = 3,4	16	15		

Note: Chi-square analyses were used to confirm that matching variables were equivalent between BPSA and no-BPSA groups. Children were not matched for race, but the distribution was similar between groups. GMFCS, Gross Motor Function Classification System.

Table 2. Descriptive statistics for children who underwent hip reconstruction or posterior spinal fusion, whether they had a biopsychosocial assessment (BPSA) administered, the number of comorbidities, and whether they were readmitted within 30 days.

Surgery Type	BPSA	Comorbidities	n	LOS Days Median	LOS Days IQR	CI	30-Day Readmission
Hip	No	None	4	5.5	1.75	2.72	0
Hip	No	Small	16	6.5	4	1.76	2
Hip	No	Large	8	6.5	7.75	4.07	2
Spine	No	None	2	11	3	38.1	1
Spine	No	Small	8	11	2.5	21.2	0
Spine	No	Large	8	21	31	21.8	0
Hip	Yes	None	6	6	1.5	21.6	0
Hip	Yes	Small	16	5.5	2.25	1.06	1
Hip	Yes	Large	6	8	1.5	3.8	0
Spine	Yes	None	2	9	1	12.7	0
Spine	Yes	Small	7	10	5	3.16	1
Spine	Yes	Large	9	7	1	1.96	2

IQR, interquartile range; LOS, length of stay.

3.1. Group Analysis

3.1.1. Length of Stay

The median LOS for the children in the PSF group was 10 days. The difference in LOS in this group was statistically significant between the BPSA (median [CI] = 7.0 [1.4]) and no-BPSA groups (median [CI] = 12.5 [12.2]; $p = 0.00023$). The median LOS for the children in the HR group was six days. After HR, there was no significant difference in LOS between the BPSA (median [CI] = 6.0 [3.7]) and no-BPSA groups (median [CI] = 7.0 [1.5]) ($p = 0.51$; Figure 1).

3.1.2. Extended Length of Stay

Three of the eighteen children who had a BPSA in the PSF group had an ELOS, compared with twelve out of eighteen children who did not have a BPSA. Chi-squared analysis showed a significant difference between these groups ($p = 0.0023$). In the HR group, 3 out of 28 (BPSA) and 7 out of 28 patients (no BPSA) had an ELOS ($p = 0.16$).

3.1.3. Thirty-Day Readmission

Three of the eighteen children in the PSF surgery group who had a BPSA were readmitted within 30 days, while one of the eighteen children who did not have a BPSA was readmitted within 30 days ($p = 0.29$). One of the twenty-eight children in the HR surgery group who had a BPSA was readmitted within 30 days and five of the twenty-eight children who did not have a BPSA were readmitted within 30 days ($p = 0.084$). Reasons for 30-day readmission can be found in Table 3.

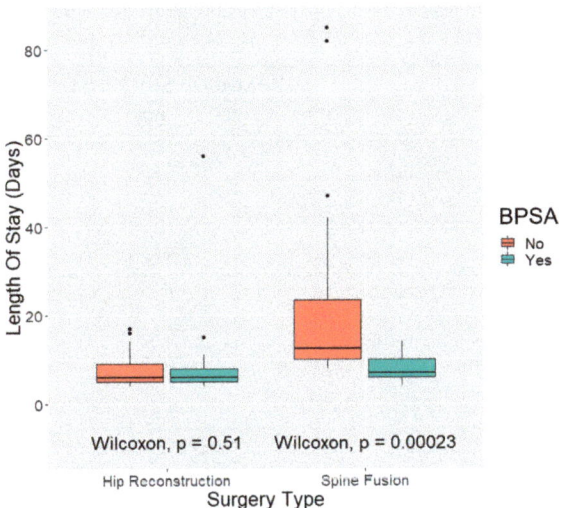

Figure 1. Differences in length of stay in days between biopsychosocial assessment (BPSA) and no-BPSA groups following hip reconstruction and spine fusion.

Table 3. Reasons for 30-day readmission.

Subject Number	Surgery	Reason for 30-Day Readmission
1	HR	Oropharyngeal dysphagia, diabetes insipidus
2	HR	Postoperative pain management
3	HR	Vomiting, constipation
4	HR	Decubitus ulcer
5	PSF	Urinary retention
6	HR	Wound infection
7	PSF	Urinary tract infection
8	PSF	Wound infection
9	PSF	Wound infection

HR, hip reconstruction; PSF, posterior spinal fusion.

3.2. Multivariate Analyses

3.2.1. Length of Stay

In the LOS model for PSF, statistically significant effects were found for the following factors: the inclusion of a preoperative BPSA was associated with a shorter LOS ($p < 0.001$); an additional number of comorbidities, both small (1,2) ($p = 0.03$) and large (3,4) ($p < 0.001$), was associated with a longer LOS; and a higher GMFCS level was associated with a longer LOS ($p = 0.005$). Older children tended to have an increased LOS, but this did not reach significance levels ($p = 0.06$).

In the LOS model for HR, statistically significant effects were found for the following factors: an additional number of small medical issues was associated with a shorter LOS ($p < 0.001$), and a longer LOS was observed for male children ($p = 0.019$). For this group, the inclusion of a preoperative BPSA was not relevant to the LOS ($p > 0.05$). Table 4 shows the summary of the multivariate analysis for children who underwent PSF and HR.

Table 4. Summary of the length of stay multivariate model for children in the PSF and hip reconstruction groups.

	Length of Stay Models Fit			
	PSF			
χ^2 (5)			186.96	
p			0.00	
Pseudo-R^2 (McFadden)			0.29	
Standard errors: MLE				
	Est.	S.E.	z val.	p
(Intercept)	0.17	0.64	0.27	0.78
BPSA (yes)	−1.08	0.10	11.16	<0.001
additional comorbidities (small)	0.37	0.17	2.16	0.03
additional comorbidities (large)	0.63	0.19	3.27	<0.001
Age	0.05	0.02	1.90	0.06
GMFCS	0.41	0.12	3.48	0.005
	Hip Reconstruction			
χ^2 (3)			22.56	
p			0.00	
Pseudo-R^2 (McFadden)			0.06	
Standard errors: MLE				
	Est.	S.E.	z val.	p
(Intercept)	2.23	0.12	19.24	0.00
Additional comorbidities (small)	−0.46	0.12	−3.89	<0.001
Additional comorbidities (large)	−0.13	0.13	−1.03	0.30
Sex (male)	0.23	0.1	2.34	0.019

BPSA, biopsychosocial assessment; GMFCS, Gross Motor Function Classification System.

3.2.2. Extended Length of Stay

For children who underwent PSF, the ELOS model was statistically significant for a median or shorter LOS in patients with a BPSA ($p = 0.004$). For children who underwent HR, the ELOS model found statistically significant effects for BPSA and a median or lower LOS ($p = 0.03$), higher GMFCS level, and extended LOS ($p = 0.04$). Male patients tended to have an ELOS but this did not reach significance levels ($p = 0.05$). Table 5 shows the summary of the multivariate analysis for children who underwent PSF and hip reconstruction.

Table 5. Summary of the length of stay multivariate model for children in the PSF and hip reconstruction groups.

	Extended Length of Stay Models Fit			
	PSF			
χ^2 (1)			9.77	
p			0.00	
Pseudo-R^2 (McFadden)			0.20	
Standard errors: MLE				
	Est.	S.E.	z val.	p
(Intercept)	0.69	0.5	1.39	0.17
BPSA (Yes)	−2.3	0.81	−2.86	0.004
	Hip Reconstruction			
χ^2 (3)			11.66	
p			0.01	
Pseudo-R^2 (McFadden)			0.22	
Standard errors: MLE				

Table 5. Cont.

	Extended Length of Stay Models Fit			
	Est.	S.E.	z val.	p
(Intercept)	−13.99	6.07	−2.31	0.02
BPSA (yes)	−2.16	1.01	−2.13	0.03
Sex (male)	1.96	1.02	1.92	0.05
GMFCS	2.56	1.22	2.09	0.04

BPSA, biopsychosocial assessment; GMFCS, Gross Motor Function Classification System; MLE, maximum likelihood estimation.

3.2.3. Thirty-Day Readmission

There were no statistically significant relationships between any of the factors included in this study and a 30-day RR model for either the PSF or HR groups.

4. Discussion

Family stress associated with caring for a child with CP can be exacerbated by orthopaedic surgery due to pain and financial impact [19–21]. Risks associated with social determinants of health can increase caregiver stress and lead to difficulties in caring for a child with CP [11,12]. Identification of SDOH utilizing a BPSA facilitates the implementation of psychosocial interventions aimed at reducing risk and improving outcomes in care [22].

In late 2018, our hospital undertook a new initiative aimed at reducing disparities in health outcomes for youth with CP undergoing orthopaedic surgery. The social work and orthopaedic teams led a program to offer psychosocial support to families in this group. During the first year of the program, referrals for BPSA were low relative to the number of eligible families and some families did not receive the assessment. By 2021, nearly all patients having orthopaedic surgery with an anticipated hospital LOS of more than a few days completed a BPSA prior to surgery. The time frame in which the service was developing allowed us to examine the impact of the BPSA on hospital admissions.

Average hospital LOS for patients with PSF was significantly shorter for those who completed a BPSA compared with those who did not. For patients with HR, there was no difference in average LOS for those who completed a BPSA compared with those who did not. Examining LOS on a dichotomous scale, as extended (>median) or not (≤median), revealed similar results with a significant difference between BPSA and no-BPSA groups in patients who had PSF but not HR. Children tend to have longer admissions after PSF than with HR due to the greater burden of the surgery. Perhaps with this greater burden, more demand was placed on family resources, leading to a stronger (statistically significant) impact of the BPSA. Anecdotally, nursing staff and case managers report that families with a BPSA experience smoother, less chaotic hospital discharge.

The 30-day RR for the 92 patients in this analysis was 9.8% and was not statistically different between those who had a BPSA and those who did not. We observed a trend of fewer 30-day readmissions in HR patients who had a BPSA, though there was no significant difference (4% vs. 18% in patients without a BPSA). We continue to observe this trend in our clinical practice and expect to find significant differences as we analyze larger groups and examine reasons for 30-day readmissions with standardized methods.

The medical complexity of youth with CP functioning at GMFCS levels IV/V justified additional multifactorial analysis of LOS after PSF and HR. Studying a similar patient sample, Jain et al. reported a higher frequency of complications following PSF in those with more comorbidities: 49% in those with three or four comorbidities compared with 12% in those with no comorbidities [23]. When we included factors that capture medical comorbidities and motor disability, we found statistically significant results. Multifactorial analysis revealed that a preoperative BPSA, a lower GMFCS level (IV vs. V), and fewer comorbidities were associated with a shorter median LOS and less frequent ELOS following PSF and HR. A higher GMFCS level and higher number of comorbidities likely contribute to medical complications that extend hospital stay, but these same factors can also result in higher caregiving demands and stress, leading to a possible psychosocial explanation for delays in discharge.

Medical chart review for this study tried to identify explanations for ELOS and readmission within 30 days. Reasons for 30-day readmission and ELOS offered a mix of medically driven diagnoses such as infection, patient management difficulties such as postoperative pain and constipation, as well as combinations of medical/social circumstances. While it was clear that some issues could have been addressed with preventative strategies identified through a preoperative BPSA, we could not analyze reasons for ELOS and 30-day RR statistically in this work.

This study serves to capture our new clinical practice of completing a BPSA preoperatively in children with CP undergoing orthopaedic surgery who have an anticipated hospital stay of more than a few days. Given the benefit demonstrated, we advocate for clinicians in similar settings to institute this process. The BPSA standardizes the process of identifying SDOH. Our current clinical practice aims to develop methods qualifying improvement in issues identified through the preoperative BPSA. While the social work teams utilized the BPSA to identify areas of risk and guide the implementation of patient- and family-specific interventions, some issues identified through the BPSA (for example, chronic financial insecurity) may be beyond the scope of the relatively short time frames of preoperative planning and preparation. We are working with the Health Equity Office at our hospital to identify strategies to address these broader issues.

Limitations of this study include the analysis of only PSF and HR surgical groups. While these two procedures are common and highly impactful, both in health benefit to the child and reduction in caregiving needs, there are other common surgery situations in which families likely benefit but whom we did not study. The retrospective nature of the study introduces the possibility of bias in the study groups. While we tried to minimize this in our methodology, there could be differences in the early referral patterns that contributed to group differences. Some physicians were early adopters of the service, while others took longer to integrate the preoperative BPSA into their practice. We used BPSA as a marker for intervention; we did not look at the interventions and assumed that after BPSA, appropriately directed interventions were delivered. Finally, the medically complex nature of this patient population may contribute to outliers in LOS that could impact results unrelated to the BPSA.

5. Conclusions

Identifying and addressing psychosocial needs of patients and their caregivers through a preoperative BPSA is associated with positive impacts on hospital quality metrics including less time spent in the hospital after surgical admissions for spinal fusion for youth with CP.

Supplementary Materials: The following supporting information can be downloaded at: https://www.mdpi.com/article/10.3390/bs13050383/s1.

Author Contributions: Conceptualization, N.L., C.S.-R. and M.W.S.; methodology, N.L., C.S.-R. and M.W.S.; software, J.J.S.-T.; validation, N.L., C.S.-R. and J.J.S.-T.; formal analysis, N.L., C.S.-R., T.B., D.B.K. and J.J.S.-T.; investigation, N.L., C.S.-R. and T.B.; resources, N.L., C.S.-R., C.C. and M.W.S.; data curation, N.L., C.S.-R., T.B., D.B.K. and J.J.S.-T.; writing—original draft preparation, N.L., C.S.-R., T.B., C.C. and M.W.S.; writing—review and editing, N.L., C.S.-R., T.B., D.B.K., J.J.S.-T., C.C. and M.W.S.; visualization, N.L., C.S.-R., T.B. and J.J.S.-T.; supervision, N.L., C.S.-R. and M.W.S.; project administration, N.L. and C.S.-R. All authors have read and agreed to the published version of the manuscript.

Funding: This research received no external funding.

Institutional Review Board Statement: The study was conducted in accordance with the Declaration of Helsinki and approved by the Institutional Review Board of Nemours Children's Health (approval number 1763544 on 4 June 2021).

Informed Consent Statement: Patient consent was waived due to the retrospective nature of the study. All data were de-identified.

Data Availability Statement: The data presented in this study are available on request from the corresponding author.

Conflicts of Interest: The authors declare no conflict of interest.

References

1. Centers for Disease Control and Prevention. Cerebral Palsy. Available online: http://www.cdc.gov/ncbddd/dd/ddcp.htm (accessed on 30 November 2021).
2. Graham, H.K.; Rosenbaum, P.; Paneth, N.; Dan, B.; Lin, J.P.; Damiano, D.L.; Becher, J.G.; Gaebler-Spira, D.; Colver, A.; Reddihough, D.S.; et al. Cerebral palsy. *Nat. Rev. Dis. Primers* **2016**, *2*, 15082. [CrossRef]
3. Palisano, R.; Rosenbaum, P.; Walter, S.; Russell, D.; Wood, E.; Galuppi, B. Development and reliability of a system to classify gross motor function in children with cerebral palsy. *Dev. Med. Child Neurol.* **1997**, *39*, 214–223. [CrossRef] [PubMed]
4. Wimalasundera, N.; Stevenson, V.L. Cerebral palsy. *Pract. Neurol.* **2016**, *16*, 184–194. [CrossRef] [PubMed]
5. Davis, E.; Shelly, A.; Waters, E.; Boyd, R.; Cook, K.; Davern, M.; Reddihough, D. The impact of caring for a child with cerebral palsy: Quality of life for mothers and fathers. *Child Care Health Dev.* **2010**, *36*, 63–73. [CrossRef]
6. Brehaut, J.C.; Kohen, D.E.; Raina, P.; Walter, S.D.; Russell, D.J.; Swinton, M.; O'Donnell, M.; Rosenbaum, P. The health of primary caregivers of children with cerebral palsy: How does it compare with that of other Canadian caregivers? *Pediatrics* **2004**, *114*, e182–e191. [CrossRef]
7. Guillamón, N.; Nieto, R.; Pousada, M.; Redolar, D.; Muñoz, E.; Hernández, E.; Boixadós, M.; Gómez-Zúñiga, B. Quality of life and mental health among parents of children with cerebral palsy: The influence of self-efficacy and coping strategies. *J. Clin. Nurs.* **2013**, *22*, 1579–1590. [CrossRef]
8. Parkes, J.; Caravale, B.; Marcelli, M.; Franco, F.; Colver, A. Parenting stress and children with cerebral palsy: A European cross-sectional survey. *Dev. Med. Child Neurol.* **2011**, *53*, 815–821. [CrossRef]
9. Svedberg, L.E.; Englund, E.; Malker, H.; Stener-Victorin, E. Comparison of impact on mood, health, and daily living experiences of primary caregivers of walking and non-walking children with cerebral palsy and provided community services support. *Eur. J. Paediatr. Neurol.* **2010**, *14*, 239–246. [CrossRef]
10. Britner, P.A.; Morog, M.C.; Pianta, R.C.; Marvin, R.S. Stress and coping: A comparison of self-report measures of functioning in families of young children with cerebral palsy or no medical diagnosis. *J. Child Fam. Stud.* **2003**, *12*, 335–348. [CrossRef]
11. Lee, M.H.; Matthews, A.K.; Park, P. Determinants of health-related quality of life among mothers of children with cerebral palsy. *J. Pediatr. Nurs.* **2019**, *44*, 1–8. [CrossRef]
12. Tseng, M.H.; Chen, K.L.; Shieh, J.Y.; Lu, L.; Huang, C.Y.; Simeonsson, R.J. Child characteristics, caregiver characteristics, and environmental factors affecting the quality of life of caregivers of children with cerebral palsy. *Disabil. Rehabil.* **2016**, *38*, 2374–2382. [CrossRef] [PubMed]
13. Healthy People 2030. U.S. Department of Health and Human Services. Office of Disease Prevention and Health Promotion. Social Determinants of Health. Available online: https://health.gov/healthypeople/priority-areas/social-determinants-health (accessed on 12 December 2022).
14. Pruszczynski, B.; Sees, J.; Miller, F. Risk factors for hip displacement in children with cerebral palsy: Systematic review. *J. Pediatr. Orthop.* **2016**, *36*, 829–833. [CrossRef] [PubMed]
15. McGinley, J.L.; Dobson, F.; Ganeshalingam, R.; Shore, B.J.; Rutz, E.; Graham, H.K. Single-event multilevel surgery for children with cerebral palsy: A systematic review. *Dev. Med. Child Neurol.* **2012**, *54*, 117–128. [CrossRef] [PubMed]
16. Miller, D.J.; Flynn, J.J.M.; Pasha, S.; Yaszay, B.; Parent, S.; Asghar, J.; Abel, M.F.; Pahys, J.M.; Samdani, A.; Hwang, S.W.; et al. Improving health-related quality of life for patients with nonambulatory cerebral palsy: Who stands to gain from scoliosis surgery? *J. Pediatr. Orthop.* **2020**, *40*, e186–e192. [CrossRef] [PubMed]
17. Hosseinzadeh, P.; Baldwin, K.; Minaie, A.; Miller, F. Management of hip disorders in patients with cerebral palsy. *JBJS Rev.* **2020**, *8*, e0148. [CrossRef] [PubMed]
18. Koop, S.E. Scoliosis in cerebral palsy. *Dev. Med. Child Neurol.* **2009**, *51* (Suppl. S4), 92–98. [CrossRef]
19. Iversen, A.S.; Graue, M.; Clare, J. Parents' perspectives of surgery for a child who has cerebral palsy. *J. Pediatr. Health Care* **2009**, *23*, 165–172. [CrossRef]
20. Park, M.S.; Chung, C.Y.; Lee, K.M.; Sung, K.H.; Choi, I.H.; Kim, T.W. Parenting stress in parents of children with cerebral palsy and its association with physical function. *J. Pediatr. Orthop. B* **2012**, *21*, 452–456. [CrossRef]
21. Vessey, J.A.; DiFazio, R.L.; Strout, T.D.; Snyder, B.D. Impact of non-medical out-of-pocket expenses on families of children with cerebral palsy following orthopaedic surgery. *J. Pediatr. Nurs.* **2017**, *37*, 101–107. [CrossRef]
22. Shanske, S.; Arnold, J.; Carvalho, M.; Rein, J. Social workers as transition brokers: Facilitating the transition from pediatric to adult medical care. *Soc. Work Health Care* **2012**, *51*, 279–295. [CrossRef]
23. Jain, A.; Sponseller, P.D.; Shah, S.A.; Samdani, A.; Cahill, P.J.; Yaszay, B.; Njoku, D.B.; Abel, M.F.; Newton, P.O.; Marks, M.C.; et al. Subclassification of GMFCS level-5 cerebral palsy as a predictor of complications and health-related quality of life after spinal arthrodesis. *J. Bone Jt. Surg. Am.* **2016**, *98*, 1821–1828. [CrossRef] [PubMed]

24. National Association of Social Workers (NASW). NASW Standards for Social Work Practice in Health Care Settings. Washington, DC: NASW. Available online: https://www.socialworkers.org/LinkClick.aspx?fileticket=fFnsRHX-4HE%3d&portalid=0 (accessed on 19 December 2022).
25. R Core Team. *R: A Language and Environment for Statistical Computing*; R Foundation for Statistical Computing: Vienna, Austria, 2021. Available online: https://www.R-project.org/ (accessed on 19 December 2022).

Disclaimer/Publisher's Note: The statements, opinions and data contained in all publications are solely those of the individual author(s) and contributor(s) and not of MDPI and/or the editor(s). MDPI and/or the editor(s) disclaim responsibility for any injury to people or property resulting from any ideas, methods, instructions or products referred to in the content.

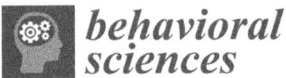

Article

Manual Abilities and Cognition in Children with Cerebral Palsy: Do Fine Motor Skills Impact Cognition as Measured by the Bayley Scales of Infant Development?

Thais Invencao Cabral [1], Xueliang Pan [2], Tanya Tripathi [1], Jianing Ma [2] and Jill C. Heathcock [1,*]

[1] School of Health and Rehabilitation Sciences, The Ohio State University, Columbus, OH 43220, USA; thais.invencaocabral@osumc.edu (T.I.C.); tanya.tripathi@mcri.edu.au (T.T.)

[2] Department of Biomedical Informatics, The Ohio State University, Columbus, OH 43210, USA; jeff.pan@osumc.edu (X.P.); jianing.ma@osumc.edu (J.M.)

* Correspondence: jill.heathcock@osumc.edu

Abstract: Manual ability may be an important consideration when measuring cognition in children with CP because many items on cognitive tests require fine motor skills. This study investigated the association of fine motor dependent (FMD) and fine motor independent (FMI) items within the cognitive domain (COG) of the Bayley Scales of Infant Development—Third Edition (Bayley-III) and Manual Ability Classification System (MACS) in children with cerebral palsy. Children aged 2 to 8 (3.96 ± 1.68) years were included in this study. MACS levels were assigned at baseline. COG was administrated at baseline (n = 61) and nine months post-baseline (n = 28). The 91 items were classified into FMD (52) and FMI (39). Total raw score, FMD, and FMI scores were calculated. The association between MACS and cognitive scores (total, FMD, and FMI) were evaluated using linear regression and Spearman correlation coefficients. We found total, FMD, and FMI scores decrease significantly as the MACS level increases at the baseline. Both FMD and FMI scores decreased as MACS levels increased (worse function). There was a significant difference between the two slopes, with the FMD scores having a steeper slope. Similar patterns were observed nine months post-baseline. Children with lower manual ability scored lower in the cognitive domain at baseline and 9 months post-baseline. The significant difference in the performance of FMD items and FMI items across MACS levels with a steeper slope of changes in FMD items suggests fine motor skills impact cognition.

Keywords: child; cognitive impairment; psychomotor performance; disability; upper extremity; manual ability

1. Introduction

Cerebral palsy (CP) is a heterogeneous group of neurodevelopmental conditions that present as impairments in movement and posture. CP is the result of brain injury during fetal or infant development. Brain injuries that cause motor impairments are permanent and non-progressive. It is often accompanied by epilepsy, secondary musculoskeletal disorders, and sensory and cognitive impairments, which cause limitations in activities and participation [1–5]. CP is commonly classified according to muscle tone topography [6], gross motor function [7], and manual function [8].

Functional impairments across developmental domains in children with CP are often evaluated using standardized assessments of cognitive and motor skills [9–12]. Many standardized cognitive assessments appropriate for children with cerebral palsy, such as the Bayley Scales of Infant Development—Third Edition (Bayley-III) and the Weschler Intelligence Scale for Children, require fine motor actions to accomplish cognitive tasks. Most cognitive assessments require reaching, pointing, grasping, manipulating objects, and other manual abilities that demand precision, speed, dexterity, and coordination [13–17].

Thus, whether the cognitive scores reflect purely cognitive performance or if cognitive performance is masked by poor fine motor skills is sometimes unclear, especially in children with limited fine motor or manual skills [17].

In children with CP, cognitive impairment is present in 50% of the cases [2,18,19]. Cognitive impairment is influenced by many components, such as the type and distribution of CP, gross motor functioning, and manual ability [18,19]. Bilateral spastic CP is common and represents 60 to 80% of the occurrences, with 40.3% of the children classified at GMFCS levels IV and V. Upper extremity functions are impacted in a range from 57 to 83% of the occurrences [2]. Additionally, impairments in manual function may cause disuse and lack of learning opportunities early in life, i.e., impairments in upper extremity function limit opportunities for manipulation and object exploration, which have an impact on cognitive development [17,20]. Also, motor and cognitive development overlap and are interrelated [21]. According to Osorio-Valencia et al. [14], the components of cognitive skill are influenced by gross and fine motor abilities acquired in the first three years of life. However, the long-term interrelation of fine motor and cognitive skills still needs to be clarified, especially for children with motor disabilities.

Children with CP might be unable to show their abilities compared to neurotypical children in the cognitive domain during the standardized assessment [20,22–24] because of the requirements in fine motor skills. They may need more time to deal with the material or might not be able to manipulate the test materials without adaptation. The study by Visser et al. [16,17] examined the validity of the Bayley-III Low Motor/Vision version and its suitability for children with motor and/or visual impairment(s). It contains accommodated items, that is, adaptations to minimize impairment bias, without altering what the test measures. The results found that the accommodations in the cognitive domain did not affect the test scores of children with neurotypical development and did improve the test scores of children with atypical development. In addition, the results indicated that most children with atypical development could show their abilities in the cognitive domain and that the accommodations were beneficial in 29 of these 52 cases. Therefore, standardized tools to evaluate cognition that consider adaptations, especially for children with manual ability impairment are important [16,17,22–24].

To evaluate cognition in children with CP, understanding the relationship between manual and cognitive abilities is important, especially when administering a standardized assessment such as Bayley-III. Measuring cognition in children with CP while considering their manual ability and the demands of the test could provide a more accurate method for tracking development, predicting outcomes, and evaluating intervention approaches to provide accurate and reliable quantifications of performance. Besides that, an accurate measure and reporting can facilitate a comprehensive discussion between parents and rehabilitation professionals on the children's cognitive abilities.

The primary purpose of this study was to identify the association between manual ability and cognition in children with CP. Our goal was to investigate if manual ability levels and cognitive performance in children with CP were related to fine motor-dependent and -independent items within the cognitive domain of Bayley-III. These categories of fine motor dependent and independent were assigned by our research team. The secondary purpose was to investigate the impact of the distribution of CP and gross motor function levels (GMFCS) and factors such as gestational age, birth weight, NICU stay, age of CP diagnosis, and CP type on the relationship between manual ability levels and cognition. We expected children with lower manual ability to have lower cognitive scores than children with higher manual ability. Additionally, we anticipated that gross motor functions would be associated with manual and cognitive abilities.

2. Materials and Methods

2.1. Participants

Participants in this prospective, observational study were children with CP who were part of a larger randomized controlled clinical trial [NCT02897024]. Sixty-one children aged between 2 and 8 years (median age: 3.50; IQR: 2.58, 4.75) participated in this study. The Ohio State University and Nationwide Children's Hospital's [NCH] Institutional Review Boards approved this study [IRB16-00492], and parental consent was obtained for all participants. Participants with uncontrollable seizures, unknown auditory or visual impairments, progressive neurological disorder, recent surgery, or participation in another daily physical therapy treatment program in the last six months were excluded from the larger trial, and only those eligible for the Bayley evaluation were included in this study. See Table 1 for demographic information.

Table 1. Baseline participant characteristics (median and interquartile for continuous variables, count and % for categorical variables).

Characteristic	Overall (n = 61)
Gestational Age (weeks)	37.0 (27.1, 39.0)
Birth Weight (kg)	2.48 (0.93, 3.41)
Birth Length (in)	18.0 (13.0, 20.0)
APGAR 1	6.00 (2.00, 8.00)
APGAR 5	6.00 (5.00, 9.00)
Total Hospital Length of Stay (days)	28.50 (0.00, 134.75)
Type of CP	
Hypotonic	10 (16.39%)
Hypertonic Spastic	45 (73.77%)
Ataxic	5 (8.20%)
Unspecified	1 (1.64%)
CP distribution	
Left hemiplegia	9 (15.52%)
Right hemiplegia	2 (3.45%)
Diplegia	9 (15.52%)
Quadriplegia	37 (63.79%)
Triplegia	1 (1.72%)
Not reported	3
GMFCS	
Level I	14 (23.33%)
Level II	8 (13.33%)
Level III	5 (8.33%)
Level IV	21 (35.00%)
Level V	12 (20.00%)
Age at enrollment (years)	3.50 (2.58, 4.75)
Gender	
Male	37 (60.66%)
Female	24 (39.34%)
Race	
White	43 (70.49%)
Black or African American	12 (19.67%)
More than One Race	4 (6.56%)
Asian	2 (3.28%)
Hispanic	1 (1.64%)

2.2. Procedure

The participants were assessed at baseline and nine months post-baseline. At baseline, the manual ability level of children with CP was classified using Mini-Manual Ability Classification System (mini-MACS) or MACS according to the participant's age. The MACS describes children with CP 4 to 18 years of age in daily manual activities. Mini-MACS is an updated version of the MACS for younger children 1 to 4 years of age but has the same concept as MACS. In this study, the term MACS will be used for both classification systems. The cognitive domain of the Bayley Scales of Infant Development—Third Edition (Bayley III) was administered at baseline (n = 61) and nine months post-baseline (n = 28).

The participants received 40 h of outpatient physical therapy during the nine months with a randomized treatment service delivery frequency: daily (high intensity periodic) or weekly (usual and customary treatment). No between-group treatment effects were expected or found between groups for cognition.

2.3. Measures

2.3.1. Manual Ability Classification System (MACS)

The Manual Ability Classification System (MACS) describes how children with CP 4 to 18 years of age use both hands together to manipulate toys and objects in daily activities. MACS is described hierarchically in five levels (I to V). The levels are based on the self-initiated ability to handle objects and the need for assistance or adaptation to perform manual activities [8]. Children in level I (highest ability) can easily and successfully handle objects. In contrast, children in level V (most limited ability) cannot handle objects or complete simple manual actions alone [8]. We used the Mini-MACS as the manual classification system for those under four.

MACS is a classification system, not an outcome measure. It was used to classify our sample of participants. Trained, reliable, and blinded assessors determined the MACS level for the participants. The intra- and inter-rater correlation coefficients were calculated for each blinded assessor every six months. All assessors needed to achieve and maintain the agreement index >85% to pass reliability. The agreement index was evaluated using inter-rater reliability (IRR) in 10% of the sample.

2.3.2. Bayley Scales of Infant and Toddler Development—Third Edition (Bayley-III)

The Bayley-III is a valid and reliable measure of a child's neurodevelopment from 1 to 42 months of age and was developed specifically for use in research and clinical practice. It is the most common assessment tool for evaluating early development and measuring delays across multiple domains of development (cognition, motor, language, and socio-emotional) [12]. Bayley-III has been validated for use in children at high risk for CP with good discriminative properties [12,23,24]. According to the manual administration's instructions, Bayley-III was administered to children out of the age range but in the developmental range appropriate for this tool [12]. The raw score was considered in the analysis. Blinded assessors completed training and intra- and inter-rater reliability testing on the Bayley-III (>85% to pass reliability).

The cognitive total raw score was based on 91 cognitive domain items. These 91 items were classified into two groups (see Appendix A Table A1): 52 items relied on fine motor abilities (reaching, pointing, grasping, and manipulating objects, with components such as precision, speed, dexterity, and coordination), which were classified as fine motor dependent (FMD); 39 items not requiring the skills listed (looking at pictures, turning the head to specific sounds, counting numbers) were classified as fine motor independent (FMI). The items were classified by two experienced researchers trained in Bayley-III, with a strong agreement between the researchers. The FMD and FMI scores were calculated as the proportion of the number of items scored, specifically, the sum of the items that received credit (score of 1) divided by the total number of items (52 and 39 for FMD and FMI, respectively). In other words, the FMD score is the total FMD items credited/52, and the FMI score is the total FMI items credited/39.

2.4. Analysis

Descriptive statistics (means and standard deviation) of the Bayley-III cognitive raw scores at baseline and nine months post-baseline were summarized for children at each MACS level. The Spearman correlation coefficient was used to evaluate the association between MACS levels and cognitive scores at baseline and nine months post-baseline. General Linear Model and Kruskal–Wallis tests were used to explore the difference in the cognitive scores (including total raw score and proportion of fine motor dependent and independent scores) among MACS levels at baseline. The change in the cognitive score from baseline to nine months post-baseline and the impact of the baseline MACS levels were explored using linear mixed models to account for the association of the baseline and nine months post-baseline data from the same participant. All 61 participants were included in these analyses while assuming data missing at random for these without post-baseline data.

In addition, using multiple regression analysis, we further investigated the impact of the distribution of CP and gross motor function level (Gross Motor Function Classification—GMFCS) and factors such as gestational age, birth weight, NICU stay, age of CP diagnosis, and CP type on the association between MACS level and Bayley-III cognitive scores (total scores, FMD, FMI) at baseline. See Table 2 for descriptive statistics (means and standard deviation) of the Bayley-III cognitive raw scores at baseline and nine months post-baseline.

Table 2. Bayley-III cognitive score at baseline and 9-month post-baseline via MACS level (mean and standard deviation).

MACS Level	Baseline (n = 61)			9-Month Post-Baseline (n = 28)		
	Total	FMD Score *	FMI Score **	Total	FMD Score *	FMI Score **
1	64.94 (14.10)	0.74 (0.20)	0.68 (0.10)	64.80 (15.28)	0.73 (0.21)	0.68 (0.11)
2	56.80 (16.40)	0.62 (0.24)	0.63 (0.11)	60.00 (12.88)	0.68 (0.17)	0.63 (0.10)
3	40.50 (14.20)	0.35 (0.23)	0.58 (0.06)	46.67 (21.36)	0.44 (0.33)	0.61 (0.10)
4	27.79 (8.14)	0.17 (0.09)	0.49 (0.10)	28.67 (10.03)	0.17 (0.14)	0.50 (0.07)
5	12.64 (8.82)	0.03 (0.07)	0.28 (0.15)	16.75 (13.30)	0.07 (0.10)	0.34 (0.23)

* FMD score = total FMD items credited/52; ** FMI score = total FMI items credited/39.

3. Results

There was a significant association between the MACS levels and the Bayley–III cognitive total raw scores of children with CP at baseline (Spearman correlation Rho = −0.84 and p values of <0.001). The higher the MACS level (lower manual ability), the lower the cognitive scores. See Figure 1 for Bayley-III cognitive total scores at baseline and 9-month post-baseline across the MACS levels. A similar relationship between cognitive score and MACS levels was observed nine months post-baseline (Rho = −0.80 and p values of <0.001).

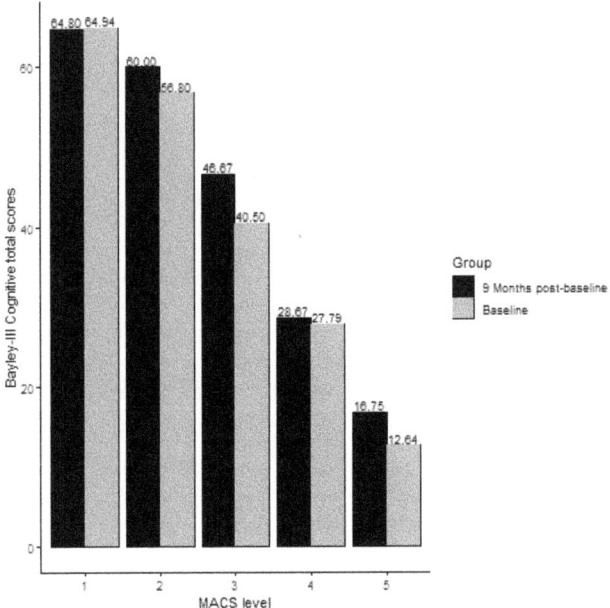

Figure 1. Bayley-III cognitive total scores at baseline and 9-month post-baseline via MACS level.

At baseline, cognitive scores of children with CP in both the FMD and FMI groups were significantly associated with their MACS levels ($Rho_{FMD} = -0.85$, $p < 0.001$ and $Rho_{FMI} = -0.81$, $p < 0.0001$). See Figure 2 for the FMD and FMI scores across the MACS levels. The decline between FMD and FMI cognitive scores over MACS levels was significantly different ($p < 0.001$). Additionally, the decline of FMD scores across MACS levels is steeper than the FMI scores (0.09 vs. 0.187 for FMD and FMI, respectively, linear regression models, Figure 2). Similar patterns in the change slope in FMD and FMI cognitive scores over MACS levels were observed nine months post-baseline.

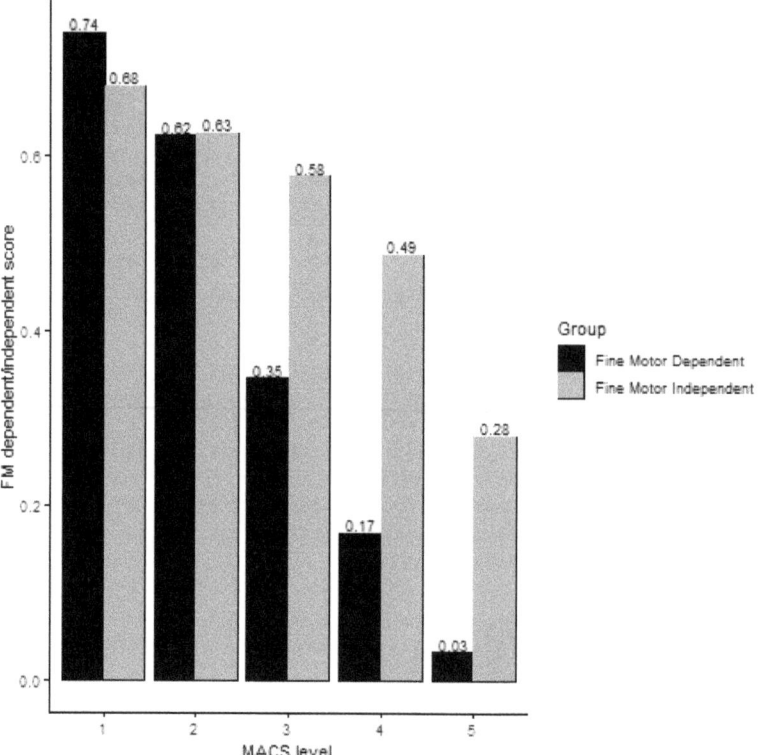

Figure 2. Fine motor dependent and fine motor independent score via MACS level (y-axis as FM dependent/independent score).

Medical and demographic factors impact manual abilities and cognition in children with CP at baseline.

A significant association was found between the CP distribution and MACS level ($p < 0.001$). Moreover, the CP distribution was significantly related to the cognitive total raw score, FMD score, and FMI score ($p < 0.001$, $p < 0.001$, and $p = 0.002$, respectively) items. We did not find significant associations at nine months post-baseline. Similarly, GMFCS levels were also associated with MACS level and cognitive scores (total, FMD, and FMI). These findings suggest that a combination of better manual ability and gross motor function corresponds to higher cognitive performance in children with CP. In addition, the gestational age, birth weight, NICU stay, age of CP diagnosis, and CP type did not significantly impact the association between MACS level and Bayley-III cognitive scores (total scores, FMD, FMI) at baseline. See Table 3 for the Bayley-III cognitive total raw score and FMD and FMI items across the MACS level amongst the CP distribution.

Table 3. Cerebral palsy distribution and GMFCS level across MACS level at baseline for the Bayley-III cognitive total raw score and fine motor dependent and independent items.

	Cerebral Palsy Distribution				GMFCS Level					
	Hemiplegia (n = 11)	Diplegia (n = 9)	Quadriplegia and Triplegia (n = 38)	p-Value	I	II	III	IV	V	p-Value
MACS Level				<0.001						NA [1]
1	6 (55%)	6 (67%)	3 (7.9%)		11 (79%)	3 (38%)	1 (20%)	1 (4.8%)	0 (0%)	
2	4 (36%)	2 (22%)	8 (21%)		3 (21%)	4 (50%)	3 (60%)	5 (24%)	0 (0%)	
3	0 (0%)	1 (11%)	3 (7.9%)		0 (0%)	1 (12%)	0 (0%)	3 (14%)	0 (0%)	
4	1 (9.1%)	0 (0%)	13 (34%)		0 (0%)	0 (0%)	1 (20%)	11 (52%)	2 (17%)	
5	0 (0%)	0 (0%)	11 (29%)		0 (0%)	0 (0%)	0 (0%)	1 (4.8%)	10 (83%)	
Cognitive total raw score	55 (44, 68)	70 (49, 75)	32 (16, 43)	<0.001	73 (62, 75)	55 (48, 64)	43 (36, 44)	34 (30, 39)	12 (8, 16)	<0.001
Fine Motor Dependent	32 (22, 42)	42 (26, 48)	10 (2, 21)	<0.001	0.87 (0.74, 0.90)	0.63 (0.49, 0.71)	0.40 (0.29, 0.42)	0.23 (0.17, 0.33)	0.00 (0.00, 0.04)	<0.001
Fine Motor Independent	23 (22, 26)	27 (23, 29)	21 (15, 22)	0.002	0.69 (0.61, 0.76)	0.58 (0.56, 0.69)	0.56 (0.54, 0.56)	0.54 (0.51, 0.56)	0.31 (0.20, 0.36)	<0.001

[1] Too many 0 s, so we cannot calculate a p-value here.

4. Discussion

This study aimed to identify the association between manual ability and cognitive performance in children with CP. In addition, the aim was to investigate if manual ability levels and cognitive performance of children with CP were related to cognitive items on the Bayley-III that require fine motor components (fine motor dependent) and items that do not require fine motor components (fine motor independent) within the cognitive domain items of the Bayley-III. The second analysis investigated the impact of the CP distribution and gross motor function levels (GMFCS) and factors such as gestational age, birth weight, NICU stay, age of CP diagnosis, and CP type on the relationship between manual ability levels and cognitive performance. Our hypotheses were partially supported.

Manual exploration affords learning opportunities that impact cognition in children with CP by manipulating objects [10,11]. Our findings show an association between manual ability and cognition in this population. Specifically, lower manual ability (higher MACS level) corresponds to lower cognitive performance. Due to the manual ability impairment (for example, not being able to grasp an object), children with CP might demonstrate difficulty in cognitive tasks, such as solving a puzzle, within the cognitive domain of Bayley-III. Our findings support the interrelationship between movement and learning [10,11,15,19,25–30], which are basic principles for building cognitive functions [18,31,32]. Our findings emphasized that the cognitive abilities of children with CP are likely underestimated in Bayley-III due to the inherent reliance on the hands and arms to complete cognitive tasks. This underestimation was particularly evident for children with severe manual impairment, as indicated by MACS levels IV and V. Returning to our initial question of whether the cognitive scores reflect purely cognitive performance or are influenced by manual ability, our findings suggest that manual ability has an impact and can mask cognitive performance in children with CP.

The manual ability level and the success in performing cognitive tasks that have or do not have fine motor components are related according to our findings. Children with CP in MACS levels IV and V had significantly lower scores in the cognitive items, dependent and independent of fine motor abilities, than those in MACS levels II and I. However, our findings suggest a large difference between FMD and FMI across MACS levels III to V, as observed in Figure 2, suggesting their cognitive performances are lower on FMD items than on FMI items. Thus, the manual ability has a higher impact on the fine motor-dependent items than on the fine motor-independent items, especially for those with severe manual impairments. In this study, children in MACS levels I and II performed better than children in MACS IV to V because in Bayley-III, children with MACS levels I to III commonly use their less-affected hand for the cognitive items and can, presumably, score within the normative reference values, regardless of the impairment with the affected hand. However, children in MACS levels IV and V, with both upper extremities impaired, will likely perform lower and consequently score lower in the cognitive domain. Although children with very low manual abilities struggled to perform well in cognitive items requiring fine motor abilities, they also struggled in cognitive items not requiring them. This finding could be attributed to the fact that child development is a product of multi-domain interactions [18,19,25,27,30–32], and thus, limitations beyond manual abilities across development impact cognitive performance. In addition, cognitive impairments are common in this population.

The findings of this study also demonstrate that cognitive performance in children with CP changes over time. In this study, despite the challenges in manual functions, children with CP at different levels of manual ability improved their cognitive performance. Considering the CP distribution factor, our findings suggest that children with hemiplegia and diplegia CP, distributed mostly on MACS levels I to III, performed better on fine motor dependent items and, consequently, had better cognition performance than children with triplegia or quadriplegia, mostly assigned to levels IV and V. Children with triplegia or quadriplegia seem to perform better on fine motor independent items. Previous studies have shown that up to 29% of children with CP may be incapable of demonstrating their actual cognitive capacity in most standardized assessments, such as the commonly used Bayley-III, due to poor fine motor skills or verbal demands involved in completing most of the testing items [5,23,24,30,32]. Our study demonstrates that 43% of our sample might have their cognitive abilities misrepresented due to their manual impairment, as seen in Table 3. Thus, this study has an emerging answer to whether cognitive scores reflect purely cognitive performance or are influenced by fine motor ability, but deep investigations are needed. These data suggest that the 52 cognitive fine motor dependent items are more appropriate for children with diplegia and hemiplegia than for those with quadriplegia and triplegia.

Cognitive total raw scores were significantly different across children's gross motor function levels. Gross motor and manual exploration support learning opportunities that further impact cognition in children with CP [10,11,25]. Our findings suggest lower cognitive performance is related to lower manual abilities (higher MACS level). Besides that, cognitive performance and manual abilities are significantly associated with gross motor function. Through the MACS and GMFCS level documentation, a snapshot of the cognitive challenges of children with CP can be anticipated. The combination of MACS and GMFCS when referring to cognitive performance is especially relevant for children with severe limitations in manual ability. This study contributes to the clinical practice field, reinforcing that a combination of classification systems, such as MACS and GMFCS, and CP distribution need to be included in the assessment and individualized treatment plans for cognition. These will provide accurate, reliable quantifications and facilitate a comprehensive discussion between parents and rehabilitation professionals on understanding real-life barriers children with CP face. In addition, raising awareness of these findings is substantial regarding the cognitive performance of children with CP, especially at MACS and GMFCS levels IV and V. Thus, when reporting cognitive performance in pediatric services, motor abilities should be accounted for interpreting cognition, especially for children with significant impairments.

To our knowledge, this is the first study to categorize the testing items in the cognitive domain of Bayley-III based on if fine motor skills are required to receive a full score and then compare the performance of children with CP who have different manual abilities (MACS level) on these item categories (fine motor dependent versus fine motor independent). This study highlights that evaluating cognitive performance in children with CP using standardized tools such as Bayley-III needs careful interpretation and modifications. For children with CP, an assessment tool for cognitive performance could consider (1) the MACS levels when interpreting the scores, (2) different attributions for FM-dependent and

FM-independent items, (3) adjustment on the requirements of the tasks such as timing the items, and/or (4) bimanual and unimanual skill necessary to complete items. Previous studies, such as Visser et al. [16,17], have demonstrated success with valid results in the accommodations made on Bayley-III. The accommodations were beneficial for a subset of children with atypical development who showed a larger raw score. Thus, our study adds that accommodations might be needed for children with CP on cognitive scales, especially in MACS IV and V. Cognitive performance affects daily functioning and predicts participation and is an important factor when addressing the treatment plan. Future research is necessary to review the current instruments available to evaluate cognitive performance and develop an appropriate standardized instrument for children with atypical development as children with CP.

There are some limitations to this current study. First, this study is an exploratory analysis of a set of data from a large clinical trial and other components of the trial may have confounded the results. Second, some children in the age range at baseline were not in the developmental range nine months later, meaning that the sample size is smaller than the baseline analysis, which might have impacted our ability to assess if differences in manual abilities account for the magnitude of change in cognitive performance. Third, our sample had unequal sample sizes among MACS levels, possibly resulting in lower power for the subgroup analysis. Fourth, although a comprehensive list of factors (birth-related, medical, and environmental) was analyzed, other demographics, such as parental education and maternal age, were not considered.

5. Conclusions

Children with CP are vulnerable to motor and cognitive impairments [1,23,24,29]. Fine motor and cognition functions develop concurrently in children with CP, where deficits in manual abilities may also indicate cognitive struggles. Categorizing the cognitive domain items of Bayley-III that require fine motor skills and comparing the performance of children with CP who have different manual abilities on the items fine motor dependent and independent is a novel approach. Understanding the relationship between manual abilities and cognition testing items may help healthcare professionals identify children's potential with CP. Our findings elaborate on the need for a deep investigation into whether cognitive scores reflect purely cognitive performances or are influenced by fine motor abilities.

Author Contributions: Conceptualization: J.C.H., T.I.C. and T.T.; Data curation: X.P., J.M. and J.C.H.; Formal analysis: X.P., J.M., J.C.H., T.I.C. and T.T.; Investigation: J.C.H.; Methodology: X.P. and J.C.H.; Supervision: J.C.H.; Visualization: J.C.H., X.P., J.M., T.I.C. and T.T.; Writing—original draft: J.C.H., T.I.C. and T.T.; Writing—review and editing: J.C.H., T.I.C., T.T., X.P. and J.M. All authors have read and agreed to the published version of the manuscript.

Funding: Funding provided by the Patient-Centered Outcomes Research Institute, [NCT02897024] and the National Institutes of Health [P2CAHD101912].

Institutional Review Board Statement: This study was conducted in accordance with the Declaration of Helsinki and approved by The Ohio State University and Nationwide Children's Hospital's (NCH) Institutional Review Boards (IRB16-00492), and parental consent was obtained for all participants.

Informed Consent Statement: Informed consent was obtained from all subjects involved in this study.

Acknowledgments: The authors thank the Nationwide Children's Hospital for their collaboration and the ACHIEVE patients and families for their availability and support with this study.

Conflicts of Interest: The authors declare no conflict of interest.

Appendix A

Individual analysis of Bayley-III cognitive domain items according to the requirement of fine motor components to complete tasks.

Table A1. Bayley-III cognitive domain items.

Item Number	Fine Motor Dependent	Item Number	Fine Motor Independent
16	Explores Object	1	Calms When Picked Up
17	Carries Object to Mouth	2	Responds to surroundings Series: Inspects
21	Persistent Reach	3	Regards Object for 3 s
23	Plays With String	4	Habituates to Rattle
24	Bangs in Play	5	Discriminates Between Objects
26	Bell Series: Manipulates	6	Recognizes Caregiver
27	Picks Up Block Series: Reaches for Second Block	7	Becomes Excited in Anticipation
28	Pulls Cloth to Obtain Object	8	Regards Object for 5 s
29	Pulls String Adaptively	9	Reacts to Disappearance of Face
30	Retains Both Blocks	10	Shifts Attention
31	Bell Series: Rings Purposely	11	Shows Visual Preference
33	Picks Up Block Series: Retains 2 or 3 Blocks	12	Habituates to Object
35	Takes Blocks out of Cup	13	Prefers Novel Object
36	Block Series: 1 Block	14	Habituates to Picture (Balloons)
37	Picks Up Block Series: 3 Blocks	15	Prefers Novel Picture (Ball)
38	Explores Holes in Pegboard	18	Inspects Own Hand
39	Pushes Car	19	Mirror Image Series: Approaches
40	Finds Hidden Object	20	Responds to Surroundings Series: Awareness of Novelty
41	Suspends Ring	22	Mirror Image Series: Responds Positively
42	Removes Pellet	25	Searches for Fallen Object
43	Clear Box: Front	32	Looks at Pictures
44	Squeezes Object	34	Searches for Missing Objects
45	Finds Hidden Object (Reversed)	59	Attends to Story
46	Removes Lid from Bottle	64	Matches Pictures
47	Pegboard Series: 2 Holes	68	Matches 3 Colors
48	Relational Play Series: Self	72	Concept Grouping: Color
49	Pink Board Series: 1 Piece	73	Concept Grouping: Size
50	Finds Hidden Object (Visible Displacement)	75	Matches size
51	Blue Board Series: 1 Piece	76	Discriminates Pictures
52	Clear Box: Slides	77	Simple Pattern
53	Relational Play Series: Others	79	Counts (One-to-One Correspondence)
54	Block Series: 9 Blocks	80	Discriminates Sizes
55	Pegboard Series: 6 Pegs	81	Identifies 3 Incomplete Pictures
56	Pink Board Series: Completes	83	Discriminates Patterns
57	Uses Pencil to Obtain Object	85	Counts (Cardinality)
58	Blue Board Series: 4 Pieces	86	Number Constancy
60	Rotated Pink Board	88	Classifies Objects
61	Object Assembly (Ball)	89	Understands Concept of More
62	Completes Pegboard: 25 s	90	Repeats Number Sequences
63	Object Assembly (Ice Cream Cone)		
65	Representational Play		
66	Blue Board Series: Completes (75 s)		
67	Imitates a Two-Step Action		
69	Imaginary Play		
70	Understands Concept of One		
71	Multischeme Combination Play		
74	Compares Masses		
78	Sorts Pegs by Color		
82	Object Assembly (Dog)		
84	Spatial Memory		
87	Laces Card		
91	Completes Patterns		

References

1. Rosenbaum, P.; Paneth, N.; Leviton, A.; Goldstein, M.; Bax, M.; Damiano, D.; Dan, B.; Jacobsson, B. A Report: The Definition and Classification of Cerebral Palsy April 2006. *Dev. Med. Child Neurol.* **2007**, *49*, 1–44. [CrossRef]
2. Kirby, R.S.; Wingate, M.S.; Braun, K.V.N.; Doernberg, N.S.; Arneson, C.L.; Benedict, R.E.; Mulvihill, B.; Durkin, M.S.; Fitzgerald, R.T.; Maenner, M.J.; et al. Prevalence and Functioning of Children with Cerebral Palsy in Four Areas of the United States in 2006: A Report from the Autism and Developmental Disabilities Monitoring Network. *Res. Dev. Disabil.* **2011**, *32*, 462–469. [CrossRef] [PubMed]
3. Tonmukayakul, U.; Shih, S.T.F.; Bourke-Taylor, H.; Imms, C.; Reddihough, D.; Cox, L.; Carter, R. Systematic Review of the Economic Impact of Cerebral Palsy. *Res. Dev. Disabil.* **2018**, *80*, 93–101. [CrossRef]
4. Boyle, C.A.; Boulet, S.; Schieve, L.A.; Cohen, R.A.; Blumberg, S.J.; Yeargin-Allsopp, M.; Visser, S.; Kogan, M.D. Trends in the Prevalence of Developmental Disabilities in US Children, 1997–2008. *Pediatrics* **2011**, *127*, 1034–1042. [CrossRef]
5. McGuire, D.O.; Tian, L.H.; Yeargin-Allsopp, M.; Dowling, N.F.; Christensen, D.L. Prevalence of Cerebral Palsy, Intellectual Disability, Hearing Loss, and Blindness, National Health Interview Survey, 2009–2016. *Disabil. Health J.* **2019**, *12*, 443–451. [CrossRef] [PubMed]
6. Richards, C.L.; Malouin, F. Cerebral Palsy: Definition, Assessment and Rehabilitation. *Handb. Clin. Neurol.* **2013**, *111*, 183–195. [CrossRef] [PubMed]
7. Palisano, R.; Rosenbaum, P.; Walter, S.; Russell, D.; Wood, E.; Galuppi, B. GMFCS–E & R Gross Motor Function Classification System Expanded and Revised. *Dev. Med. Child Neurol.* **1997**, *39*, 214–223.
8. Eliasson, A.C.; Krumlinde-Sundholm, L.; Rösblad, B.; Beckung, E.; Arner, M.; Öhrvall, A.M.; Rosenbaum, P. The Manual Ability Classification System (MACS) for Children with Cerebral Palsy: Scale Development and Evidence of Validity and Reliability. *Dev. Med. Child Neurol.* **2006**, *48*, 549–554. [CrossRef]
9. Carey, H.; Hay, K.; Nelin, M.A.; Sowers, B.; Lewandowski, D.J.; Moore-Clingenpeel, M.; Maitre, N.L. Caregiver Perception of Hand Function in Infants with Cerebral Palsy: Psychometric Properties of the Infant Motor Activity Log. *Dev. Med. Child Neurol.* **2020**, *62*, 1266–1273. [CrossRef]
10. Thelen, E. Grounded in the World: Developmental Origins of the Embodied Mind. *Dev. Perspect. Embodiment Conscious.* **2012**, *1*, 99–130. [CrossRef]
11. Thelen, E.; Schöner, G.; Scheier, C.; Smith, L.B. The Dynamics of Embodiment: A Field Theory of Infant Perseverative Reaching. *Behav. Brain Sci.* **2001**, *24*, 1–34. [CrossRef] [PubMed]
12. Bayley, N. *Bayley Scales of Infant and Toddler Development*, 3rd ed.; PsychCorp: San Antonio, TX, USA, 2006.
13. Dusing, S.C.; Harbourne, R.T.; Lobo, M.A.; Westcott-Mccoy, S.; Bovaird, J.A.; Kane, A.E.; Syed, G.; Marcinowski, E.C.; Koziol, N.A.; Brown, S.E. A Physical Therapy Intervention to Advance Cognitive and Motor Skills: A Single Subject Study of a Young Child with Cerebral Palsy. *Pediatr. Phys. Ther.* **2019**, *31*, 347–352. [CrossRef] [PubMed]
14. Osorio-Valencia, E.; Torres-Sánchez, L.; López-Carrillo, L.; Rothenberg, S.J.; Schnaas, L. Early Motor Development and Cognitive Abilities among Mexican Preschoolers. *Child Neuropsychol.* **2018**, *24*, 1015–1025. [CrossRef]
15. Veldman, S.L.C.; Santos, R.; Jones, R.A.; Sousa-Sá, E.; Okely, A.D. Associations between Gross Motor Skills and Cognitive Development in Toddlers. *Early Hum. Dev.* **2019**, *132*, 39–44. [CrossRef] [PubMed]
16. Visser, L.; Ruiter, S.A.J.; Van Der Meulen, B.F.; Ruijssenaars, W.A.J.J.M.; Timmerman, M.E. Accommodating the Bayley-III for Motor and/or Visual Impairment: A Comparative Pilot Study. *Pediatr. Phys. Ther.* **2014**, *26*, 57–67. [CrossRef]
17. Visser, L.; Ruiter, S.A.J.; Van der Meulen, B.F.; Ruijssenaars, W.A.J.J.M.; Timmerman, M.E. Validity and Suitability of the Bayley-III Low Motor/Vision Version: A Comparative Study among Young Children with and without Motor and/or Visual Impairments. *Res. Dev. Disabil.* **2013**, *34*, 3736–3745. [CrossRef]
18. Laporta-Hoyos, O.; Panek, K.; Pagnozzi, A.M. Cognitive, Academic, Executive and Psychological Functioning in Children with Spastic Motor Type Cerebral Palsy: Influence of Extent, Location, and Laterality of Brain Lesions. *Eur. J. Paediatr. Neurol.* **2022**, *38*, A1. [CrossRef]
19. Al-Nemr, A.; Abdelazeim, F. Relationship of Cognitive Functions and Gross Motor Abilities in Children with Spastic Diplegic Cerebral Palsy. *Appl. Neuropsychol. Child* **2018**, *7*, 268–276. [CrossRef]
20. Deluca, S.C.; Echols, K.; Law, C.R.; Ramey, S.L. Intensive Pediatric Constraint-Induced Therapy for Children with Cerebral Palsy: Randomized, Controlled, Crossover Trial. *J. Child Neurol.* **2006**, *21*, 931–938. [CrossRef]
21. Ryalls, B.O.; Harbourne, R.; Kelly-Vance, L.; Wickstrom, J.; Stergiou, N.; Kyvelidou, A. A Perceptual Motor Intervention Improves Play Behavior in Children with Moderate to Severe Cerebral Palsy. *Front. Psychol.* **2016**, *7*, 643. [CrossRef]
22. World Health Organization. *International Classification of Functioning Disability and Health: Children & Youth Version*; ICF-CY: Geneva, Switzerland, 2007.
23. Novak, I.; Hines, M.; Goldsmith, S.; Barclay, R. Clinical Prognostic Messages from a Systematic Review on Cerebral Palsy. *Pediatrics* **2012**, *130*, e1285–e1312. [CrossRef]
24. Morgan, C.; Honan, I.; Allsop, A.; Novak, I.; Badawi, N. Psychometric Properties of Assessments of Cognition in Infants with Cerebral Palsy or Motor Impairment: A Systematic Review. *J. Pediatr. Psychol.* **2019**, *44*, 238–252. [CrossRef] [PubMed]
25. Oudgenoeg-Paz, O.; Mulder, H.; Jongmans, M.J.; van der Ham, I.J.M.; Van der Stigchel, S. The Link between Motor and Cognitive Development in Children Born Preterm and/or with Low Birth Weight: A Review of Current Evidence. *Neurosci. Biobehav. Rev.* **2017**, *80*, 382–393. [CrossRef]

26. Adolph, K.E.; Hoch, J.E. Motor Development: Embodied, Embedded, Enculturated, and Enabling. *Annu. Rev. Psychol.* **2019**, *70*, 141–164. [CrossRef] [PubMed]
27. Molinini, R.M.; Koziol, N.A.; Marcinowski, E.C.; Hsu, L.Y.; Tripathi, T.; Harbourne, R.T.; McCoy, S.W.; Lobo, M.A.; Bovaird, J.A.; Dusing, S.C. Early Motor Skills Predict the Developmental Trajectory of Problem Solving in Young Children with Motor Delays. *Dev. Psychobiol.* **2021**, *63*, e22123. [CrossRef]
28. Karlsson, P.; Honan, I.; Warschausky, S.; Kaufman, J.N.; Henry, G.; Stephenson, C.; Webb, A.; McEwan, A.; Badawi, N. A Validation and Acceptability Study of Cognitive Testing Using Switch and Eye-Gaze Control Technologies for Children with Motor and Speech Impairments: A Protocol Paper. *Front. Psychol.* **2022**, *13*, 991000. [CrossRef] [PubMed]
29. Pahwa, P.K.; Mani, S. Current Profile of Physical Impairments in Children with Cerebral Palsy in Inclusive Education Settings: A Cross-Sectional Study. *J. Neurosci. Rural Pract.* **2022**, *13*, 424–430. [CrossRef]
30. Ballester-Plané, J.; Laporta-Hoyos, O.; Macaya, A.; Póo, P.; Meléndez-Plumed, M.; Toro-Tamargo, E.; Gimeno, F.; Narberhaus, A.; Segarra, D.; Pueyo, R. Cognitive Functioning in Dyskinetic Cerebral Palsy: Its Relation to Motor Function, Communication and Epilepsy. *Eur. J. Paediatr. Neurol.* **2018**, *22*, 102–112. [CrossRef]
31. Lobo, M.A.; Harbourne, R.T.; Dusing, S.C.; McCoy, S.W. Grounding Early Intervention: Physical Therapy Cannot Just Be about Motor Skills Anymore. *Phys. Ther.* **2013**, *93*, 94–103. [CrossRef]
32. Sherwell, S.; Reid, S.M.; Reddihough, D.S.; Wrennall, J.; Ong, B.; Stargatt, S. Measuring Intellectual Ability in Children with Cerebral Palsy: Can We Do Better? *Res. Dev. Disabil.* **2014**, *35*, 2558–2567. [CrossRef]

Disclaimer/Publisher's Note: The statements, opinions and data contained in all publications are solely those of the individual author(s) and contributor(s) and not of MDPI and/or the editor(s). MDPI and/or the editor(s) disclaim responsibility for any injury to people or property resulting from any ideas, methods, instructions or products referred to in the content.

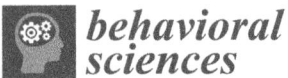

Article

Factors Influencing Receipt and Type of Therapy Services in the NICU

Christiana D. Butera [1], Shaaron E. Brown [2], Jennifer Burnsed [3], Jodi Darring [4], Amy D. Harper [5], Karen D. Hendricks-Muñoz [6], Megan Hyde [7], Audrey E. Kane [2], Meagan R. Miller [2], Richard D. Stevenson [6], Christine M. Spence [8], Leroy R. Thacker [9] and Stacey C. Dusing [1,2,*]

1. Division of Biokinesiology and Physical Therapy, University of Southern California, Los Angeles, CA 90033, USA; cbutera@usc.edu
2. Motor Development Lab, Department of Physical Therapy, Virginia Commonwealth University, Richmond, VA 23298, USA; mrmiller2@vcu.edu (M.R.M.)
3. Departments of Pediatrics and Neurology, Division of Neonatology, University of Virginia, Charlottesville, VA 22903, USA; jcw5b@hscmail.mcc.virginia.edu
4. Department of Pediatrics, Division of Neurodevelopmental and Behavioral Pediatrics, University of Virginia School of Medicine, Charlottesville, VA 22903, USA
5. Department of Neurology, Virginia Commonwealth University, Richmond, VA 23284, USA
6. Department of Pediatrics, Children's Hospital of Richmond at VCU, Virginia Commonwealth University School of Medicine, Richmond, VA 23284, USA; karen.hendricks-munoz@vcuhealth.org (K.D.H.-M.)
7. Department of Physical Therapy, University of Virginia, Charlottesville, VA 22903, USA; mh5gt@hscmail.mcc.virginia.edu
8. Department of Counseling and Special Education, Virginia Commonwealth University, Richmond, VA 23284, USA
9. Department of Biostatistics, Virginia Commonwealth University School of Medicine, Richmond, VA 23284, USA
* Correspondence: stacey.dusing@pt.usc.edu

Abstract: Understanding the type and frequency of current neonatal intensive care unit (NICU) therapy services and predictors of referral for therapy services is a crucial first step to supporting positive long-term outcomes in very preterm infants. This study enrolled 83 very preterm infants (<32 weeks, gestational age mean 26.5 ± 2.0 weeks; 38 male) from a longitudinal clinical trial. Race, neonatal medical index, neuroimaging, and frequency of therapy sessions were extracted from medical records. The Test of Infant Motor Performance and the General Movement Assessment were administered. Average weekly sessions of occupational therapy, physical therapy, and speech therapy were significantly different by type, but the magnitude and direction of the difference depended upon the discharge week. Infants at high risk for cerebral palsy based on their baseline General Movements Assessment scores received more therapy sessions than infants at low risk for cerebral palsy. Baseline General Movements Assessment was related to the mean number of occupational therapy sessions but not physical therapy or speech therapy sessions. Neonatal Medical Index scores and Test of Infant Motor Performance scores were not predictive of combined therapy services. Medical and developmental risk factors, as well as outcomes from therapy assessments, should be the basis for referral for therapy services in the neonatal intensive care unit.

Keywords: therapy services; preterm infants; therapy frequency; neonatal intensive care unit

1. Introduction

In 2020, the incidence of preterm birth (before 37 weeks of gestation) impacted one in every ten infants born in the United States [1]. Compared with term infants, the medical cost associated with preterm birth is almost doubled from birth to 2 years of age [2] and is highest for those with early preterm births [3]. Rates of preterm birth differ by race and ethnicity with the preterm birth rate at 14.4% among African American women, and 9.1%

and 9.8% among white and Hispanic women, respectively [1]. Infants who are born preterm are at a significantly higher risk of developmental disability including cerebral palsy, intellectual disability, autism spectrum disorders, learning disabilities, and other general developmental delays [4–7]. These risks, along with attention deficit hyperactivity disorder (ADHD), brain injury, visual and hearing impairment, and cognitive impairment [8–14] lead to the need for specialized services such as physical therapy (PT), occupational therapy (OT), speech and language therapy services (ST), and special education services as well as many other medical subspecialty services [15]. Developmental difficulties can appear as early as term equivalent age, even before infants leave the Neonatal Intensive Care Unit (NICU) [16–19].

Therapies consisting of physical, occupational, or speech–language therapies in the NICU aim to improve the neurobehavioral, sensory, feeding behavior, state regulation, and neuromotor function of infants who were born less than 37 weeks of gestational age [20]. The American Academy of Pediatrics (AAP) recommends specialized OT, PT, and ST therapy services while infants are still in the NICU [21]. Each of these disciplines (OT, PT, and ST) has specific competency recommendations for training in order to provide specialized services to infants born preterm within the NICU [22–24]. There is evidence that therapy interventions beginning in the NICU have benefits on motor skills, oral motor skills, feeding volume, prevention of scapular–humeral tightness and shoulder retraction, exploratory problem-solving behaviors, and can result in less asymmetry of reflexes and movement [25–30]. Further, one systematic review demonstrates that parent-delivered motor interventions, as guided by a physical or occupational therapist, may improve both cognitive and motor outcomes in infants born preterm [30]. Engaging parents early throughout the NICU stay fosters relationship building between a therapist and parent, and provides parent education about the infant including how to developmentally support the infant [31]. This engagement is especially important towards the end of the NICU stay to support the transition from NICU to home.

Given the short and long-term developmental challenges associated with preterm birth, there is increased emphasis on training therapists to deliver interventions to preterm infants. Research on the effectiveness of targeted early interventions in the NICU is needed but should be considered when compared with the current standard of practice. Understanding the current state of therapy in the NICU, the type and amount of therapy being administered as usual care, and which demographic, behavioral, and medical risk factors are associated with access to therapy services will help with intervention research and public policy. Despite the importance of these questions, to the best of our knowledge, only one study to date has examined the type and frequency of therapy services provided for preterm infants in a single-level IV NICU [32]. They found that all included preterm infants in the NICU received OT and PT services, and 51% received ST [32]. Infants received OT, PT, and ST therapy an average of between one to two times per week for each service. Initial referral for PT or OT was due to positioning evaluation and intervention, then the routine continuation of therapy services was noted at 30 weeks of gestational age [32]. Sicker infants (those on respiratory supports, who had sepsis, or had a brain injury) received more therapy services before discharge and had an earlier initiation of OT and PT services. ST services were initiated at 36 weeks, coinciding with feeding/swallowing issues [32]. Though PT, OT, and ST services had some overlap in their interventions, there was a clear delineation between the services provided [32].

Here, we aim to add to this literature by using primary medical data that documented the frequency of therapy visits between baseline assessment and NICU discharge for infants born <32 weeks gestational age and who were part of the Supporting Play Exploration and Early Development Intervention (SPEEDI2) clinical trial (NCT03518736). SPEEDI is a three-arm randomized clinical trial, with participants enrolled at three sites. One arm (SPEEDI_Early) provides an intervention that starts in the NICU and aims to provide an enriched environment and increased opportunities for infant-initiated movements through collaborative parent, therapist, and infant interactions during the first months of life [33].

The objectives of this paper are to (1) describe the therapy services that very preterm infants received in the NICUs and evaluate if the frequency or type of services changed over time as infants moved closer to NICU discharge, and (2) evaluate if medical, behavioral, and sociodemographic infant risk factors (race, NMI, TIMP score, abnormal GMA) influenced amount or type of therapy services received in the NICU.

2. Methods

2.1. Recruitment and Consenting

Every infant admitted to participating Level IV NICUs during the enrollment period was screened for eligibility. Initially, only infants <29 weeks of gestation were enrolled from one of two hospitals; however, following the COVID-19 pandemic, the inclusion criteria were changed to <32 weeks of gestation and a NICU stay of greater than 28 days. These criteria are consistent with the state criteria for automatic eligibility for early intervention ensuring all infants were eligible for the same early intervention services. In addition, a community hospital with a level III NICU was added as an enrollment site, but all infants enrolled were counted toward the primary site's enrollment as all study visits were completed by the primary hospital's research team. Infants were offered enrollment if they were between 35 and 42 weeks of gestation, medically stable, off invasive or non-invasive ventilation, lived within 100 miles of the hospital, and spoke English. Exclusion criteria included a diagnosis of a genetic syndrome or musculoskeletal deformity.

2.2. Sample

Participants included 83 infants (mean gestational age of 26.5 (2) weeks) enrolled in a therapeutic clinical trial and were randomly assigned to one of 3 groups, Usual Care, SPEEDI_early, and SPEEDI_Late (NCT02153736). While only the infants in SPEEDI_Early were receiving NICU-based intervention visits, all 3 groups were monitored, and able to continue their usual clinical care including therapy services (Table 1). The usual care group received business-as-usual clinical care for the duration of the study, and the SPEEDI_Late group received additional intervention after being discharged from the NICU. The combined sample's mean age at baseline assessment was 11.21 (3.57) weeks of chronological age or 37.35 (4.61) weeks of gestation (Table 1). More than 50 percent were considered to be at high risk for cerebral palsy or other neurodevelopmental disability based on having a brain injury demonstrated on cranial ultrasound or poor repertoire, cramped synchronized, or chaotic general movements at baseline. Of the participants, 46% percent were male, 52% were Caucasian, 31% were Black, and 14% identified as more than one race. Three percent identified as Hispanic (Table 1).

Table 1. Descriptives.

	Total (n = 83)	Usual Care (n = 27)	SPEEDI—Early (n = 27)	SPEEDI—Late (n = 29)
High-Risk Strata	65% (54)	63% (17)	67% (18)	66% (19)
Low-Risk Strata	35% (29)	37% (10)	33% (9)	34% (10)
Gender (Male)	46% (38)	52% (14)	44% (12)	41% (12)
Race				
Asian	1% (1)	4% (1)	0% (0)	0% (0)
Black/AA	31% (26)	33% (9)	26% (7)	34% (10)
White	52% (43)	44% (12)	63% (17)	48% (14)
Multiple	14% (12)	19% (5)	11% (3)	14% (4)
Unknown/Not Reported	1% (1)	0% (0)	0% (0)	3% (1)
Ethnicity				
Hispanic/Latino	4% (3)	4% (1)	4% (1)	3% (1)
Not Hispanic/Latino	93% (77)	93% (25)	93% (25)	93% (27)
Not Reported	4% (3)	4% (1)	4% (1)	3% (1)

Table 1. Cont.

	Total (n = 83)	Usual Care (n = 27)	SPEEDI—Early (n = 27)	SPEEDI—Late (n = 29)
Gestational Age—Birth (Mean (Std))	26.49 (1.99)	25.56 (1.42)	26.89 (2.03)	26.07 (2.36)
NMI				
3	18% (15)	22% (6)	19% (5)	14% (4)
4	10% (8)	15% (4)	4% (1)	10% (3)
5	72% (60)	63% (17)	77% (21)	76% (22)
PSI (Mean (Std)) [1]	64.05 (15.96)	63.17 (14.61)	62.39 (16.56)	66.24 (17.04)

Caption: Sample Descriptive Statistics. ([1]) Twenty-six (26) infants missing PSI score at baseline (9 in control, 9 in SPEEDI—Early, 8 in SPEEDI—Late); NMI = Neonatal Medical Index; PSI = Parent Stress Index—Short Form; Std = standard deviation; AA = African American; and SPEEDI = Supporting Play Exploration and Early Developmental Intervention.

2.3. Primary Outcome Measures

All outcome measures used in this analysis were part of the research protocol and completed by highly trained research therapists. At baseline, the Test of Infant Motor Performance (TIMP), General Movement Assessment, and an initial medical record review were completed. Ongoing medical record reviews were completed by the site's clinical research coordinator who was familiar with the site's medical record system. Each hospital had similar policies for therapy documentation of any completed therapy visit.

Test of Infant Motor Performance (TIMP). The TIMP is an assessment of posture and movement for infants from 32 weeks of gestational age to 4 months of corrected age ([34] Campbell et al., 1995). Testing combines observation of spontaneous movements and placement in various positions to assess activities such as head centering, reaching, finger movements, and head and trunk control. The TIMP is a reliable and valid measure of motor performance [35] and is sensitive to age-related changes (r = 0.83) [36].

Prechtl's Assessment of General Movements (GMA). The GMA is a standardized, noninvasive method of observation of spontaneous, complex movements to evaluate the typical maturation of the nervous system [37]. Prior studies have shown high sensitivity and specificity of the GMA to predict which children are at the highest risk for developing cerebral palsy (CP) [38,39]. Videos were scored for writhing movements by a certified and experienced investigator. Writhing movements were scored as normal or abnormal (poor repertoire, cramp synchronized, or chaotic). We used GMA classification to identify which infants were at high or low risk for CP for our risk strata variable.

Medical Record. Electronic medical records were reviewed weekly from the time of enrollment to NICU discharge. Weeks were considered Sunday to Saturday and thus the last Saturday the infant was in the NICU ended the final week of data extraction. If babies were given a baseline assessment and discharged within 24 h, their data were not included in the analysis. Data from full weeks were considered in all analyses. The length of NICU stay after the baseline assessment ranged from 0 days to more than 100 days (median 14 days, range 0–110 days). However, only 2 infants were still in the hospital 10 weeks after baseline; therefore, data provided in this paper are presented by week post baseline, including the infants who were in the hospital the entire week (Table 2). The frequency of sessions per therapy discipline was calculated and quantified based on the presence of a therapy note describing the usual care intervention session in the documentation. Neither site had a standard order set for therapy, so therapy visits were based on individual physician referral. Medical, behavioral, and sociodemographic infant risk factors (race, sex, NMI, and neuroimaging findings) were collected or calculated from the infant medical records and parent report surveys.

Table 2. Services Count All Weeks—Week of Discharge Removed.

	OT Visits		PT Visits		ST Visits		All Services	
	N	Mean (Std)	n	Mean (Std)	n	Mean (Std)	n	Mean (Std)
Week 1 Post Enrollment	73 *	1.16 (0.99)	73	1.27 (0.96)	71	1.93 (1.28)	73	4.37 (2.19)
Week 2 Post Enrollment	51	1.37 (0.94)	51	1.45 (0.97)	51	2.75 (1.13)	51	5.57 (1.66)
Week 3 Post Enrollment	38	1.76 (1)	38	1.68 (0.9)	38	2.58 (1.24)	38	6.03 (1.99)
Week 4 Post Enrollment	28	1.96 (1.07)	28	1.71 (1.12)	28	2.29 (1.3)	28	5.96 (1.75)
Week 5 Post Enrollment	18	2.00 (0.77)	18	1.67 (0.84)	18	2.17 (0.92)	18	5.83 (1.54)
Week 6 Post Enrollment	13	2.00 (1.08)	13	1.62 (1.04)	13	1.77 (1.17)	13	5.38 (1.8)
Week 7 Post Enrollment	11	1.91 (0.94)	11	1.45 (0.69)	11	1.91 (1.38)	11	5.27 (2.69)
Week 8 Post Enrollment	9	1.89 (1.45)	9	0.89 (1.05)	9	1.00 (0.5)	9	3.78 (2.33)
Week 9 Post Enrollment	4	0.50 (0.58)	4	1.50 (0.58)	4	1.75 (1.26)	4	3.75 (2.06)

Caption: Services Count All Weeks—With Week of Discharge Removed. OT = occupational therapy; PT = physical therapy; ST = speech therapy; Std = standard deviation. * A total of 10 babies were discharged within 24 h of baseline assessment and had no opportunity for therapy services in the NICU.

2.4. Statistics

Service Type Over Time. To describe the therapy services that very preterm infants received in the NICU, we fit a generalized linear model to the data for each week post baseline in which the infant was in the NICU, utilizing a Poisson distribution to model the mean number of services. The model included an effect for service Type (OT, PT, and ST), the number of weeks since baseline (1 to 9), and the interaction between Type and Week as well as a random effect for participant. We tested to see if we could treat Week as a continuous variable (with the built-in assumption of linearity), as opposed to treating Week as categorical (and thus a non-linear effect), and found that the less complex model using Week as a continuous variable was sufficient (likelihood ratio = 2.99, 21 d.f., $p = 0.9999$).

Service Type Before Discharge. To specifically explore the weeks leading up to hospital discharge, we fit a generalized linear model to the data for the three weeks prior to discharge, utilizing a Poisson distribution to model the mean number of services. The model included an effect for service Type (OT, PT, and ST), Discharge Relative Week (-3, -2, -1), and the interaction between Type and Discharge Relative Week as well as a random effect for participant. We tested to see if we could treat Week as a continuous variable (with the built-in assumption of linearity), as opposed to treating Week as categorical (and thus a non-linear effect), and found that similar to the above, the less complex model was sufficient (likelihood ratio = 2.48, 3 d.f., $p = 0.4789$).

Predictors of All Services. To evaluate if sociodemographic, neurological function, or medical risk factors, which can be measured by the medical team who make the referrals, influenced access to therapy in the NICU, we refit the initial service model ("Service Type Over Time") described above and added in fixed effects for race (Caucasian yes/no), baseline NMI, and GMA (normal/abnormal).

Predictors of Individual Services. In order to determine if medical risk or standardized therapy assessment results influenced the frequency of individual therapy service, we repeated the analysis by adding the TIMP, which is typically completed by therapists and for each therapy service, rather than aggregate. We used three separate generalized linear models (baseline NMI, baseline TIMP, and baseline GMA) of the data for the frequency of therapy services from baseline through discharge or 9 weeks post baseline, whichever was shorter, utilizing a Poisson distribution to model the mean number of services. The models included a fixed effect for (NMI, TIMP, or GMA) as well as a random effect for participant. Parameter estimates were examined and post hoc tests performed with a Tukey HSD correction were calculated when relevant for pairwise comparisons (OT, PT, and ST).

3. Results

3.1. Service Type

We fit a generalized linear model including an effect for service Type (OT, PT, and ST), Week (one to nine), and the interaction between Type and Week as well as a random effect for participant. The interaction effect for Type by Week was significant ($F_{1,729} = 7.6$, $p = 0.0005$). This significant interaction indicates that services provided were significantly different, but the magnitude and significance of the difference depend upon the discharge week (Figure 1a.)

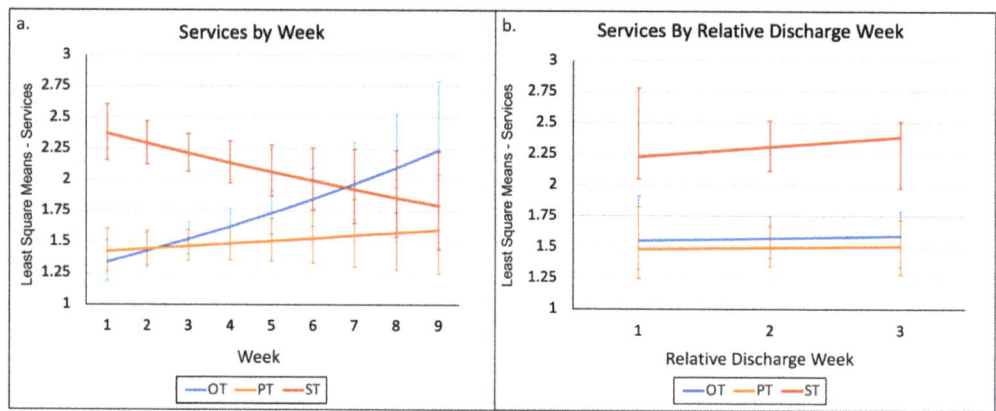

Figure 1. Service Types Over Time. Caption: Plots of the least square (LS) means for services over time. (**a**) A plot of least square means for the generalized linear model including an effect for service Type (OT, PT, and ST) and Week (1 to 9). (**b**) A plot of least square means for the generalized linear model including an effect for service Type (OT, PT, and ST), only on the week of discharge and the three weeks before discharge. OT = occupational therapy; PT = physical therapy; and ST = speech therapy.

First, we focused only on the week of discharge and the three weeks before discharge to see if therapy services increased to get infants ready to be discharged (means and standard deviation, Table 3). In this model, the interaction effect for Type by Week was not significant ($F_{1,480} = 0.06$, $p = 0.9428$) and the model was refit to exclude the interaction effect. The Service Type effect was significant ($F_{2,482} = 25.22$, $p < 0.0001$) but the Week effect was not significant ($F_{1,482} = 0.34$, $p = 0.5622$). Post hoc tests revealed that ST services are significantly different from both OT ($t_{482} = -5.61$, adjusted $p < 0.0001$) and PT ($t_{482} = -6.24$, adjusted $p < 0.0001$) services, but there was no difference between OT and PT ($t_{482} = 0.65$, adjusted $p = 0.7926$) in terms of the frequency of services (Figure 1b).

Table 3. Services During Week of Discharge and Three Prior Weeks.

	OT Visits		PT Visits		ST Visits	
	n	Mean (Std)	n	Mean (Std)	n	Mean (Std)
3 Weeks Prior to Discharge	38	1.55 (1.01)	38	1.47 (0.95)	38	2.37 (1.17)
2 Weeks Prior to Discharge	51	1.63 (1.17)	51	1.55 (1.08)	51	2.33 (1.34)
1 Week Prior to Discharge	73	1.53 (1.11)	73	1.47 (0.9)	73	2.22 (1.2)

Caption: To specifically explore the weeks leading up to hospital discharge, we fit a generalized linear model to the data for the three weeks prior to discharge, utilizing a Poisson distribution to model the mean number of services. OT = occupational therapy; PT = physical therapy; ST = speech therapy; and Std = standard deviation.

3.2. Predictors of All Services—Medical, Race, and Severity Strata/GMA

In examining the significant parameter estimates, we found that when holding all things equal, infants at high risk for CP (abnormal GMA) received an average of 0.12 more therapy sessions than did infants at low risk for CP (Table 4). In addition, while holding all things equal, Caucasian infants received on average 0.11 fewer therapy sessions than did non-Caucasian infants. The medical risk was non-significant (Table 4).

Table 4. Final Poisson Mixed Model Results.

Effect	Numerator d.f.	Denominator d.f.	F-Statistic	p-Value	Adjusted Effect Size Cohen's f (95% CI)
Service Type	2	726	29.41	<0.0001 **	0.279 (0.219, 0.344)
Week	1	726	0.33	0.5673	0 (0, 0.081)
Service Type*Week	2	726	7.79	0.0005 **	0.136 (0.078, 0.203)
GMA	1	726	4.88	0.0276	0.073 (0.02, 0.143)
Baseline NMI Score	1	726	2.09	0.1491	0.039 (0, 0.115)
Caucasian	1	726	5.21	0.0228 *	0.076 (0.023, 0.146)

Caption: To evaluate if sociodemographic, neurological function, or medical risk factors, which can be measured by the medical team who make the referrals, influenced access to therapy in the NICU, we refit the initial service model ("Service Type Over Time") described above and added in fixed effects for race (Caucasian yes/no), baseline NMI, and GMA (normal/abnormal). * = $p < 0.05$; ** = $p < 0.001$. d.f = degrees of freedom; and CI = confidence interval.

3.3. Predictors of Individual Services—Severity Strata/GMA

Baseline GMA was related to the mean number of OT sessions over the 9 weeks of NICU time ($t_{54} = 2.86$, $p = 0.006$). Examination of the parameter estimate for GMA indicates that infants who had an abnormal baseline GMA had a higher mean number of OT sessions (0.51 more). The baseline GMA score was not statistically significantly associated with PT sessions ($t_{64} = 0.08$, $p = 0.9356$) or ST sessions ($t_{60} = 0.02$, $p = 0.9827$).

3.4. Predictors of Individual Services—Baseline NMI

Baseline NMI was related to the mean number of OT sessions over the nine weeks of NICU time ($t_{64} = 3.19$, $p = 0.0022$). Examination of the parameter estimate for NMI indicates that as the baseline NMI score increases, the mean number of OT sessions increases. With regards to the mean number of PT sessions, the baseline NMI score is not statistically significantly associated with PT sessions ($t_{64} = -1.07$, $p = 0.2894$). With regards to the mean number of ST sessions, we see that baseline NMI is related to the mean number of ST sessions over the 9 weeks of NICU time ($t_{889} = -2.16$, $p = 0.0346$). Examination of the parameter estimate for NMI indicates that as the baseline NMI score increases, the mean number of ST sessions decreases.

3.5. Predictors of Individual Services—Baseline TIMP

The baseline TIMP score was not associated with the mean number of OT sessions ($t_{44} = -0.74$, $p = 0.4643$), the mean number of PT sessions ($t_{53} = 0.08$, $p = 0.9379$), or the mean number of ST sessions ($t_{889} = 0.03$, $p = 0.9795$).

4. Discussion

This study found that services provided in the NICU were significantly different by type, but the magnitude and significance of the difference depended upon the time since enrollment week. Across weeks 1–9, OT and PT services increased over time, and ST decreased over time when the NICUs were combined. In weeks 1–6, infants received the most ST services, and in weeks 7–9 infants received the most OT services. Considering that the median length of stay was 14 days after the baseline assessment, the infants who remained in the NICU after 6 weeks were likely to have had a new onset of medical instability, prolonged feeding difficulty warranting placement of a G-tube, and reduced attempts at oral feeding, thus requiring less ST. However, the prolonged admission and increasing age are consistent with the need for more intervention focusing on social and play interaction that may have been provided by OT. Given the nature of the data used in this analysis, we are unable to determine the impact of medical stability and feeding outcomes.

In the three weeks leading up to discharge (Table 3), ST services were significantly greater than both OT and PT services, but there was no difference between OT and PT in the frequency of services. Infants at high risk for CP based on an abnormal GMA received more combined therapy sessions than did infants at low risk for CP. This relationship seemed largely driven by the mean number of OT sessions as the baseline GMA score was not statistically significantly associated with the number of PT or ST sessions. As the baseline NMI score increased, the mean number of OT sessions increased, PT sessions were not changed, and the mean number of ST sessions decreased. The baseline TIMP score was not associated with the mean number of OT, PT, or ST sessions. These findings must be considered within the context of the data, and NICU admission and staffing. The data reflect documented visits for clinical care. However, in acute care hospitals, the focus of therapy is often on supporting the discharge process for all patients resulting in staffing being pulled from the NICU to other areas to ensure discharge of older patients is not delayed. Thus, data on the planned or recommended therapeutic dose by the clinical care team are not included in this analysis; only data on the delivered sessions were analyzed. In addition, a portion of this study was completed during the COVID-19 pandemic, which influenced many aspects of care, from staffing to visitation in NICUs [40].

Our findings support the work of Ross et al. [32] by demonstrating that OTs, PTs, and STs have a role in providing therapeutic interventions early in gestation to high-risk infants in the NICU with concurrent medical interventions. The previous study found that sicker infants (those on respiratory supports, who had sepsis, or had a brain injury) received more therapy services before discharge and had an earlier initiation of OT and PT services. Our paper adds to this by showing that an abnormal GMA (a predictor of high risk for developing cerebral palsy) is also associated with more therapy services in the NICU and that NMI and TIMP scores are not within this sample. It should be noted that this paper [32] started collecting data earlier than the current study (30 weeks vs. 35 weeks of gestation).

Although infants at high risk for CP based on an abnormal GMA received more therapy sessions than did infants at low risk for CP, when looking at the service type, this relationship was only significant for the number of OT sessions. Similarly, the baseline NMI score predicted greater OT sessions only. The baseline TIMP score was not associated with the mean number of any type of therapy session. These results highlight the lack of valuable clinical and developmental information being used to guide therapy referrals. While GMA is well known as a strong predictor of CP, the TIMP score has also been associated with longitudinal cognitive, motor, and language outcomes [41]. The TIMP could be uniquely important for guiding the referral of PT services—a less consistently utilized profession in this sample—with content expertise in motor development, motor disorders, and movement therapies. The lack of relationship seen in this study could also be related to the earlier onset of PT in the NICU prior to the baseline for this study. Thus the family may have already received training and information for PT clinically.

The number of staff per bed in a NICU can vary depending on the level of NICU and location of the NICU within the U.S. [42]. The adequate number of full-time therapists in a Level III/IV NICU with high acuity can be determined via a formula developed by Craig and Smith [43]. Ross et al. [32] reported a level of adequate coverage of a high acuity Level IV NICU according to this formula. In a national survey of NICUs, 97% of Level-IV NICUs and 83% of Level-III NICUs reported having dedicated therapy teams [42]. Based on this previous work, it may be feasible to increase therapy services for children who need it, particularly OT and PT services given that ST sessions occurred most frequently within three weeks of discharge in our sample.

Limitations

This study had some limitations which should be considered. Data were collected manually through weekly review of the medical record, and it is possible that we may have missed valuable information that was not documented in the medical record (e.g., therapist speaking with parents at a non-scheduled visit or reasons for missed therapy visits such as medical instability). Further, we did not document therapy coverage for the NICUs (i.e., how many therapists per discipline provide services), or the individual hospital distribution of roles and responsibilities between therapy disciplines. Moreover, we did not collect the recommended frequency of therapy services by each discipline, and staffing may have impacted the actual frequency, which may not have been consistent with the recommended amount in each case. This study also did not track parent presence in therapy sessions, which impacts the efficacy and carryover of therapy services. We did not record the duration of therapy sessions, or exactly what a therapist did in any given session. Data were not collected regarding the timing to full oral feeds, which is likely highly related to the need and timing of therapy services. These data may not be representative of other types of NICU settings or for samples with different socio-demographic compositions. Future work may compare referral practices to elucidate optimal referral protocols for the best service outcomes. Our work highlights that improvement is still needed in utilizing medical and developmental risk factors, as well as outcomes from therapy assessments, as the basis for referral for therapy services in the NICU.

5. Conclusions

This study found that services provided in the NICU were significantly different by type, but the magnitude and significance of the difference depended upon the time since enrollment week. Our study adds to previous research by demonstrating that an abnormal GMA (a predictor of high risk for developing cerebral palsy) is associated with more therapy services in the NICU, and that NMI and TIMP scores are not. These results highlight the lack of valuable clinical and developmental information being used to guide therapy referrals. The clinical impact of this work recommends that medical and developmental risk factors, as well as outcomes from therapy assessments, should be the basis for referral for therapy services in the neonatal intensive care unit.

Author Contributions: Conceptualization, S.C.D., S.E.B., M.R.M., J.D., J.B., R.D.S. and L.R.T.; methodology, S.C.D. and M.R.M.; formal analysis, L.R.T.; resources, S.C.D., C.M.S., J.B. and R.D.S.; data curation, M.R.M.; writing—original draft preparation, C.D.B.; writing—review and editing, C.D.B., S.C.D., C.M.S., S.E.B., J.B., J.D., A.D.H., K.D.H.-M., M.H., A.E.K., M.R.M., R.D.S. and L.R.T.; visualization, L.R.T. and C.D.B.; supervision, S.C.D.; project administration, M.R.M.; funding acquisition, S.C.D. All authors have read and agreed to the published version of the manuscript.

Funding: This research and the APC were funded by Eunice Kennedy Shriver National Institute of Child Health and Human Development, grant number R01 HD093624.

Institutional Review Board Statement: The study was conducted according to the guidelines of the Declaration of Helsinki, and approved as a single IRB by the Institutional Review Board of Virginia Commonwealth University (protocol code HM20013026 approved 26 April 2018).

Informed Consent Statement: Informed consent was obtained from all parents of infants involved in the study.

Data Availability Statement: The data presented in this study are available on request from the corresponding author. The data are not publicly available due to ongoing parent clinical trial.

Acknowledgments: We thank all the participants and their families who made this work possible.

Conflicts of Interest: The authors declare no conflict of interest.

References

1. Osterman, M.; Hamilton, B.; Martin, J.A.; Driscoll, A.K.; Valenzuela, C.P. Births: Final data for 2020. *Natl. Vital Stat. Rep.* **2021**, *70*, 1–50.
2. Bérard, A.; Le Tiec, M.; De Vera, M. Study of the costs and morbidities of late-preterm birth. *Arch. Dis. Child. Fetal Neonatal Ed.* **2012**, *97*, F329–F334. [CrossRef] [PubMed]
3. Jacob, J.; Lehne, M.; Mischker, A.; Klinger, N.; Zickermann, C.; Walker, J. Cost effects of preterm birth: A comparison of health care costs associated with early preterm, late preterm, and full-term birth in the first 3 years after birth. *Eur. J. Health Econ.* **2016**, *18*, 1041–1046. [CrossRef]
4. Aylward, G.P. Neurodevelopmental Outcomes of Infants Born Prematurely. *J. Dev. Behav. Pediatr.* **2014**, *35*, 394–407. [CrossRef]
5. Johnson, S.; Fawke, J.; Hennessy, E.; Rowell, V.; Thomas, S.; Wolke, D.; Marlow, N. Neurodevelopmental Disability Through 11 Years of Age in Children Born Before 26 Weeks of Gestation. *Pediatrics* **2009**, *124*, e249–e257. [CrossRef]
6. Marlow, N.; Wolke, D.; Bracewell, M.A.; Samara, M. Neurologic and Developmental Disability at Six Years of Age after Extremely Preterm Birth. *N. Engl. J. Med.* **2005**, *352*, 9–19. [CrossRef]
7. Schieve, L.A.; Tian, L.H.; Rankin, K.; Kogan, M.D.; Yeargin-Allsopp, M.; Visser, S.; Rosenberg, D.; Schieve, L.A.; Tian, L.H.; Rankin, K.; et al. Population impact of preterm birth and low birth weight on developmental disabilities in US children. *Ann. Epidemiol.* **2016**, *26*, 267–274. [CrossRef]
8. Delobel-Ayoub, M.; Arnaud, C.; White-Koning, M.; Casper, C.; Pierrat, V.; Garel, M.; Burguet, A.; Roze, J.-C.; Matis, J.; Picaud, J.-C.; et al. Behavioral Problems and Cognitive Performance at 5 Years of Age After Very Preterm Birth: The EPIPAGE Study. *Pediatrics* **2009**, *123*, 1485–1492. [CrossRef]
9. DiSalvo, D. The correlation between placental pathology and intraventricular hemorrhage in the preterm infant. The Developmental Epidemiology Network Investigators. *Pediatr. Res.* **1998**, *43*, 15–19. [CrossRef] [PubMed]
10. Linnet, K.M.; Wisborg, K.; Agerbo, E.; Secher, N.J.; Thomsen, P.H.; Henriksen, T.B. Gestational age, birth weight, and the risk of hyperkinetic disorder. *Arch. Dis. Child.* **2006**, *91*, 655–660. [CrossRef] [PubMed]
11. McCormick, M.C.; Litt, J.S.; Smith, V.C.; Zupancic, J.A. Prematurity: An Overview and Public Health Implications. *Annu. Rev. Public Health* **2011**, *32*, 367–379. [CrossRef] [PubMed]
12. Moster, D.; Lie, R.T.; Markestad, T. Long-term medical and social consequences of preterm birth. *N. Engl. J. Med.* **2008**, *359*, 262–273. [CrossRef] [PubMed]
13. Rezaie, P.; Dean, A. Periventricular leukomalacia, inflammation and white matter lesions within the developing nervous system. *Neuropathology* **2002**, *22*, 106–132. [CrossRef] [PubMed]
14. Saigal, S.; Doyle, L.W. An overview of mortality and sequelae of preterm birth from infancy to adulthood. *Lancet* **2008**, *371*, 261–269. [CrossRef] [PubMed]
15. Nwabara, O.; Rogers, C.; Inder, T.; Pineda, R. Early Therapy Services Following Neonatal Intensive Care Unit Discharge. *Phys. Occup. Ther. Pediatr.* **2016**, *37*, 414–424. [CrossRef]
16. Brown, N.C.; Doyle, L.W.; Bear, M.J.; Inder, T.E. Alterations in Neurobehavior at Term Reflect Differing Perinatal Exposures in Very Preterm Infants. *Pediatrics* **2006**, *118*, 2461–2471. [CrossRef]
17. Pineda, R.G.; Tjoeng, T.H.; Vavasseur, C.; Kidokoro, H.; Neil, J.J.; Inder, T. Patterns of Altered Neurobehavior in Preterm Infants within the Neonatal Intensive Care Unit. *J. Pediatr.* **2013**, *162*, 470–476.e1. [CrossRef]
18. Pitcher, J.B.; Schneider, L.A.; Drysdale, J.L.; Ridding, M.C.; Owens, J.A. Motor System Development of the Preterm and Low Birthweight Infant. *Clin. Perinatol.* **2011**, *38*, 605–625. [CrossRef]
19. Smith, G.C.; Gutovich, J.; Smyser, C.; Pineda, R.; Newnham, C.; Tjoeng, T.H.; Vavasseur, C.; Wallendorf, M.; Neil, J.; Inder, T. Neonatal intensive care unit stress is associated with brain development in preterm infants. *Ann. Neurol.* **2011**, *70*, 541–549. [CrossRef]
20. Barbosa, V.M. Teamwork in the Neonatal Intensive Care Unit. *Phys. Occup. Ther. Pediatr.* **2013**, *33*, 5–26. [CrossRef]
21. Kilpatrick, S.J.; Papile, L.A.; Macones, G.A.; Watterberg, K.L. AAP Committee on Fetus and Newborn, ACOG Committee on Obstetric Practice. *Guidel. Perinat. Care*. 2017. Available online: https://www.acog.org/clinical-information/physician-faqs/-/media/3a22e153b67446a6b31fb051e469187c.ashx (accessed on 30 May 2023).
22. Craig, J.W.; Carroll, S.; Ludwig, S.; Sturdivant, C. Occupational Therapy's Role in the Neonatal Intensive Care Unit. *Am. J. Occup. Ther.* **2018**, *72*, 1–9.
23. Sweeney, J.K.; Heriza, C.B.; Blanchard, Y. Neonatal Physical Therapy. Part I: Clinical Competencies and Neonatal Intensive Care Unit Clinical Training Models. *Pediatr. Phys. Ther.* **2009**, *21*, 296–307. [CrossRef] [PubMed]
24. Ad Hoc Committee on Speech-Language Pathology Practice in the Neonatal Intensive Care Unit (NICU). Knowledge and Skills Needed by Speech-Language Pathologists Providing Services to Infants and Families in the NICU Environment. *Ameri-can Speech-Language-Hearing Association*. 2004. Available online: https://www.asha.org/policy/KS2004-00080/ (accessed on 10 April 2023).
25. Case-Smith, J. An Efficacy Study of Occupational Therapy with High-Risk Neonates. *Am. J. Occup. Ther.* **1988**, *42*, 499–506. [CrossRef] [PubMed]
26. Dusing, S.C.; Thacker, L.R. Supporting mother-infant interaction in the NICU may enhance oral motor skills, weight gain, and feeding volume: A pilot study. *Dev. Med. Child Neurol.* **2016**, *58*, 13–14. [CrossRef]

27. Dusing, S.C.; Tripathi, T.; Marcinowski, E.C.; Thacker, L.R.; Brown, L.F.; Hendricks-Muñoz, K.D. Supporting play exploration and early developmental intervention versus usual care to enhance development outcomes during the transition from the neonatal intensive care unit to home: A pilot randomized controlled trial. *BMC Pediatr.* **2018**, *18*, 46. [CrossRef]
28. Madlinger-Lewis, L.; Reynolds, L.; Zarem, C.; Crapnell, T.; Inder, T.; Pineda, R. The effects of alternative positioning on preterm infants in the neonatal intensive care unit: A randomized clinical trial. *Res. Dev. Disabil.* **2013**, *35*, 490–497. [CrossRef]
29. Monfort, K.; Case-Smith, J. The Effects of a Neonatal Positioner on Scapular Rotation. *Am. J. Occup. Ther.* **1997**, *51*, 378–384. [CrossRef]
30. Khurana, S.; Kane, A.E.; Brown, S.E.; Tarver, T.; Dusing, S.C. Effect of neonatal therapy on the motor, cognitive, and behavioral development of infants born preterm: A systematic review. *Dev. Med. Child Neurol.* **2020**, *62*, 684–692. [CrossRef]
31. Dusing, S.C.; Van Drew, C.M.; Brown, S.E. Instituting Parent Education Practices in the Neonatal Intensive Care Unit: An Administrative Case Report of Practice Evaluation and Statewide Action. *Phys. Ther.* **2012**, *92*, 967–975. [CrossRef]
32. Ross, K.; Heiny, E.; Conner, S.; Spener, P.; Pineda, R. Occupational therapy, physical therapy and speech-language pathology in the neonatal intensive care unit: Patterns of therapy usage in a level IV NICU. *Res. Dev. Disabil.* **2017**, *64*, 108–117. [CrossRef]
33. Dusing, S.C.; Burnsed, J.C.; Brown, S.E.; Harper, A.D.; Hendricks-Munoz, K.D.; Stevenson, R.D.; Thacker, L.R.; Molinini, R.M. Efficacy of Supporting Play Exploration and Early Development Intervention in the First Months of Life for Infants Born Very Preterm: 3-Arm Randomized Clinical Trial Protocol. *Phys. Ther.* **2020**, *100*, 1343–1352. [CrossRef] [PubMed]
34. Campbell, S.K.; Kolobe, T.H.; Osten, E.T.; Lenke, M.; Girolami, G.L. Construct Validity of the Test of Infant Motor Performance. *Phys. Ther.* **1995**, *75*, 585–596. [CrossRef] [PubMed]
35. Campbell, S.K. Test-Retest Reliability of the Test of Infant Motor Performance. *Pediatr. Phys. Ther.* **1999**, *11*, 60–66. [CrossRef]
36. Campbell, S.K.; Kolobe, T.H.A. Concurrent Validity of the Test of Infant Motor Performance with the Alberta Infant Motor Scale. *Pediatr. Phys. Ther.* **2000**, *12*, 2. [CrossRef]
37. Prechtl, H. Qualitative changes of spontaneous movements in fetus and preterm infant are a marker of neurological dysfunction. *Early Hum. Dev.* **1990**, *23*, 151–158. [CrossRef]
38. Einspieler, C.; Marschik, P.B.; Bos, A.F.; Ferrari, F.; Cioni, G.; Prechtl, H.F. Early markers for cerebral palsy: Insights from the assessment of general movements. *Futur. Neurol.* **2012**, *7*, 709–717. [CrossRef]
39. Noble, Y.; Boyd, R. Neonatal assessments for the preterm infant up to 4 months corrected age: A systematic review. *Dev. Med. Child Neurol.* **2011**, *54*, 129–139. [CrossRef]
40. Brown, S.E.; Darring, J.D.; Miller, M.; Inamdar, K.; Salgaonkar, A.; Burnsed, J.C.; Stevenson, R.D.; Shall, M.S.; Harper, A.D.; Hendricks-Munoz, K.D.; et al. Impact of the COVID-19 Pandemic on a Clinical Trial: A Qualitative Report on Study Engagement. *Pediatr. Phys. Ther.* **2023**, in press.
41. Peyton, C.; Schreiber, M.D.; Msall, M.S. The Test of Infant Motor Performance at 3 months predicts language, cognitive, and motor outcomes in infants born preterm at 2 years of age. *Dev. Med. Child Neurol.* **2018**, *60*, 1239–1243. [CrossRef]
42. Pineda, R.G.; Lisle, J.; Ferrara, L.; Knudsen, K.; Kumar, R.; Fernandez-Fernandez, A. Neonatal Therapy Staffing in the United States and Relationships to Neonatal Intensive Care Unit Type and Location, Level of Acuity, and Population Factors. *Am. J. Perinatol.* **2021**, eFirst. [CrossRef]
43. Craig, J.W.; Smith, C.R. Risk-adjusted/neuroprotective care services in the NICU: The elemental role of the neonatal therapist (OT, PT, SLP). *J. Perinatol.* **2020**, *40*, 549–559. [CrossRef] [PubMed]

Disclaimer/Publisher's Note: The statements, opinions and data contained in all publications are solely those of the individual author(s) and contributor(s) and not of MDPI and/or the editor(s). MDPI and/or the editor(s) disclaim responsibility for any injury to people or property resulting from any ideas, methods, instructions or products referred to in the content.

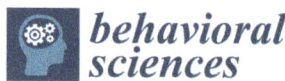

Article

Information Available to Parents Seeking Education about Infant Play, Milestones, and Development from Popular Sources

Julie M. Orlando [1], Andrea B. Cunha [2], Zainab Alghamdi [1] and Michele A. Lobo [1,3,*]

[1] Biomechanics & Movement Science Program, University of Delaware, Newark, DE 19711, USA; jorlando@udel.edu (J.M.O.); zainabgh@udel.edu (Z.A.)
[2] Physical Therapy Department, Munroe Meyer Institute, University of Nebraska Medical Center, Omaha, NE 68105, USA; abaraldicunha@unmc.edu
[3] Physical Therapy Department, University of Delaware, Newark, DE 19713, USA
* Correspondence: malobo@udel.edu

Abstract: Parents commonly seek information about infant development and play, yet it is unclear what information parents find when looking in popular sources. Play, Milestone, and Development Searches in Google identified 313 sources for content analysis by trained researchers using a standardized coding scheme. Sources included websites, books, and apps created by professional organizations, commercial entities, individuals, the popular press, and government organizations/agencies. The results showed that for popular sources: (1) author information (i.e., qualifications, credentials, education/experience) is not consistently provided, nor is information about the developmental process, parents' role in development, or determining an infant's readiness to play; (2) milestones comprise a majority of the content overall; (3) search terminology impacts the information parents receive; (4) sources from the Milestone and Development Searches emphasized a passive approach of observing developmental milestones rather than suggesting activities to actively facilitate learning and milestone development. These findings highlight the need to discuss parents' online information-gathering process and findings. They also highlight the need for innovative universal parent-education programs that focus on activities to facilitate early development. This type of education has potential to benefit all families, with particular benefits for families with children who have unidentified or untreated developmental delays.

Keywords: child development; internet; infancy; parenting practices; play and playthings; health education; information seeking; content analysis; milestones

Citation: Orlando, J.M.; Cunha, A.B.; Alghamdi, Z.; Lobo, M.A. Information Available to Parents Seeking Education about Infant Play, Milestones, and Development from Popular Sources. *Behav. Sci.* **2023**, *13*, 429. https://doi.org/10.3390/bs13050429

Academic Editor: Scott D. Lane

Received: 6 April 2023
Revised: 12 May 2023
Accepted: 17 May 2023
Published: 19 May 2023

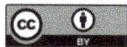

Copyright: © 2023 by the authors. Licensee MDPI, Basel, Switzerland. This article is an open access article distributed under the terms and conditions of the Creative Commons Attribution (CC BY) license (https://creativecommons.org/licenses/by/4.0/).

1. Introduction

A key problem in pediatric rehabilitation is the lack of provision of early intervention (EI) services to young children requiring those services to mitigate developmental delays. Less than 10% of eligible children receive EI services in the United States [1,2]. Traditional approaches to address this challenge include working within the medical and EI systems to improve surveillance, screening, assessment tools, and procedures, as well as addressing barriers to service provision [3–7]. In parallel, we propose that an innovative and effective way to address this challenge would be through the development of high-quality universal education programs that teach parents how to engage and support infants in ways shown to promote learning and development. Universal parent education programs that provide information via the sources parents prefer to access have the potential to positively impact parental knowledge [8], parent–child interaction [9,10], child development [11], and discussions between parents and care providers [12]. These outcomes would be beneficial for all children, while being especially beneficial for children with unidentified and/or untreated developmental delays. This study analyzes the existing content universally available to parents in popular sources to identify what information is already being shared with parents and to determine whether this information aligns with current developmental science.

Parental knowledge about infant development was originally defined as a "parent's understanding of developmental norms and milestones, processes of child development, and familiarity with caregiving skills" (p. 1187, [13]). This definition continues to be used today [14,15]. Parental knowledge is positively related to parent–child interaction [16–19] and infant development [13,14,20]. These relations have been demonstrated among parents of differing ages [14], varying socioeconomic status [16], across cultures [15,21,22], and with infants with typical development as well as those born preterm and at increased risk for developmental delay [20]. Importantly, there is the potential to improve parental knowledge [8], parent–child interaction [10,23,24], and infant development [11,25,26] through parent education interventions [27,28].

In contrast to developmental knowledge, parental knowledge about infant play has not been as thoroughly studied. Damast, Tamis-LeMonda, and Bornstein determined that mothers who had greater knowledge about play were more likely to offer higher-level play activities for their young children, potentially leading to advanced development [29]. Parents who participated in an early positioning and handling education program with their infants had infants who demonstrated short-term advances in prone skills and longer term advancements in crawling, standing, and walking compared to a control group [11]. Similarly, educating parents to encourage infants' general arm movements (i.e., using wrist tethers to control toys) advanced the ability to reach for objects in two-month-olds with typical development [30]. Thus, parental knowledge about play and the information that parents receive about how to interact with their infants can impact parent–child interaction and infant development.

Parents and pediatric clinicians actively seek information about infant development and play [31]. In a national survey of 2200 parents conducted by Zero to Three®, most parents agreed that new research about child development could improve their parenting; about half of the parents wanted more information about how to be a better parent and/or wished they had known more about brain development when their child was younger [32]. Pediatricians and other pediatric clinicians often recommend resources about infant development and play to parents [12,31,33,34]. In a survey of 112 parents of children under two years of age, a majority of parents reported searching for information about development (88.4%) or play (68.8%). Similarly, a majority (92.8%) of the 138 EI clinicians surveyed reported recommending resources about infant development and play to parents [31]. Importantly, parents exposed to the Learn the Signs Act Early Campaign by the Centers for Disease Control (CDC), a program that aims to help families learn about and participate in developmental surveillance and improve early identification of delays [35], had a greater understanding of milestones and engaged in more discussion about development during pediatrician visits [12,36]. These findings suggest that the education that parents receive about development and play may also impact the way that parents engage with healthcare providers, which may impact the early identification of delays.

Parents around the world have reported using the internet and other mass media to find information about infant development [31,37–39]. In a systematic review, Kubb et al. identified that there is a high prevalence of parents using the internet to find health information, including information about specific health conditions, treatment options, and general health information about their children [40]. Notably, the authors describe that "Google was the most common starting point for general health information" (p. 177, [40]). In addition to internet searches, parents also turn to books and mobile applications (apps) for parenting advice [32] and information about infant development and play [31]. It is important for pediatric clinicians to understand the content that parents encounter when searching for information about infant development and play.

Content analyses provide insight into the resources that are available for a target population and can provide recommendations for improved future content creation. For instance, to determine if the needs of parents of children with cerebral palsy were being appropriately addressed, Lau S.K. examined the content on cerebral palsy agency websites and concluded that the agency websites were meeting the needs of parents [41]. Only two content analyses have evaluated the information available to parents regarding infant development, and none have evaluated content regarding infant play. Williams et al. analyzed sources discovered after searching Google and Yahoo search engines for information about child development, parenting, and developmental milestones [42]. The authors reviewed 44 websites and described the accuracy of their content in comparison to the American Academy of Pediatrics' book, *From Birth to Five Years*. They concluded that many of the resources reviewed were accurate, yet they often lacked clarity, were incomplete, or were difficult to navigate. Dewitt et al. evaluated the functionality and content of apps about development from birth through 5 years [43]. They found that few app development teams described the inclusion of a subject matter expert, and only 15% of the apps included content about developmental milestones. Overall, little is known about the information parents may encounter when they look to popular sources for information about infant development and play. This study aimed to fill that knowledge gap by systematically evaluating the content of popular sources about infant play, milestones, and development available to parents searching in the United States (US). Specifically, we aimed to describe: (1) the types of sources available and the authors of these materials; (2) the source content (i.e., number of play activities, milestones, and toys suggested); (3) the information shared with parents regarding developmental processes, the role that parents play in development, and how to determine when an infant is ready to play. These data were collected to describe the information available to parents as well as to identify whether the information presented emphasizes infants' daily experiences and environment in a manner that aligns with current developmental theories. An understanding of the educational materials currently available is critical to evaluate the need for and to inform the development of early parent education programs that can serve as innovative, universal rehabilitation tools to benefit all children with specific benefits for children with or at risk for developmental delays.

2. Materials and Methods

2.1. Source Selection

Searches were conducted using the Google search engine between October 2019 and March 2021 with the following search phrases: (1) "How to play with baby" (i.e., referred to in this paper as the Play Search); (2) "Baby milestones first year" (i.e., the Milestone Search); or (3) "Your baby's development first year" (i.e., the Development Search). Each search was conducted one time during this period. The search terms were selected to replicate searches that a parent may perform. The search results included videos, websites, books, and apps and were saved and exported as a CSV file using the SEOquake plugin (Boston, MA, USA) for Google Chrome. The top 150 results from each search were screened based on the inclusion and exclusion criteria described below. We selected 150 as our cut-off for screening based on the decreased relevance of the search results between 100 and 150. Sources were included in the content analysis if they: (1) involved infants within the 0–12-month age range; (2) were written in English; (3) included content related to infant development and/or play (examples of sources that did not meet this inclusion criterion were keepsake items, growth charts, and sources with only feeding or nutrition content). Sources were excluded if they: (1) were not accessible; or (2) only served a commercial purpose (i.e., promoting a product). Content for each source that met the screening criteria was archived at the time of screening for future analysis. In addition, sources that parents reported referencing for information about infant development and play from an online survey *(n* = 112 participants) conducted by the authors were also screened [31]. Parents were specifically asked to list examples of sources they had accessed for information about infant development or play. We included these sources in our screening process to ensure that our content analysis broadly represented sources accessed by parents.

Our initial search (between October 2019 and March 2021) resulted in 268 sources. To ensure the sample reflected current information, the content for these sources was reviewed in November 2022, and recoding was performed in cases where a new edition was published for a book or where content had been altered for a website. We found that only 19 sources (7.06% of the total number of sources) had modified content; 25 sources (9.33% of the total) had updated the date the source was last reviewed without changing any of the relevant content. The updated coding for the 19 sources with modified content resulted in changes to only 3.6% of the play activities recommended, 2.47% of the milestones listed, and 1.61% of the toys recommended, suggesting that this content remains relatively stable across time. To further update the dataset, we also repeated the Play, Milestone, and Development Searches in September of 2022. We screened the top 50 results from each search for inclusion in order to identify examples of the most relevant additional sources. We added an additional 22 Play, 8 Milestone, and 14 Development sources (44 total) to the content analysis from this more recent search.

2.2. Content Coding Procedures

The codebook was developed by a team of experts in child development and early intervention (Supplementary Materials S1). It aimed to gather information about each source, including information about the authors and about the depth and type of information within each source. The *source type* was classified as book, website, or app. The *author type* was classified as commercial entity, government organization/agency, individual, popular press, or professional organization. *Author credentials* were coded as being present if there was a description of the degree(s) (e.g., PhD, MD, RN, LSW), certifications, or licenses earned by the author. *Author qualifications* were coded as being present if there was a description about the author's experience or expertise, including being a parent. Although sources from professional organizations did not often identify the authors of their content, we credited them as having provided credentials and qualifications based on the noted affiliation with the professional organization. *Author education/experience* was coded based on descriptions provided within the sources as falling into the categories of early childhood education, healthcare, human services (e.g., social worker, therapist, psychologist), parental experience, other (e.g., media relations, editor), or unspecified (e.g., listing "Dr." without further description); multiple selections were possible.

The depth (i.e., amount of content) and type of information within each source was comprised of the inclusion (1 = yes, 0 = no) of play activities, milestones, and toy recommendations as well as the quantity (i.e., the count of all of the play activities, milestones, and toy recommendations described within the source). A play activity was defined as something that a person could do with an infant or something that the infant could do on their own (e.g., hold your baby and dance to their favorite song; give your baby a container filled with scarves and toys and let them explore; talk with your baby). If multiple activities were described within one sentence, each activity was coded separately. A milestone was defined as a behavior that an infant would be expected to perform by a specified timepoint (e.g., your baby will sit without support by nine months). A toy recommendation was coded when an object was recommended to parents for use by the infant or parent (e.g., rattles, spoons, plastic water bottles, scarves, books).

We also coded whether the source shared information about: (1) developmental processes (i.e., information describing how development happens, such as developmental theories or factors influencing development); (2) a parent's role in development (i.e., information describing the role that parents can play in impacting developmental outcomes for their infants); (3) how to determine if an infant is ready to play (i.e., directing parents to infants' signs of readiness to play signs or signs of overstimulation). Any text related to these topics was copied into the coding files. Text content related to the developmental process, parents' role in development, and infants' readiness to play was independently evaluated for themes by two researchers. The researchers then converged to review, discuss, and come to agreement about the emergent themes from this coding.

The content for each source was coded in Google Sheets by research assistants trained to reach greater than 90% inter-rater agreement. The content within each source was coded by two independent coders. The primary coder first extracted and coded all relevant information from the source. The secondary coder then coded the relevant material from the same source and added any material that may have been missed. The primary and secondary coding sheets were compared using a custom MATLAB program (Natick, MA, USA). Only 8.28% of the data were found to disagree. All disagreements were reviewed by the first, second, or third author, all of whom were involved in developing the coding scheme or a senior research assistant with additional training. The review involved returning to the source content to ensure the accuracy and completeness of the dataset. The final data (Supplementary Materials S2) were then compiled and stored in a custom Claris FileMaker Pro (Cupertino, CA, USA) relational database.

2.3. Statistical Analysis

Data were analyzed using descriptive statistics, including frequencies and percentages. The source medium, author type, author credentials, and author qualifications were described as a percentage of the total number of unique sources (i.e., eliminating redundancies in cases where a source was encountered through more than one search) in order to describe the materials available to parents as a whole. In contrast, since one purpose of this study was to characterize the information parents would encounter from each type of search (i.e., Play, Milestone, or Development), when analyzing author education/experience and outcomes related to depth and type of information, data from individual sources that were found through more than one search type (n = 47, 15.01% of all sources) were included in the analyses for each of their associated searches.

Statistical analyses were conducted using SPSS version 29 (Armonk, NY, USA). To determine whether author characteristics and information shared varied based on the search type (i.e., Play, Milestone, or Development), Pearson's Chi-Square Test of Independence was used to evaluate whether there were relations between search type and: (1) author type; (2) author credentials; (3) author qualifications; (4) the inclusion of source content (i.e., play activities, milestones, and toy recommendations); (5) the inclusion of information related to developmental process, parent's role in development, and readiness to play; (6) themes identified related to developmental process, parent's role in development, and infant readiness to play. To determine whether the authors of the content from the Play, Milestone, or Development Searches differed, relations among author education/experience and the type of search conducted were evaluated with Fisher's Exact Test. Author education/experience was a multiple selection variable (e.g., parental experience and healthcare). Only author education/experience combinations with greater than five responses in total among the Play, Milestone, and Development Searches were included in analyses. Fisher's Exact Test accounts for instances when the observed frequency of an author education/experience variable was greater than five overall but less than five within a specific search (i.e., Play, Milestone, or Development). The significance level was set to alpha = 0.05. Post-hoc analyses were conducted using standardized adjusted residuals and Bonferroni adjustments with the null hypothesis that all observed values were equally distributed [44–46].

3. Results

The Play Search resulted in 122 sources published between 1995 and 2022 (median: 2019). The Milestone Search resulted in 126 sources published between 2005 and 2022 (median: 2019). The Development Search resulted in 112 sources published between 2000 and 2022 (median: 2020). In total, 313 unique sources were analyzed; 47 sources were found through more than one search. Examples of the sources reviewed included books, such as *Your Baby's First Year* by the American Academy of Pediatrics [47] and *What to Expect the First Year* by Heidi Murkoff [48]; websites, such as Pathways.org® [49], ZerotoThree.org® [50], BabyCenter.com® [51] (accessed on 5 April 2023), and Learn The Signs Act Early by the Centers for Disease Control and Prevention [52]; and apps, such as BabySparks® [53] and

Kinedu® [54]. The complete list of sources reviewed is available within the final data (Supplementary Materials S2).

3.1. Description of the Sources

3.1.1. Source Medium and Author Type

The majority of the sources ($n = 289$, 92.33%) were websites which may be a reflection of the search process being conducted online. However, books ($n = 14$, 4.47%) and apps ($n = 10$, 3.19%) discovered through online searches and/or through the parent survey were also included. Of the 313 unique sources, most were created by professional organizations ($n = 176$, 56.23%), followed by commercial entities ($n = 50$, 15.97%), individuals ($n = 42$, 13.42%), the popular press ($n = 33$, 10.54%), and government organizations/agencies ($n = 12$, 3.83%). Within each search type, most of the sources were from professional organizations (Play: $n = 51$, 41.80%; Milestone: $n = 85$, 67.46%, Development: $n = 76$, 67.86%). There was a significant relation between the type of search conducted and the author type ($X^2(8) = 38.77$, $p < 0.001$). Individual authors were significantly more likely to create content discovered from the Play Search ($Z = 4.97$, $p < 0.001$) while professional organizations were significantly less likely to create content discovered from the Play Search ($Z = -4.72$, $p < 0.001$).

3.1.2. Author Credentials, Qualifications, and Education

Of the 313 unique sources, author credentials ($n = 213$, 67.73%) and author qualifications ($n = 225$, 71.88%) were often included. There was a significant relation between the search type and the presence of author credentials ($X^2(2) = 11.75$, $p = 0.003$) and qualifications ($X^2(2) = 47.30$, $p < 0.001$). Author credentials were significantly less likely to be present in the sources discovered in the Play Search ($Z = -3.41$, $p < 0.001$). Author qualifications were significantly more likely to be present in the sources from the Milestone ($Z = 3.33$, $p < 0.001$) and Development Searches ($Z = 3.6$, $p < 0.001$) and less likely to be present in the sources from the Play Search ($Z = -6.87$, $p < 0.001$).

Author education/experience was reported by 137 sources (38.02% of the unique sources), and there were 17 combinations of author education/experience selections (Supplementary Materials S3). *Healthcare* education/experience was most frequently reported ($n = 54$, 39.42%), followed by *healthcare and parental education/experience* ($n = 15$, 10.95%) and *parental experience and other* ($n = 11$, 8.03%). Sources authored by individuals from healthcare were often discovered in the Milestone ($n = 22$, 52.38%) or Development ($n = 19$, 48.72%) Searches. Authors who were described solely as parents were only 5.11% of the sample ($n = 7$) and were most often discovered from the Play Search ($n = 6$, 85.71%). Interestingly, authors who identified as parents with healthcare education/experience were discovered most often from the Play Search ($n = 10$, 66.67% of healthcare and parents). Only healthcare, healthcare/parent, parent/other, early childhood education, human services, parent, parent/human services and "other" received greater than five total responses and were therefore included in the analyses. There was a significant relation between search type and author education; Fishers Exact test ($X^2(14) = 30.09$, $p = 0.002$) and post-hoc analyses identified that individuals with healthcare education/experience were less likely to have authored sources from the Play Search ($Z = -3.22$, $p = 0.001$).

3.2. Description of the Source Content

3.2.1. Inclusion of Play Activities, Milestones, and Toy Recommendations

The presence of play activity, milestone, and toy recommendation content was evaluated within each search type. Play activity content was found within 95.90% ($n = 117$) of the sources from the Play Search, 41.27% ($n = 52$) of the sources from the Milestone Search, and 59.82% ($n = 67$) of the sources from the Development Search. There was a significant relation between the presence of play activity content and the search type ($X^2(2) = 85.30$, $p \leq 0.001$). Post-hoc analyses identified that sources discovered from the Play Search were significantly more likely to include play activity content ($Z = 8.68$, $p < 0.001$), while sources from the Milestone Search were significantly less likely to include play activity content ($Z = -7.12, p < 0.001$).

Milestone content was found within 65.57% ($n = 80$) of the sources from the Play Search, 98.41% ($n = 124$) of the sources from the Milestone Search, and 94.64% ($n = 106$) of the sources from the Development Search. There was a significant relation between the presence of milestone content and the search type ($X^2(2) = 65.78, p \leq 0.001$). Post-hoc analyses identified that sources discovered from the Development and Milestone Searches were significantly more likely to include milestone content (Development: $Z = 3.15, p = 0.002$; Milestone: $Z = 4.95, p < 0.001$), while sources from the Play Search were significantly less likely to include milestone content ($Z = -8.07, p < 0.001$).

Toy recommendations were found within 90.16% ($n = 110$) of the sources from the Play Search, 42.86% ($n = 54$) of the sources from the Milestone Search, and 58.93% ($n = 66$) of the sources from the Development Search. There was also a significant relation between the presence of toy recommendations and the search type ($X^2(2) = 61.86, p \leq 0.001$). Post-hoc analysis identified that sources discovered from the Play Search were significantly more likely to include toy recommendations ($Z = 7.43, p < 0.001$), while sources from the Milestone Search were significantly less likely to include them ($Z = -6.1, p < 0.001$).

3.2.2. Quantity of Play Activities, Milestones, and Toy Recommendations

The Play Search had a total of 5064 combined items (2254 play activities, 1551 milestones, 1259 toy recommendations), the Milestone Search had 10,085 combined items (1377 play activities, 7898 milestones, 810 toy recommendations), and the Development Search had 8854 combined items (1602 play activities, 5650 milestones, 1602 toy recommendations; Figure 1).

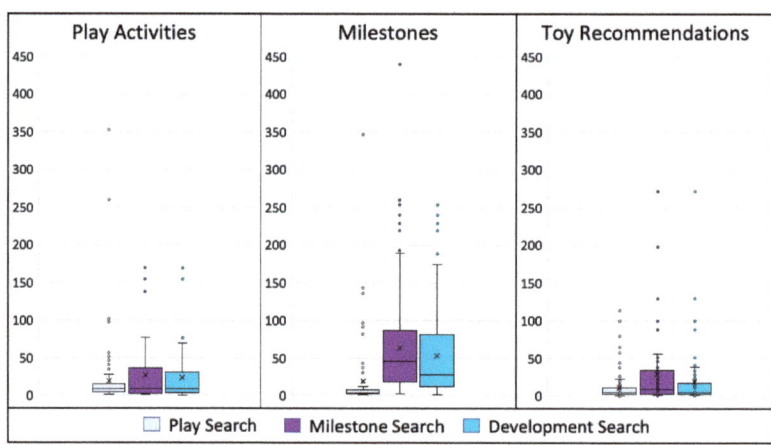

Figure 1. Number of play activities, milestones, and toy recommendations identified in the content from the Play, Milestone, and Development Searches. Box and whisker plots with the horizontal line denoting the median, X indicating the mean, and the bottom and top borders of the box representing the first and third quartiles. The whiskers extend to the minimum and maximum values while additional points indicate outliers that are greater than 1.5 times the interquartile range.

3.3. Description of the Content Related to Developmental Process, Parents' Roles in Development, and Infants' Readiness to Play

Information about the developmental process was present in 37.70% ($n = 46$) of the sources from the Play Search, 49.21% ($n = 62$) of the sources from the Milestone Search, and 38.39% ($n = 43$) of the sources from the Development Search. There was no significant relation between the presence of information about developmental process and the search type ($p = 0.122$).

Information about parents' role in development was present in 46.72% ($n = 57$) of the sources from the Play Search, 41.27% ($n = 52$) of the sources from the Milestone Search, and 35.71% ($n = 40$) of the sources from the Development Search. There was no significant relation between the presence of information about parents' role in the development and the search type ($p = 0.233$).

Information about infant readiness for play was present in 22.13% ($n = 27$) of the sources from the Play Search, 7.94% ($n = 10$) of the sources from the Milestone Search, and 8.93% ($n = 10$) of the sources from the Development Search. There was a significant relation between the presence of information about infant readiness to play and the search type ($X^2(2) = 13.44$, $p = 0.001$). Post-hoc analysis identified that sources discovered from the Play Search were significantly more likely to include information about infant readiness for play ($Z = 3.66$, $p < 0.001$).

The themes identified in the content regarding developmental process, parents' roles, and infants' readiness to play can be seen in Figure 2. Among the developmental process themes, three varied in relation to the search type. There was a significant relation between the type of search and the presence of information stating that *milestones occur at their own pace* ($X^2(2) = 35.20$, $p < 0.001$). Post-hoc analyses identified that sources from the Milestone Search were more likely to include this theme ($Z = 5.61$, $p < 0.001$), while sources from the Play Search were less likely to include it ($Z = -4.6$, $p < 0.001$). There was also a significant relation between the search type and the theme that *infants learn through play* ($X^2(2) = 28.78$, $p < 0.001$), which was more likely to be present in sources from the Play Search ($Z = 5.31$, $p < 0.001$) and less likely to be present in sources from the Milestone Search ($Z = -3.43$, $p < 0.001$). Further, there was a significant relation between the search type and content about *development occurring in a specific order* ($X^2(2) = 9.75$, $p = 0.008$), with post-hoc analyses identifying that sources from the Milestone Search were more likely ($Z = 2.63$, $p = 0.009$) and sources from the Play Search were less likely ($Z = -2.83$, $p = 0.005$) to discuss this.

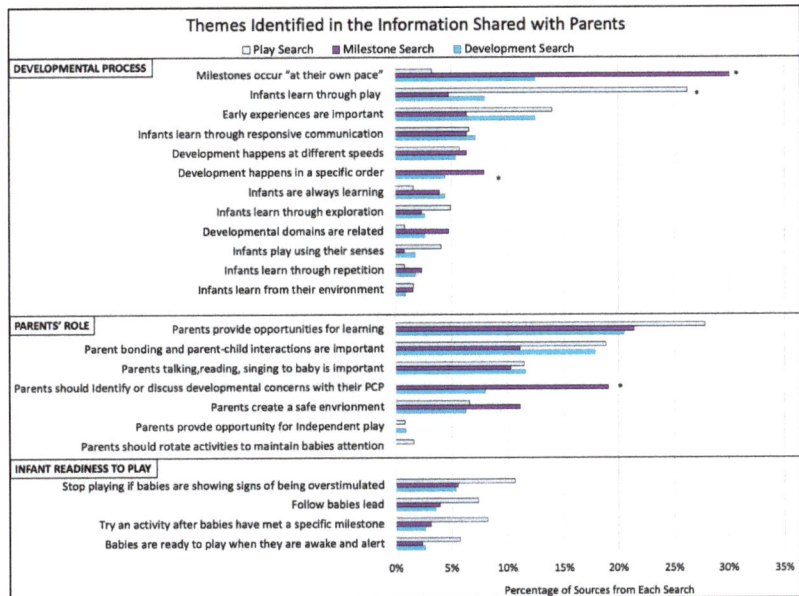

Figure 2. Themes identified in the information shared with parents. The percentage of sources from the Play, Milestone, and Development Searches that mentioned each theme identified regarding the developmental process, parents' role in development, and infant readiness to play; themes are shown from highest to lowest rate of occurrence within these topic areas. * Denotes significant findings. PCP = Primary Care Provider.

Within the themes related to the parents' role in development, one varied in relation to search type. There was a significant relation between the search type and the theme that *parents should identify or discuss concerns about development with their child's primary care provider*; $X^2(2) = 27.26$, $p < 0.001$). Sources from the Milestone Search were more likely ($Z = 4.77$, $p < 0.001$) to include information about the importance of identifying and bringing up concerns with the primary care provider, while sources from the Play Search were less likely ($Z = -4.32$, $p < 0.001$) to include this information.

4. Discussion

There were several interesting findings from this content analysis of the popular sources of information available to parents searching for education about infant play, milestones, and development. Information was shared with parents via a variety of media, including websites, books, and apps. While author credentials or qualifications were provided in most cases, for about a third of the content, it remained unclear who authored the materials and/or what qualified them to do so. Moreover, author's education or experience was described for just over a third of the sources. Information about the developmental process and about parents' roles in development was shared in less than half of the sources, and information about determining whether an infant was ready to play or overstimulated was provided in less than a quarter of the sources. Below, we discuss the key findings of the content analysis along with their implications.

An important novel finding from this content analysis is that, overall, parents who perform searches such as the ones conducted here are most likely to learn about milestones when looking for information about infant play, milestones, and development. Milestones outnumbered play activities by about three to one and toy recommendations by about four to one across all of the content analyzed. Developmental science is a relatively new scientific field, and its early decades focused primarily on documenting developmental products—noting which behaviors emerged and the timeline in which they were observed [55–57]. More recent decades have been marked by efforts to better understand the processes through which developmental milestones emerge [57–59]. Parent education programs have existed in the US for almost as long as the field of developmental science itself. For example, the Parent Teacher Association (PTA) was founded in 1897 and has published a variety of materials to educate parents [60]. The preponderance of milestones in the educational materials available to parents may reflect that the content is delayed in keeping pace with the science of development.

Another novel finding from this study is that parents will likely encounter distinct types of information created by different groups of authors when they perform searches for information specifically about infant play, milestones, or development. When seeking information about infant play using search terms such as those employed in this study, parents are likely to find information about play activities they can engage in with infants and recommendations for toys and common objects to use in play. On the contrary, when seeking information about milestones using search terms such as those employed in this study, parents are likely to encounter lists of developmental milestones infants are expected to achieve. Interestingly, if parents search for information about infant development using search terms such as those employed in this study, the content closely mirrors that found through the Milestone Search. This perpetuates the concept that development is characterized by the milestones that infants achieve rather than the processes involved in supporting the development of those milestones [56]. Historically, infant development has been widely defined as a series of changes in developmental milestones [55,61], but it is now recognized that infant development is a cascading process that is shaped by a variety of factors, including environmental factors and experiences [62]. Current developmental theory and interventions aimed at advancing development acknowledge that factors such as early experiences [63], postural stability [64], and the environment [65] (e.g., the physical environment [66] and parent–child interaction [67]) can serve as drivers for developmental change. With a strong focus on milestones and less focus on activities and objects that can be used to drive the advancement of those milestones, popular sources share information that reflects an outdated view of development and misses the opportunity to educate parents about how to promote development for young children.

The results of this study are the first to our knowledge to highlight that, although some healthcare professionals have developed educational content for parents of young children that is accessible via online searches (i.e., they authored about a quarter of the sources reviewed), the content created by healthcare providers and other authors should be updated to reflect more current, empirically supported developmental theories [62,68,69]. Those with healthcare education/experience were more likely to author content that was found through the Milestone Search. Importantly, this content primarily listed developmental milestones and advised parents to observe for these milestones as they occur at their own pace and in a specific order. This approach reflects more outdated developmental theories, such as neural-maturation theory, that focused on the typical progression of milestone emergence with a primary driver, such as maturation of the nervous system, causing those changes [56]. Further, content from the Milestone Search was less likely to include play activity suggestions, to recommend toys, or to highlight that infants learn through play. Therefore, like more outdated developmental theories, this content placed less emphasis on the infant's environment and daily experiences. One potential benefit of this content was that it was more likely to advise parents to communicate with their primary care providers should they note delays in the emergence of developmental milestones. This may support the early identification of delays and utilization of EI services, as children whose parents have developmental concerns may be more likely to receive an EI evaluation and be identified as eligible for services compared to children whose parents who did not have developmental concerns [70].

An innovative approach for healthcare providers and child development experts to optimize development for young children may be through the creation of universal parent education materials that reflect current developmental science. Interestingly, in the current study, most authors who identified as healthcare providers alone published content found through the Milestone and Development Searches, while most authors who identified as healthcare providers and parents published content found through the Play Search. Furthermore, parents and other individuals, rather than professional organizations, were more likely to author content found through the Play Search. This suggests that parents as a whole, including those with healthcare education/experience, recognize the value of and the need for educational content related to infant play. It also suggests that the importance of play and daily activity may not be understood by the professional organizations currently engaged in educating parents. Most parents reportedly seek information about how to play with their infants [31]. Current empirically supported developmental theories, including ecological systems theory and dynamic systems theory, emphasize the critical role of experiences in constructing and shaping children's developmental trajectories. They claim that milestones do not emerge due to time or maturation, rather they are learned through children's ongoing, daily experiences [71–73]. With parents eager to learn about how to play with their infants and with daily parent–child activity serving as the foundation for milestone development, there is a prime opportunity for healthcare providers and child development experts to generate high-quality educational content for parents with the aim of advancing children's developmental trajectories [74]. This content should teach parents ways to shape the environment and to enhance learning opportunities for infants [11,75,76].

The results of this study can help pediatric healthcare providers and educators understand what information parents likely encounter through popular sources. The results also highlight the need for updated educational materials for parents. Professionals should engage in discussions with parents about their online information search processes and results. Professionals may direct parents to utilize different search terms to better direct them to the type of information they desire. For example, if parents are interested in learning about play activities or toys, replicating the Play Search would be most effective. If parents are interested in learning about milestones, this content was readily available within all of the searches, however, replicating the Milestone Search would produce the highest volume of milestone content. Future research should further explore the content parents receive when they use a greater variety of search terminology.

The results should be Interpreted"Iit' a consideration of the study's limitations. One limitation may be that the majority of sources analyzed were found online. While this likely reflects the search practices of most parents in the US [40], it may not reflect the search practices of all. In addition, the searches were conducted in one location in the US and were limited to English. Geographic location can impact search engine optimization and therefore, future research may benefit from a broader search region. Future research should expand the search locations and compare the results of searches conducted in different countries and languages. Another limitation is that the study reports only on the quantity of play activities, milestones, and toy recommendations shared with parents. It remains unclear whether directing parents to this information would benefit an infant's development because the quality of the information was not evaluated. Future research should evaluate the quality of the information shared with parents to identify high-quality sources.

The clinical implications of this study are that current, accessible, popular sources available to parents emphasize developmental products (i.e., the milestones that an infant should achieve) and a more passive approach to development. When seeking information about milestones or development, parents are more likely to find a large amount of information listing expected milestones along with instructions to wait for the milestones to emerge and to alert healthcare providers if a developmental concern is noted. Less than a quarter of the content suggested interactions with infants and objects to facilitate infants' development. In contrast, when seeking information about how to play with infants, parents are likely to find a greater number of activity and toy suggestions along with an emphasis on the importance of parents' role in development to support early learning. It is important for clinicians who interact with parents of infants to critically review and understand the available resources in order to counsel parents about information seeking practices. Additionally, professionals should engage in discussions with parents about how to critically review the content they access. Professionals should also familiarize themselves with the popular content in order to direct parents to sources that will effectively meet their educational needs. Furthermore, rehabilitation and child development experts should be developing innovative approaches to meet parents' educational needs that better align with current developmental science. This could be achieved through consultation to improve existing resources along with the creation of novel websites, books, and/or apps geared towards parents. Specifically, universal parent education programs that highlight not only which milestones are expected in development, but also the activities that parents can implement and objects they can use to advance the development of those milestones might serve as effective early intervention tools.

Supplementary Materials: The following supporting information can be downloaded at: https://www.mdpi.com/article/10.3390/bs13050429/s1, Supplementary Materials S1: Codebook; Supplementary Materials S2: Popular Source Dataset; Supplementary Materials S3: Author Education/Experience.

Author Contributions: Conceptualization, J.M.O., A.B.C., Z.A. and M.A.L.; methodology, J.M.O., A.B.C., Z.A. and M.A.L.; formal analysis, J.M.O. and A.B.C.; data curation, J.M.O., A.B.C., Z.A. and M.A.L.; writing—original draft preparation, J.M.O.; writing—review and editing, A.B.C., Z.A. and M.A.L.; visualization, J.M.O. and M.A.L.; project administration, M.A.L. All authors have read and agreed to the published version of the manuscript.

Funding: This manuscript is based upon work supported by the University of Delaware Graduate College through the Unidel Distinguished Graduate Scholar Award (Orlando). Any opinions, findings, and conclusions or recommendations expressed in this material are those of the authors.

Institutional Review Board Statement: Not applicable.

Informed Consent Statement: Not applicable.

Data Availability Statement: The data presented in this study are available in the Supplementary Materials.

Acknowledgments: We would like to acknowledge the amazing research assistants who contributed to this study.

Conflicts of Interest: The authors declare no conflict of interest. The funders had no role in the design of the study; in the collection, analyses, or interpretation of data; in the writing of the manuscript; or in the decision to publish the results.

References

1. McManus, B.M.; Richardson, Z.; Schenkman, M.; Murphy, N.J.; Everhart, R.M.; Hambidge, S.; Morrato, E. Child characteristics and early intervention referral and receipt of services: A retrospective cohort study. *BMC Pediatr.* **2020**, *20*, 84. [CrossRef] [PubMed]
2. Rosenberg, S.A.; Robinson, C.C.; Shaw, E.F.; Ellison, M.C. Part C Early Intervention for Infants and Toddlers: Percentage Eligible Versus Served. *Pediatrics* **2013**, *131*, 38–46. [CrossRef] [PubMed]
3. Bright, M.A.; Zubler, J.; Boothby, C.; Whitaker, T.M. Improving Developmental Screening, Discussion, and Referral in Pediatric Practice. *Clin. Pediatr.* **2019**, *58*, 941–948. [CrossRef] [PubMed]
4. Duby, J.C.; Lipkin, P.H.; Macias, M.M.; Wegner, L.M.; Duncan, P.; Hagan, J.F.; Cooley, W.C.; Swigonski, N.; Council Children, D.; Section Dev Behav, P.; et al. Identifying infants and young children with developmental disorders in the medical home: An algorithm for developmental surveillance and screening. *Pediatrics* **2006**, *118*, 405–420. [CrossRef]
5. Lobo, M.A.; Paul, D.A.; Mackley, A.; Maher, J.; Galloway, J.C. Instability of delay classification and determination of early intervention eligibility in the first two years of life. *Res. Dev. Disabil.* **2014**, *35*, 117–126. [CrossRef]
6. Zuckerman, K.E.; Chavez, A.E.; Wilson, L.; Unger, K.; Reuland, C.; Ramsey, K.; King, M.; Scholz, J.; Fombonne, E. Improving autism and developmental screening and referral in US primary care practices serving Latinos. *Autism* **2021**, *25*, 288–299. [CrossRef]
7. Lipkin, P.H.; Macias, M.M.; Norwood, K.W.; Brei, T.J.; Davidson, L.F.; Davis, B.E.; Ellerbeck, K.A.; Houtrow, A.J.; Hyman, S.L.; Kuo, D.Z. Promoting optimal development: Identifying infants and young children with developmental disorders through developmental surveillance and screening. *Pediatrics* **2020**, *145*, e20193449. [CrossRef]
8. Gozali, A.; Gibson, S.; Lipton, L.R.; Pressman, A.W.; Hammond, B.S.; Dumitriu, D. Assessing the effectiveness of a pediatrician-led newborn parenting class on maternal newborn-care knowledge, confidence and anxiety: A quasi-randomized controlled trial. *Early Hum. Dev.* **2020**, *147*, 105082. [CrossRef]
9. Roby, E.; Miller, E.B.; Shaw, D.S.; Morris, P.; Gill, A.; Bogen, D.L.; Rosas, J.; Canfield, C.F.; Hails, K.A.; Wippick, H.; et al. Improving Parent-Child Interactions in Pediatric Health Care: A Two-Site Randomized Controlled Trial. *Pediatrics* **2021**, *147*, e20201799. [CrossRef]
10. White-Traut, R.; Norr, K.F.; Fabiyi, C.; Rankin, K.M.; Li, Z.Y.; Liu, L. Mother-infant interaction improves with a developmental intervention for mother-preterm infant dyads. *Infant Behav. Dev.* **2013**, *36*, 694–706. [CrossRef]
11. Lobo, M.A.; Galloway, J.C. Enhanced Handling and Positioning in Early Infancy Advances Development Throughout the First Year. *Child Dev.* **2012**, *83*, 1290–1302. [CrossRef]
12. Gadomski, A.M.; Riley, M.R.; Scribani, M.; Tallman, N. Impact of "Learn the Signs. Act Early." Materials on Parental Engagement and Doctor Interaction Regarding Child Development. *J. Dev. Behav. Pediatr.* **2018**, *39*, 693–700. [CrossRef]
13. Benasich, A.A.; BrooksGunn, J. Maternal attitudes and knowledge of child-rearing: Associations with family and child outcomes. *Child Dev.* **1996**, *67*, 1186–1205. [CrossRef]
14. Jahromi, L.B.; Guimond, A.B.; Umana-Taylor, A.J.; Updegraff, K.A.; Toomey, R.B. Family Context, Mexican-Origin Adolescent Mothers' Parenting Knowledge, and Children's Subsequent Developmental Outcomes. *Child Dev.* **2014**, *85*, 593–609. [CrossRef]
15. Yue, A.; Wu, M.; Shi, Y.; Luo, R.; Wang, B.; Kenny, K.; Rozelle, S. The relationship between maternal parenting knowledge and infant development outcomes: Evidence from rural China. *Chin. J. Sociol.* **2017**, *3*, 193–207. [CrossRef]
16. Stevens, J.H. Child-Development Knowledge and Parenting Skills. *Fam. Relat.* **1984**, *33*, 237–244. [CrossRef]
17. Hess, C.R.; Teti, D.M.; Hussey-Gardner, B. Self-efficacy and parenting of high-risk infants: The moderating role of parent knowledge of infant development. *J. Appl. Dev. Psychol.* **2004**, *25*, 423–437. [CrossRef]
18. Conrad, B.; Gross, D.; Fogg, L.; Ruchala, P. Maternal confidence, knowledge, and quality of mother toddler interactions—A preliminary-study. *Infant Ment. Health J.* **1992**, *13*, 353–362. [CrossRef]
19. Mermelshtine, R.; Barnes, J. Maternal Responsive-didactic Caregiving in Play Interactions with 10-month-olds and Cognitive Development at 18 months. *Infant Child Dev.* **2016**, *25*, 296–316. [CrossRef]
20. Veddovi, M.; Gibson, F.; Kenny, D.T.; Bowen, J.; Starte, D. Preterm Behavior, Maternal Adjustment, and Competencies in the Newborn Period: What Influence Do They Have at 12 Months Postnatal Age? *Infant Ment. Health J.* **2004**, *25*, 580–599. [CrossRef]
21. Zhong, J.D.; He, Y.; Gao, J.J.; Wang, T.Y.; Luo, R.F. Parenting Knowledge, Parental Investments, and Early Childhood Development in Rural Households in Western China. *Int. J. Environ. Res. Public Health* **2020**, *17*, 2792. [CrossRef] [PubMed]
22. Huang, K.Y.; Caughy, M.O.B.; Genevro, J.L.; Miller, T.L. Maternal knowledge of child development and quality of parenting among White, African-American and Hispanic mothers. *J. Appl. Dev. Psychol.* **2005**, *26*, 149–170. [CrossRef]

23. Steinhardt, A.; Hinner, P.; Kuhn, T.; Roehr, C.C.; Rudiger, M.; Reichert, J. Influences of a dedicated parental training program on parent-child interaction in preterm infants. *Early Hum. Dev.* **2015**, *91*, 205–210. [CrossRef] [PubMed]
24. Byrne, E.M.; Sweeney, J.K.; Schwartz, N.; Umphred, D.; Constantinou, J. Effects of Instruction on Parent Competency During Infant Handling in a Neonatal Intensive Care Unit. *Pediatr. Phys. Ther.* **2019**, *31*, 43–49. [CrossRef] [PubMed]
25. Chang, S.M.; Grantham-McGregor, S.M.; Powell, C.A.; Vera-Hernandez, M.; Lopez-Boo, F.; Baker-Henningham, H.; Walker, S.P. Integrating a Parenting Intervention With Routine Primary Health Care: A Cluster Randomized Trial. *Pediatrics* **2015**, *136*, 272–280. [CrossRef]
26. Dusing, S.C.; Tripathi, T.; Marcinowski, E.C.; Thacker, L.R.; Brown, L.F.; Hendricks-Munoz, K.D. Supporting play exploration and early developmental intervention versus usual care to enhance development outcomes during the transition from the neonatal intensive care unit to home: A pilot randomized controlled trial. *BMC Pediatr.* **2018**, *18*, 46. [CrossRef]
27. Roberts, M.Y.; Curtis, P.R.; Sone, B.J.; Hampton, L.H. Association of Parent Training With Child Language Development: A Systematic Review and Meta-analysis. *JAMA Pediatr.* **2019**, *173*, 671–680. [CrossRef]
28. Jeong, J.; Franchett, E.E.; de Oliveira, C.V.R.; Rehmani, K.; Yousafzai, A.K. Parenting interventions to promote early child development in the first three years of life: A global systematic review and meta-analysis. *PLoS Med.* **2021**, *18*, e1003602. [CrossRef]
29. Damast, A.M.; Tamis-LeMonda, C.S.; Bornstein, M.H. Mother-child play: Sequential interactions and the relation between maternal beliefs and behaviors. *Child Dev.* **1996**, *67*, 1752–1766. [CrossRef]
30. Lobo, M.A.; Galloway, J.C.; Savelsbergh, G.J.P. General and task-related experiences affect early object interaction. *Child Dev.* **2004**, *75*, 1268–1281. [CrossRef]
31. Orlando, J.; Cunha, A.; Alghamdi, Z.; Lobo, M. How do parents and early intervention professionals utilize educational resources about infant development and play? *Early Hum. Dev.* **2023**, *180*, 105763. [CrossRef]
32. Zero to Three. National Parent Survey Report. Available online: https://www.zerotothree.org/resource/national-parent-survey-report/ (accessed on 22 March 2023).
33. Raspa, M.; Levis, D.M.; Kish-Doto, J.; Wallace, I.; Rice, C.; Barger, B.; Green, K.K.; Wolf, R.B. Examining Parents' Experiences and Information Needs Regarding Early Identification of Developmental Delays: Qualitative Research to Inform a Public Health Campaign. *J. Dev. Behav. Pediatr.* **2015**, *36*, 575–585. [CrossRef]
34. Kretch, K.S.; Willett, S.L.; Hsu, L.Y.; Sargent, B.A.; Harbourne, R.T.; Dusing, S.C. "Learn the Signs. Act Early.": Updates and Implications for Physical Therapists. *Pediatr. Phys. Ther.* **2022**, *34*, 440–448. [CrossRef]
35. Centers for Disease Control and Prevention. About the Program. Available online: https://www.cdc.gov/ncbddd/actearly/about.html (accessed on 18 March 2023).
36. Daniel, K.L.; Prue, C.; Taylor, M.K.; Thomas, J.; Scales, M. 'Learn the signs. Act early': A campaign to help every child reach his or her full potential. *Public Health* **2009**, *123*, e11–e16. [CrossRef]
37. Aldayel, A.S.; Aldayel, A.A.; Almutairi, A.M.; Alhussain, H.A.; Alwehaibi, S.A.; Almutairi, T.A. Parental Knowledge of Children's Developmental Milestones in Riyadh, Saudi Arabia. *Int. J. Pediatr.* **2020**, *2020*, 8889912. [CrossRef]
38. Scarzello, D.; Arace, A.; Prino, L.E. Parental practices of Italian mothers and fathers during early infancy: The role of knowledge about parenting and child development. *Infant Behav. Dev.* **2016**, *44*, 133–143. [CrossRef]
39. Harvey, S.; Memon, A.; Khan, R.; Yasin, F. Parent's use of the Internet in the search for healthcare information and subsequent impact on the doctor-patient relationship. *Ir. J. Med. Sci.* **2017**, *186*, 821–826. [CrossRef]
40. Kubb, C.; Foran, H.M. Online Health Information Seeking by Parents for Their Children: Systematic Review and Agenda for Further Research. *J. Med. Internet Res.* **2020**, *22*, e19985. [CrossRef]
41. Lau, S.K. Are Concerns and Needs of Parents Addressed? An Analysis of Cerebral Palsy Agencies Websites in Australia. In Proceedings of the 2013 46th Hawaii International Conference on System Sciences, Wailea, HI, USA, 7–10 January 2013; pp. 2425–2434.
42. Williams, N.; Mughal, S.; Blair, M. 'Is my child developing normally?': A critical review of web-based resources for parents. *Dev. Med. Child Neurol.* **2008**, *50*, 893–897. [CrossRef]
43. DeWitt, A.; Kientz, J.; Liljenquist, K. Quality of Mobile Apps for Child Development Support: Search in App Stores and Content Analysis. *JMIR Pediatr. Parent.* **2022**, *5*, e38793. [CrossRef]
44. Beasley, T.M.; Schumacker, R.E. Multiple regression approach to analyzing contingency tables: Post hoc and planned comparison procedures. *J. Exp. Educ.* **1995**, *64*, 79–93. [CrossRef]
45. Garcia-Perez, M.A.; Nunez-Anton, V. Cellwise residual analysis in two-way contingency tables. *Educ. Psychol. Meas.* **2003**, *63*, 825–839. [CrossRef]
46. Sharpe, D. Chi-Square Test is Statistically Significant: Now What? *Pract. Assess. Res. Eval.* **2015**, *20*, 8. [CrossRef]
47. Shelov, S.P. *Your Baby's First Year*; Bantam Books: New York, NY, USA, 2015.
48. Murkoff, H.E.; Eisenberg, A.; Hathaway, S.E.; Mazel, S. *What to Expect® the First Year*; Workman Publishing: New York, NY, USA, 2009.
49. Track Your Baby's Milestones! Available online: https://pathways.org/ (accessed on 12 November 2019).
50. Available online: https://www.zerotothree.org/ (accessed on 12 November 2019).
51. BabyCenter. Available online: https://www.babycenter.com/ (accessed on 1 October 2019).
52. CDC. CDC's Developmental Milestones. Available online: https://www.cdc.gov/ncbddd/actearly/milestones/index.html (accessed on 15 September 2022).

53. BabySparks Inc. BabySparks. Apple App Store, Vers 4.7.29. 2019. Available online: https://apps.apple.com/us/app/babysparks/id794574199?ls=1 (accessed on 5 April 2023).
54. Kinedu Inc. Kinedu. Apple App Store, Vers 5.35.7. 2022. Available online: https://apps.apple.com/us/app/kinedu-baby-development-plan/id741277284 (accessed on 5 April 2023).
55. Gesell, A. The ontogenesis of infant behavior. In *Manual of Child Psychology*; John Wiley & Sons, Inc.: Hoboken, NJ, USA, 1946; pp. 295–331.
56. Gesell, A. Reciprocal interweaving in neuromotor development. A principle of spiral organization shown in the patterning of infant behavior. *J. Comp. Neurol.* **1939**, *70*, 161–180. [CrossRef]
57. Whitall, J.; Schott, N.; Robinson, L.E.; Bardid, F.; Clark, J.E. Motor development research: I. The lessons of history revisited (the 18th to the 20th century). *J. Mot. Learn. Dev.* **2020**, *8*, 345–362. [CrossRef]
58. Kamm, K.; Thelen, E.; Jensen, J.L. A Dynamical Systems Approach to Motor Development. *Phys. Ther.* **1990**, *70*, 763–775. [CrossRef]
59. Colombo, J. Visual Attention in Infancy: Process and Product in Early Cognitive Development. In *Cognitive Neuroscience of Attention*; The Guilford Press: New York, NY, USA, 2004; pp. 329–341.
60. Schlossman, S. Before home start: Notes toward a history of parent education in America, 1897–1929. *Harv. Educ. Rev.* **1976**, *46*, 436–467. [CrossRef]
61. McGraw, M.B. *Growth: A Study of Johnny and Jimmy (Preface by F. Tilney; Introduction by J. Dewey)*; Appleton-Century: Oxford, UK, 1935; p. 319.
62. Adolph, K.E.; Hoch, J.E. Motor Development: Embodied, Embedded, Encultured, and Enabling. *Annu. Rev. Psychol.* **2019**, *70*, 141–164. [CrossRef]
63. Harbourne, R.T.; Dusing, S.C.; Lobo, M.A.; McCoy, S.W.; Koziol, N.A.; Hsu, L.-Y.; Willett, S.; Marcinowski, E.C.; Babik, I.; Cunha, A.B.; et al. START-Play Physical Therapy Intervention Impacts Motor and Cognitive Outcomes in Infants With Neuromotor Disorders: A Multisite Randomized Clinical Trial. *Phys. Ther.* **2021**, *101*, pzaa232. [CrossRef]
64. Franchak, J.M. Changing Opportunities for Learning in Everyday Life: Infant Body Position over the First Year. *Infancy* **2019**, *24*, 187–209. [CrossRef]
65. Saccani, R.; Valentini, N.C.; Pereira, K.R.G.; Müller, A.B.; Gabbard, C. Associations of biological factors and affordances in the home with infant motor development. *Pediatr. Int.* **2013**, *55*, 197–203. [CrossRef]
66. Franchak, J.M. The ecology of infants' perceptual-motor exploration. *Curr. Opin. Psychol.* **2020**, *32*, 110–114. [CrossRef]
67. Jensen-Willett, S.; Miller, K.; Jackson, B.; Harbourne, R. The Influence of Maternal Cognitions Upon Motor Development in Infants Born Preterm: A Scoping Review. *Pediatr. Phys. Ther.* **2021**, *33*, 137–147. [CrossRef]
68. Thelen, E. Motor development: A new synthesis. *Am. Psychol.* **1995**, *50*, 79–95. [CrossRef]
69. Iverson, J.M. Developing language in a developing body, revisited: The cascading effects of motor development on the acquisition of language. *Wiley Interdiscip. Rev. Cogn. Sci.* **2022**, *13*, e1626. [CrossRef]
70. Solgi, M.; Feryn, A.; Chavez, A.E.; Wilson, L.; King, M.; Scholz, J.; Fombonne, E.; Zuckerman, K.E. Parents' Concerns Are Associated with Early Intervention Evaluation and Eligibility Outcomes. *J. Dev. Behav. Pediatr.* **2022**, *43*, E145–E152. [CrossRef]
71. Thelen, E. Dynamic systems theory and the complexity of change. *Psychoanal. Dialogues* **2005**, *15*, 255–283. [CrossRef]
72. Spencer, J.P.; Perone, S.; Buss, A.T. Twenty Years and Going Strong: A Dynamic Systems Revolution in Motor and Cognitive Development. *Child Dev. Perspect.* **2011**, *5*, 260–266. [CrossRef]
73. Bronfenbrenner, U. Ecological systems theory. In *Six Theories of Child Development: Revised Formulations and Current Issues*; Jessica Kingsley Publishers: London, UK, 1992; pp. 187–249.
74. Lobo, M.A.; Harbourne, R.T.; Dusing, S.C.; McCoy, S.W. Grounding Early Intervention: Physical Therapy Cannot Just Be About Motor Skills Anymore. *Phys. Ther.* **2013**, *93*, 94–103. [CrossRef]
75. Bartlett, D.J.; Kneale Fanning, J.E. Relationships of Equipment Use and Play Positions to Motor Development at Eight Months Corrected Age of Infants Born Preterm. *Pediatr. Phys. Ther.* **2003**, *15*, 8–15. [CrossRef]
76. Gabbard, C.; Caçola, P.; Spessato, B.; Santos, D.C.C. The home environment and infant and young children's motor development. In *Advances in Psychology Research, Volume 90*; Advances in Psychology Research; Nova Science Publishers: Hauppauge, NY, USA, 2012; pp. 105–123.

Disclaimer/Publisher's Note: The statements, opinions and data contained in all publications are solely those of the individual author(s) and contributor(s) and not of MDPI and/or the editor(s). MDPI and/or the editor(s) disclaim responsibility for any injury to people or property resulting from any ideas, methods, instructions or products referred to in the content.

MDPI
St. Alban-Anlage 66
4052 Basel
Switzerland
www.mdpi.com

Behavioral Sciences Editorial Office
E-mail: behavsci@mdpi.com
www.mdpi.com/journal/behavsci

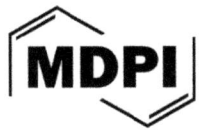

Disclaimer/Publisher's Note: The statements, opinions and data contained in all publications are solely those of the individual author(s) and contributor(s) and not of MDPI and/or the editor(s). MDPI and/or the editor(s) disclaim responsibility for any injury to people or property resulting from any ideas, methods, instructions or products referred to in the content.

www.ingramcontent.com/pod-product-compliance
Lightning Source LLC
LaVergne TN
LVHW070401100526
838202LV00014B/1362